2015
The Year Book of PULMONARY DISEASE®

Editor-in-Chief
James A. Barker, MD, CPE, FACP, FCCP, FAASM
VP and Medical Director, Clinical Services, University Health System; Adjunct Professor, UT Health Science Center at San Antonio, San Antonio, Texas

ELSEVIER
MOSBY

ELSEVIER
MOSBY

Vice President, Global Medical Reference: Mary E. Gatsch
Developmental Editor: Casey Jackson
Production Supervisor, Electronic Year Books: Donna M. Skelton
Electronic Article Manager: Mike Sheets
Illustrations and Permissions Coordinator: Dawn A. Vohsen

2015 EDITION

Printed in the United States of America
Composition by TNQ Books and Journals Pvt Ltd, India
Printing/binding by Sheridan Books, Inc

Editorial Office:
Elsevier, Inc.
Suite 1800
1600 John F. Kennedy Blvd
Philadelphia, PA 19103-2899

International Standard Serial Number: 8756-3452
International Standard Book Number: 978-0-323-35553-7

Associate Editors

Shirley F. Jones, MD, FCCP, FAASM
Medical Director, Scott and White Sleep Institute, Assistant Professor of Medicine, Scott and White Healthcare/Texas A&M Health Science Center; Division of Pulmonary, Critical Care and Sleep Medicine, Temple, Texas

Janet R. Maurer, MD, MBA
Clinical Professor of Medicine, University of Arizona College of Medicine, Phoenix, Phoenix, Arizona

Christopher D. Spradley, MD, FACP, FCCP
Medical Director, Pulmonary Hypertension Clinic, Assistant Professor of Internal Medicine, Division of Pulmonary, Critical Care and Sleep Medicine Scott & White Memorial Hospital/Texas A&M Health Science Center, Temple, Texas

Lynn T. Tanoue, MD
Professor of Medicine, Vice-Chair for Clinical Affairs, Department of Internal Medicine; Clinical Chief, Section of Pulmonary, Critical Care and Sleep Medicine, Yale School of Medicine, New Haven, Connecticut

Sandra K. Willsie, DO, MA
Staff Pulmonologist, KC Care Clinic, Kansas City, Missouri

Table of Contents

Journals Represented

Journals represented in this YEAR BOOK are listed below.

Academic Emergency Medicine
Acta Anaesthesiologica Scandinavica
Air Medical Journal
Allergy
American Journal of Emergency Medicine
American Journal of Obstetrics and Gynecology
American Journal of Respiratory and Critical Care Medicine
American Journal of Transplantation
Anaesthesia
Anaesthesia and Intensive Care
Annals of Allergy, Asthma & Immunology
Annals of Internal Medicine
Annals of the American Thoracic Society
Annals of Thoracic Surgery
Annals of Vascular Surgery
Archives of Disease in Childhood
British Medical Journal
CA: A Cancer Journal for Clinicians
Canadian Journal of Anaesthesia
Chest
Clinical Infectious Diseases
European Respiratory Journal
Injury
Intensive Care Medicine
International Journal of Cardiology
Journal of Allergy and Clinical Immunology
Journal of Clinical Microbiology
Journal of Clinical Oncology
Journal of Clinical Sleep Medicine
Journal of Heart and Lung Transplantation
Journal of Infectious Diseases
Journal of Molecular Diagnostics
Journal of Pain and Symptom Management
Journal of Surgical Research
Journal of the American College of Cardiology
Journal of the American College of Surgeons
Journal of the American Medical Association
Journal of the American Medical Association Internal Medicine
Journal of Thoracic and Cardiovascular Surgery
Journal of Trauma and Acute Care Surgery
Lung Cancer
Mayo Clinic Proceedings
New England Journal of Medicine
Otolaryngology-Head and Neck Surgery
Pediatrics
Radiology
Respiratory Medicine

Sleep
Thorax
Transplantation
Transplantation Proceedings

Standard Abbreviations

The following terms are abbreviated in this edition: acquired immunodeficiency syndrome (AIDS), cardiopulmonary resuscitation (CPR), central nervous system (CNS), cerebrospinal fluid (CSF), computed tomography (CT), deoxyribonucleic acid (DNA), electrocardiography (ECG), health maintenance organization (HMO), human immunodeficiency virus (HIV), intensive care unit (ICU), intramuscular (IM), intravenous (IV), magnetic resonance (MR) imaging (MRI), ribonucleic acid (RNA), and ultrasound (US).

Note

The Year Book of Pulmonary Disease is a literature survey service providing abstracts of articles published in the professional literature. Every effort is made to assure the accuracy of the information presented in these pages. Neither the editors nor the publisher of the Year Book of Pulmonary Disease can be responsible for errors in the original materials. The editors' comments are their own opinions. Mention of specific products within this publication does not constitute endorsement.

To facilitate the use of the Year Book of Pulmonary Disease as a reference tool, all illustrations and tables included in this publication are now identified as they appear in the original article. This change is meant to help the reader recognize that any illustration or table appearing in the Year Book of Pulmonary Disease may be only one of many in the original article. For this reason, figure and table numbers will often appear to be out of sequence within the Year Book of Pulmonary Disease.

1 Asthma, Allergy, and Cystic Fibrosis

Introduction

This year's highlighted publications about asthma and cystic fibrosis (CF) were chosen from scores of articles, and those appearing in this chapter reflect investigations that we believe hold particular significance for the practicing clinician.

Asthma remains the culprit of inordinate use of healthcare resources and a significant cause for morbidity, regardless of the age of the patient. A very provocative investigation published in 2014 by Raedler and colleagues[1] highlighted extensive work on allergic and non-allergic asthma phenotypes. The results of this research shed light on immune-regulatory cellular mechanisms at work in childhood asthma. The potential for identification of new pathways to provide the basis for individualized strategies for asthma prevention is promising and appears not too far away—exciting!

A very practical and clinically important manuscript chosen for highlighting in the 2015 Review includes "Management of acute loss of asthma control in the yellow zone: a practice parameter,"[2] which represents an evidence-based practice parameter calling for focus on the yellow zone by practitioners and education of patients on how to manage this zone. The intervention to be recommended for patients who reach the yellow zone will depend upon what type of dosing the subject is taking with regard to inhaled corticosteroid (ICS), eg, scheduled dosing of ICS alone; using ICS with short-acting, quick-onset reliever; using ICS with long-acting beta agonist). Due to the current paucity of research on how best to handle the yellow zone, and the fact that intervention in the yellow zone has the potential to prevent morbidity (emergency department visits, missed school, hospitalization), it seems high time that a practice parameter has been written. Kudos to the three organizations involved: American College of Allergy, Asthma, and Immunology; Joint Council on Allergy, Asthma, and Immunology; American Academy of Allergy, Asthma, and Immunology! It is my strong recommendation that all healthcare providers caring for asthmatics take a careful look at this practice parameter and implement it immediately!

Several studies of asthma therapeutics were published this year, including a randomized, double-blind, placebo-control, parallel group, multi-center study of benralizumab (B), an anti-interleukin 5 receptor alpha monoclonal antibody.[3] B reduced asthma exacerbation rates over 12 weeks by 49% (P =.01) and exacerbations resulting in hospitalization by 60% (P =.02). Additionally, several studies were published studying a long-acting muscarinic antagonist, umeclidinium (UMEC), in asthma, both with and without ICS.[4,5] UMEC led to significant improvements in change from baseline trough FEV1.[1] UMEC was rapidly absorbed and showed evidence of some accumulation. In the absence of ICS, there appeared no therapeutic benefit in the asthmatics studied.[5]

A study published by Bergert et al,[6] demonstrated successful reduction of hospital readmission rates by using a multidisciplinary asthma task force employing the patient-centered medical home model. This dedicated group of clinicians worked for years to finetune their model to intervene and ensure return to the medical home for follow-up visit following hospitalization of children for asthma and documented successful reduction in hospital readmission rates!

Several CF investigations were chosen for inclusion in this 2015 YEAR BOOK, including a review of gene therapy for the treatment of CF.[7] As might be expected, this represents a very complex subject due to the tremendous numbers of known mutations that exist, and not all mutations respond to the same therapeutic interventions. Nevertheless, there has been tremendous advancement in the field of genetics of CF to date. In addition, a registry-based study[8] now allows us to more accurately predict longevity in patients with CF: Median survival of children born with CF in 2010 is projected to be 37 years (CI, 35-39 years) for females and 40 years (CI, 39-42 years) for males, if mortality remains at 2010 levels. The CF Foundation published clinical care guidelines in December 2014 for the prevention of *Pseudomonas aeruginosa* (PA) infection, treatment of initial PA infection, and the use of bronchoscopy for obtaining routine airway cultures in individuals with CF.[9]

Finally, we hope that you enjoy reviewing this selection of publications as much as we enjoyed selecting them for you.

Best regards professionally,
Sandra K. Willsie, DO, MA

References

1. Raedler D, Ballenberger N, Klucker E, et al. Identification of novel immune phenotypes for allergic and nonallergic childhood asthma. *J Allergy Clin Immunol.* 2015;135:81-91.
2. Dinakar C, Oppenheimer J, Portnoy J, et al. Management of acute loss of asthma control in the yellow zone: a practice parameter. *Ann Allergy Asthma Immunol.* 2014;113:143-159.
3. Nowak RM, Parker JM, Silverman RA, et al. A randomized trial of benralizumab, an antiinterleukin 5 receptor alpha monoclonal antibody after acute asthma. *Am J Emerg Med.* 2015;33:14-20.
4. Lee LA, Briggs A, Edwards LD, Yang S, Pascoe S. A randomized, three-period crossover study of umeclidinium as monotherapy in adult patients with asthma. *Respir Med.* 2015;109:63-73.
5. Lee LA, Yang S, Kerwin E, Trivedi R, Edwards LD, Pascoe S. The effect of fluticasone furoate/umeclidinium in adult patients with asthma: a randomized, dose-ranging study. *Respir Med.* 2015;109:54-62.

6. Bergert L, Patel SJ, Kimata C, Zhang G, Matthews WJ Jr. Linking patient-centered medical home and asthma measures reduces hospital readmission rates. *Pediatrics*. 2014;134:e249-e256.
7. Armstrong DK, Cunningham S, Davies JC, Alton EW. Gene therapy in cystic fibrosis. *Arch Dis Child*. 2014;99:465-468.
8. MacKenzie T, Gifford AH, Sabadosa KA, et al. Longevity of patients with cystic fibrosis in 2000 to 2010 and beyond: survival analysis of the cystic fibrosis foundation patient registry. *Ann Intern Med*. 2014;161:233-241.
9. Mogayzel PJ, Naureckas ET, Robinson KA, et al. Cystic fibrosis foundation pulmonary guideline. Pharmacologic approaches to prevention and eradication of initial Pseudomonas aeruginosa infection. *Ann Am Thorac Soc*. 2014;11:1640-1650.

Asthma

Trends in the age of diagnosis of childhood asthma

Radhakrishnan DK, Dell SD, Guttmann A, et al (Children's Hosp, London, Ontario, Canada; Hosp for Sick Children, London, Ontario, Canada; Univ of Toronto, London, Ontario, Canada)
J Allergy Clin Immunol 134:1057-1062, 2014

Background.—The cause of rising asthma incidence over time remains unexplained. Examining trends in the age of diagnosis across successive birth cohorts may offer insights into asthma etiology.

Objective.—To examine trends in the age at asthma diagnosis and the age and proportion of children hospitalized at first asthma diagnosis in Ontario, Canada.

Methods.—Eight consecutive birth cohorts of children (1993-2000) were observed using administrative data from a universal health insurance plan in Ontario, Canada (population 13 million). Trends in the need for hospitalization and age at asthma diagnosis were examined with descriptive and survival analyses.

Results.—The records of 1,059,511 children were examined, of whom 201,958 developed asthma in the first 8 years of life, with an average cumulative incidence of 19.1%. Mean age at asthma diagnosis decreased from 4.7 ± 1.5 years in birth year 1993 to 2.6 ± 2.0 years in birth year 2000 ($P < .0001$), with a higher adjusted risk of asthma diagnosis (hazard ratio, 6.7; 95% CI, 6.5-6.9) in the first 3 years of life for children born after 1996 versus children born in the period 1993 to 1995 (hazard ratio, 1.4; 95% CI, 1.3-1.4). The proportion of children hospitalized at asthma diagnosis stayed stable while the age at first asthma hospitalization decreased over time ($P < .0001$).

Conclusions.—This study demonstrates a significant increase in asthma incidence and a decrease in the age of asthma diagnosis across multiple birth cohorts. Changes in asthma incidence over time are primarily explained by variations in asthma rates in children younger than 3 years (Fig 2, Table 1).

▶ This study evaluated all children born between 1993 and 2001 in the single province of Ontario, a single-payor system, evaluating the incidence of childhood

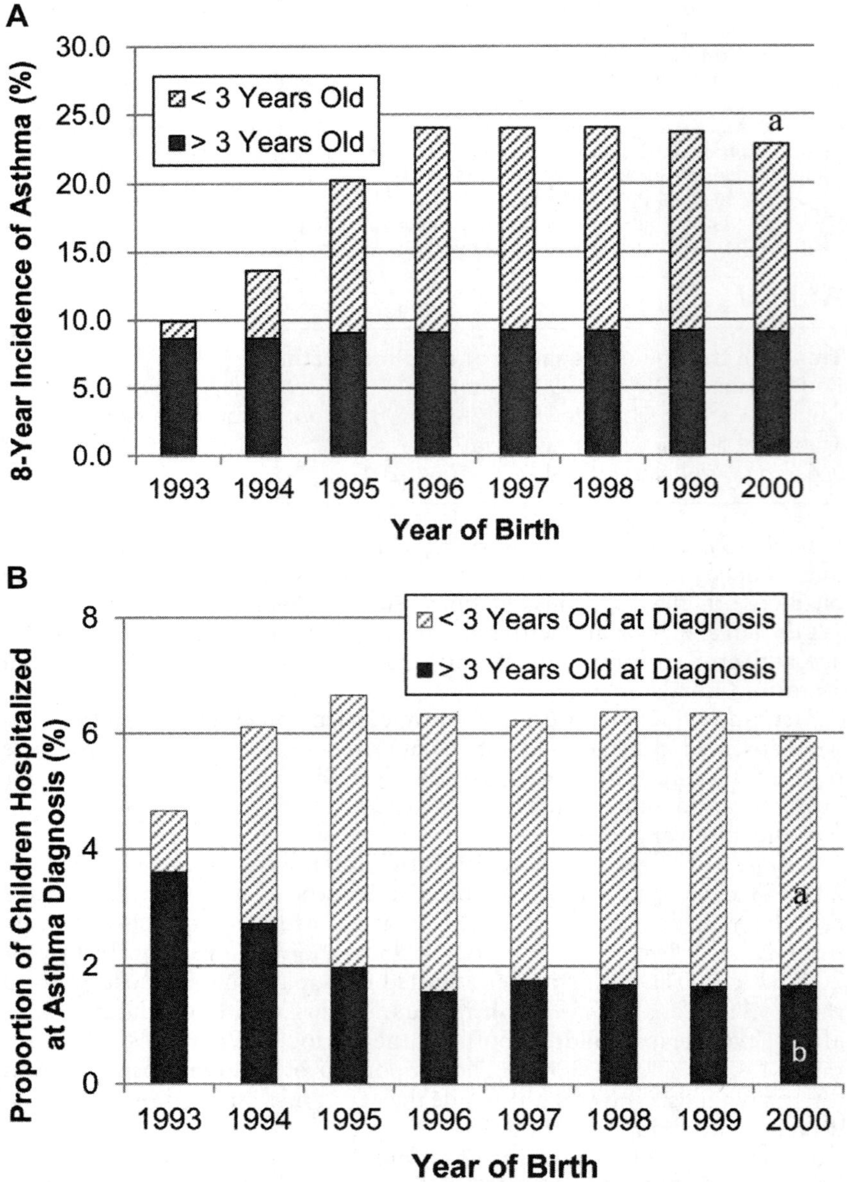

FIGURE 2.—A, Incidence of asthma in the first 8 years of life per cohort, stratified by age at diagnosis. Total sample size: N = 1,059,511 children in total and 201,958 children with asthma. [a]$P < .0001$ for significant increase in overall asthma incidence and asthma incidence in children younger than 3 years by Cochrane Armitage trend test. B, Proportion of children with asthma hospitalized at diagnosis, stratified by age at diagnosis. Total sample size: N = 201,958 children with asthma. [a]$P < .001$ for significant increase over time in proportion of children younger than 3 years hospitalized at first asthma diagnosis. [b]$P < .001$ for significant reduction over time in proportion of children 3 years or older hospitalized at first asthma diagnosis. (Reprinted from Radhakrishnan DK, Dell SD, Guttmann A, et al. Trends in the age of diagnosis of childhood asthma. J Allergy Clin Immunol. 2014;134:1057-1062, Copyright 2014, with permission from Elsevier.)

TABLE 1.—Mean Age of Asthma Diagnosis by Birth Cohort

	Birth Year							
Age (y)	1993	1994	1995	1996	1997	1998	1999	2000
Mean ± SD	4.7 ± 1.5	3.9 ± 1.8	2.9 ± 2.0	2.5 ± 2.1	2.5 ± 2.1	2.6 ± 2.1	2.6 ± 2.1	2.6* ± 2.0

Total N used for analysis = 201,962 (asthma cases).
*$P < .0001$ for significant reduction in mean age of asthma diagnosis over time.
Reprinted from The Journal of Allergy and Clinical Immunology. Radhakrishnan DK, Dell SD, Guttmann A, et al. Trends in the age of diagnosis of childhood asthma. J Allergy Clin Immunol. 2014;134:1057-1062, Copyright 2014, with permission from Elsevier.

asthma and the age at diagnosis, and observing their care, admissions, and treatment over time. Table 1 shows the mean age of asthma diagnosis by birth year cohort (1993—2000; total of 201 962 cases of asthma). The mean age of diagnosis in 1993 was 4.7 years, 1.5 (SD) and in 2000, 2.6 years, 2.0 (SD) ($P < .001$). Fig 2 depicts the incidence of asthma in the first 8 years of life, stratified by age of diagnosis and the proportion of children with asthma hospitalized at the time of diagnosis. There was a significant increase ($P < .0001$ in overall asthma incidence and asthma incidence in children younger than 3 years) and a significant reduction, over time, in the proportion of children 3 years or older hospitalized at the time of diagnosis of asthma ($P < .001$). The investigators cite previous studies indicating that childhood asthma that persists into adulthood is more likely to develop before the age of 3 years[1] and that this trend may equate to a greater burden for the healthcare system in the long run. Importantly, in this investigational population, the increased burden of asthma among preschool children warrants modification of healthcare delivery and treatments to target this youngest age group. Future research into primary prevention of asthma in the early years following birth must become a priority.

S. K. Willsie, DO, MA

Reference

1. Martinez FD, Wright AL, Taussig LM, Holberg CJ, Halonen M, Morgan WJ. Asthma and wheezing in the first six years of life. The Group Health Medical Associates. *N Engl J Med.* 1995;332:133-138.

Asthma: pathogenesis and novel drugs for treatment

Olin JT, Wechsler ME (Natl Jewish Health, Denver, CO)
BMJ 349:g5517, 2014

Asthma affects almost 20 million people in the United States and more than 300 million people worldwide. Of these, 10-15% have severe asthma, which is refractory to commonly available drugs. New drugs are needed because those that are currently available cannot control symptoms and exacerbations in all patients and can cause adverse reactions. In the past 10 years, there have been substantial advances in the understanding of

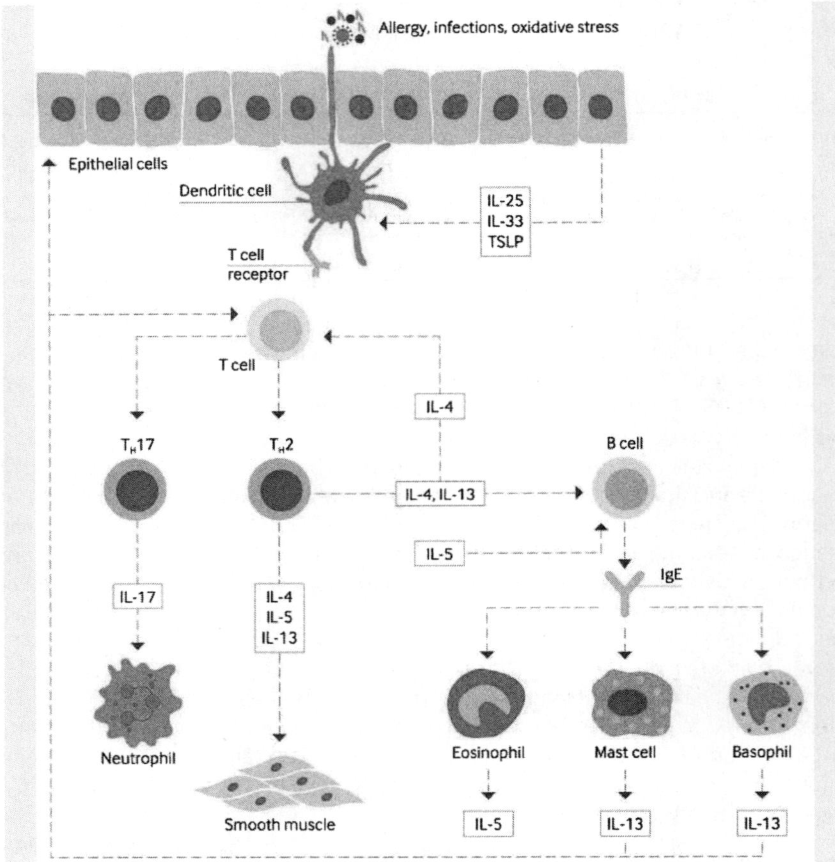

FIGURE 1.—Important host responses in the pathogenesis of asthma. Several asthma drugs in clinical trials target the cytokines (or their receptors) that are central to these pathways, including interleukin 4 (IL-4), IL-5, IL-13, and IL-17. TSLP = thymic stromal lymphopoietin. (Reprinted from Olin JT, Wechsler ME. Asthma: pathogenesis and novel drugs for treatment. *BMJ*. 2014;349:g5517, with permission from the BMJ Publishing Group Ltd.)

asthma genetics, airway biology, and immune cell signaling. These advances have led to the development of small molecule therapeutics and biologic agents that may improve asthma care in the future. Several new classes of asthma drugs—including ultra long acting β agonists and modulators of the interleukin 4 (IL-4), IL-5, IL-13, and IL-17 pathways—have been evaluated in randomized controlled trials. Other new drug classes—including dissociated corticosteroids, CXC chemokine receptor 2 antagonists, toll-like receptor 9 agonists, and tyrosine kinase inhibitors—remain in earlier phases of development. Despite some preliminary efficacy data, there is insufficient evidence to make strong recommendations about the use of these newer agents. Future research on the clinical efficacy of these biologic agents, the effect of newer agents on severe

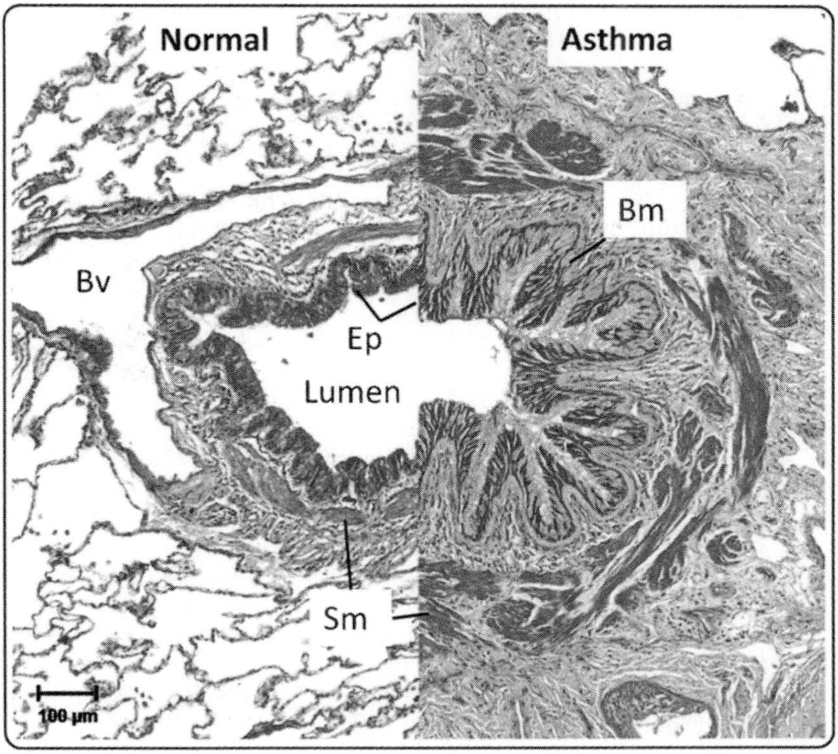

FIGURE 2.—The airways in asthma undergo substantial structural remodeling. Histological section of a medium sized airway from a person without asthma and a patient with severe asthma stained with Movat's pentachrome stain. In asthma the epithelium (Ep) shows mucus hyperplasia and hypersecretion (blue), and thickening of the basement membrane (Bm). Smooth muscle (Sm) volume is also increased in asthma. Bv = blood vessel. Reproduced, under an open access agreement, from Wadsworth and colleagues. IL-13, asthma, and glycosylation in airway epithelial repair. In: Chang C, ed. Carbohydrates—comprehensive studies on glycobiology and glycotechnology. InTech, 2012[67]. *Editor's Note*: Please refer to original journal article for full references. For interpretation of the references to color in this figure legend, the reader is referred to web version of this article. (Reprinted from Olin JT, Wechsler ME. Asthma: pathogenesis and novel drugs for treatment. *BMJ*. 2014;349:g5517, with permission from the BMJ Publishing Group Ltd.)

asthma in pediatric patients, and the biology of non-eosinophilic and corticosteroid resistant asthma is needed to reduce the morbidity of asthma worldwide (Figs 1 and 2).

▶ This state-of-the-art review is a must read for all clinicians caring for patients with asthma. Figs 1 and 2 provide an update on currently understood mechanisms for pathophysiology of asthma and potential new target for antiasthma therapeutics. Succinct and well written, this review makes a good case as to why additional therapeutics are needed.

S. K. Willsie, DO, MA

New Risk Factors for Adult-Onset Incident Asthma: A Nested Case–Control Study of Host Antioxidant Defense

Larkin EK, Gao Y-T, Gebretsadik T, et al (Vanderbilt Univ, Nashville, TN; Shanghai Cancer Inst, People's Republic of China; et al)

Am J Respir Crit Care Med 191:45-53, 2015

Rationale.—Host antioxidant defense, consisting of enzymatic antioxidant activity and nonenzymatic antioxidant micronutrients, is implicated in asthma pathogenesis. Studies of antioxidant defense and adult incident asthma have either used measures of antioxidants estimated from questionnaires or not considered enzymatic aspects of host defense.

Objectives.—We conducted the first study designed and powered to investigate the association of antioxidant defenses on adult incident asthma.

Methods.—In a nested case–control study, we followed Shanghai women (aged 40–70 years) without prevalent asthma at baseline, over 8 years. Subjects with incident asthma were ascertained prospectively by gold standard testing of symptomatic women and matched to two asymptomatic control subjects.

Measurements and Main Results.—Baseline urinary F_2-isoprostanes, plasma concentrations of antioxidant micronutrients (tocopherols, xanthines, carotenes, and lycopene), and antioxidant enzyme activity (platelet-activating factor acetylhydrolase [PAF-AH] and superoxide dismutase) were measured from samples collected before disease onset. Among 65,372 women, 150 (0.24%) developed asthma. F_2-isoprostane levels before asthma onset were not different between cases and control subjects. Doubling of α-tocopherol concentrations and PAF-AH activity was associated with 50 and 37% decreased risk of incident asthma (α-tocopherol: adjusted odds ratio = 0.52; 95% confidence interval, 0.32–0.84; PAF-AH: adjusted odds ratio = 0.63; 95% confidence interval, 0.42–0.93).

Conclusions.—In this prospective study, α-tocopherol, within normal reference ranges, and PAF-AH enzymatic activity were associated with decreased asthma development. These modifiable risk factors may be an effective strategy to test for primary asthma prevention.

▶ Theories abound and have for years that the use of antioxidant therapy may be a viable way to prevent and/or treat a variety of diseases. In the first prospective study specifically powered to evaluate quantifiable plasma biomarkers of antioxidants using a nested, case-controlled design, the investigators have shown convincingly that normal or elevated levels of alpha tocopherol (nonenzymatic) and platelet activating factor acetylhydrolase (PAF)-AH (enzymatic) antioxidants have a protective association against the development of asthma in women. Based on the results of this study, which followed 65 372 women in the Shanghai Women's Health Study for 8 years, targeting the enzymatic and nonenzymatic antioxidant defense system presents a promising strategy for the future for asthma prevention.

S. K. Willsie, DO, MA

Identification of novel immune phenotypes for allergic and nonallergic childhood asthma

Raedler D, Ballenberger N, Klucker E, et al (Univ Children's Hosp Munich, Germany; et al)

J Allergy Clin Immunol 135:81-91, 2015

Background.—Childhood asthma is classified into allergic asthma (AA) and nonallergic asthma (NA), yet both are treated identically, with only partial success.

Objective.—We sought to identify novel immune phenotypes for childhood AA and NA.

Methods.—The Clinical Asthma Research Association cohort study includes 275 steroid-naive 4- to 15-year-old German children (healthy control subjects [HCs], patients with AA, and patients with NA). In PBMCs both quantitative and functional analysis of regulatory T (Treg) and T_H17 cells (flow cytometry/Treg cell suppression) before/after anti-CD3/CD28, lipid A, and peptidoglycan stimulation were performed. Cytokines and gene expression, as assessed by using Luminex or transcriptomics/quantitative real-time RT-PCR, were analyzed by means of regression analysis. Linear discriminant analysis was applied to discriminate between phenotypes.

Results.—The 3 phenotypes were immunologically well discriminated by means of microarray and protein analysis with linear discriminant analysis. Patients with AA were characterized by increased Treg cells compared with those in HCs but not those in patients with NA. Treg cells from patients with AA, but not patients with NA, significantly suppressed IL-5, IL-13, and IFN-γ secretion. Patients with AA had decreased expression of chloride intracellular channel 4 *(CLIC4)* and tuberous sclerosis 1 *(TSC1)*, important innate immunity regulators. Patients with NA were characterized by increased proinflammatory IL-1β levels, neutrophil counts, and IL-17–shifted immunity. In parallel, expressions of anti-inflammatory *IL37*, proline-serine-threonine phosphatase–interacting protein 2 *(PSTPIP2)*, and the neutrophil-associated genes *CD93*, triggering receptor expressed on myeloid cells 1 *(TREM1)*, and regulator of G-protein signaling 13 *(RGS13)* were increased in patients with NA. A shared T_H2 immunity was present in both asthma phenotypes.

Conclusion.—Novel immune-regulatory mechanisms in childhood asthma identified increased Treg cells in patients with AA compared with those in HCs but not those in NA and decreased innate immunity genes for patients with AA, the first potentially indicating a counterregulatory mechanism to suppress cytokines yet not sufficient to control allergic inflammation. Very distinctly, patients with NA showed an IL-17–shifted proinflammatory immunity, promoting neutrophil inflammation and less functional Treg cells. Identification of these unique pathways provides a profound basis for future strategies for individualized prediction of asthma development, disease course, and prevention (Fig 2).

▶ This complex manuscript sheds significant light on the immune phenotypes (as opposed to clinical phenotypes) of allergic (AA) and nonallergic (NA) childhood asthma. Sophisticated testing of peripheral blood mononuclear cells was performed to isolate genetic material. Fig 2 displays microarray and cytokine linear discriminant analysis plots of group discrimination. AA, NA, and healthy controls (HC) are clearly depicted. NA had significantly increased expression of pro-inflammatory interleukin (IL)-1beta compared with HC. Treg

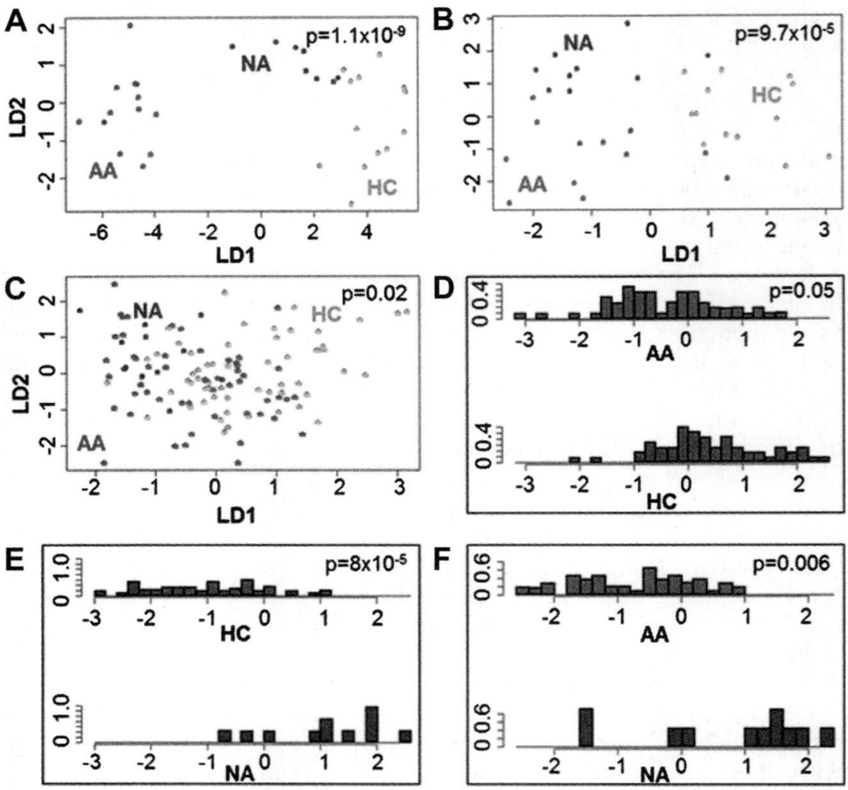

FIGURE 2.—Microarray and cytokine LDA plots of group discrimination. A scatterplot (A-C; patients with AA/patients with NA/HCs) with the first 2 linear discriminants *(LD1/2)* depicted on the *x-axis* and *y-axis* and a histogram (D-F, 2 groups) with the first linear discriminant depicted on the *x-axis* and density on the *y-axis* are shown. Fig 2, *A*, Top 600 microarray genes. Fig 2, *B*, Thirty-one microarray genes validated by means of qRT-PCR. Fig 2, *C*, Cytokines. Cytokine levels were compared between 2 groups: patients with AA versus HCs (Fig 2, *D*); patients with NA versus HCs (Fig 2, *E*); and patients with NA versus patients with AA (Fig 2, *F*). PCR: HCs/patients with AA/patients with NA, n = 14/14/8. Cytokines: HCs/patients with AA/patients with NA, n = 72/60/11. (Reprinted from The Journal of Allergy and Clinical Immunology. Raedler D, Ballenberger N, Klucker E, et al. Identification of novel immune phenotypes for allergic and nonallergic childhood asthma. *J Allergy Clin Immunol.* 2015;135:81-91, Copyright 2015, with permission from Elsevier.)

cells in NA were functionally insufficient as they did not suppress IL-5, IL-13, T_H2, and interferon-gamma, T_H1, compared with levels seen in AA. NA subjects also had increased neutrophils compared with AA ($P = .03$), increased CD93 expression, and increased TREM1, which amplifies neutrophil-mediated inflammation and IL-1B secretion. T_H1/T_H2 cytokine levels were similar between AA and NA subjects. Subjects with AA, characterized by airway obstruction and allergic inflammation, are associated with increased eosinophil counts and specific immunoglobulin E levels and also exhibit increased Treg cells, similar to NA, but with efficient suppression of T_H2 and T_H1 cytokines. AA is also associated with decreased innate immunity gene expression. What does this mean outside the research center? Probably not much to an average healthcare provider who is quite able to treat asthma according to guidelines. But the future portends that this information will revolutionize the way we treat asthma. The big mystery is how and when. We will have to wait and see what happens. Consider this the tip of the iceberg, for now.

S. K. Willsie, DO, MA

Management of acute loss of asthma control in the yellow zone: A practice parameter

Dinakar C, Oppenheimer J, Portnoy J, et al ()
Ann Allergy Asthma Immunol 113:143-159, 2014

Asthma action plans have been recommended for all patients with asthma since the 1991 publication of the first National Heart, Lung, and Blood Institute (NHLBI) guidelines for the diagnosis and management of asthma. Establishment of a patient-provider partnership was a key component of the guidelines and the asthma action plan helped create this relationship by empowering patients to monitor their asthma status and take action when control deteriorated. The most recent iteration of the guidelines, the Expert Panel Report 3 (EPR3): Guidelines for the Diagnosis and Management of Asthma (EPR3), was developed by an expert panel commissioned by the National Asthma Education and Prevention Program Coordinating Committee, coordinated by the NHLBI of the National Institutes of Health. The EPR3 emphasized attainment of asthma control and recommended strategies to treat variations in symptoms that occur over a timeframe of months.

In addition to long-term variability of asthma control, most patients with asthma experience intermittent loss of control in response to exposure to acute triggers occurring over a shorter timeframe, such as hours to days. An asthma action plan is the logical tool to instruct patients on how to recognize and respond to such rapid changes in control that occur in a setting outside a supervised medical facility, such as the home. A typical asthma action plan includes written instructions regarding treatment recommendations in the green zone (asthma doing well), the yellow zone (asthma deterioration detected, intervention needed), and the red zone (asthma exacerbation requiring urgent treatment). Responding to the symptoms of acute loss of control in the yellow zone with effective interventions can help prevent deterioration to the red zone, necessitating use of systemic corticosteroids and/or urgent medical care.

The EPR3 recommends increasing administration of inhaled SABA (such as 2–6 puffs of albuterol) every 3 to 4 hours for 24 to 48 hours to treat home exacerbations of asthma. If there is insufficient improvement, it recommends adding a short course of oral systemic corticosteroids (Figure 5–4 of the EPR3). In other words, the intervention recommended in the yellow zone by the EPR3 is to increase the frequency of reliever SABA therapy. Guidelines providing evidence-based therapeutic options to manage patients who experience short-term loss of control are therefore lacking, and this practice parameter was written with the intent of addressing the gap. This document attempts to define criteria that indicate acute loss of control into the yellow zone and reviews therapeutic maneuvers to regain asthma control and prevent further progression into the red zone. These recommendations are based on a meticulous and critical review of the medical literature, and in situations where data are lacking, options are presented.

The first recommendation in this practice parameter is that patients with asthma should be given a written and/or electronic asthma action plan. Although the format may vary, action plans most commonly follow the traffic light model. The green zone indicates asthma that is controlled, the yellow zone forewarns acute loss of control and an impending exacerbation, and the red zone indicates onset of a severe exacerbation requiring a course of systemic corticosteroids and contact with a healthcare provider. The action plans may be based on symptoms or on symptoms and peak expiratory flow (PEF), depending on the preference of the provider and the patient.

The second summary statement describes criteria for recognition of a yellow zone episode. In particular, patients should be advised to take action when they experience an increase in asthma symptoms, increased use of reliever medications, a decrease in their PEF (if they monitor it), or the onset of nocturnal symptoms. In addition, patients with a history of loss of control in response to respiratory tract infections (RTIs) are advised to take action.

The specific action to be taken is dependent on the severity of the episode and the individual response to previous episodes with those interventions. The ideal intervention should provide quick relief of symptoms, prevent progression to the red zone, be safe enough to initiate at home, be convenient and practical for self-administration, be portable so that it is always available, and be cost effective. Obviously, the perfect intervention does not exist; however, some potential interventions have been studied and are discussed below.

Potential interventions for yellow zone treatment include repetitive use of inhaled SABA administered through a metered dose inhaler or nebulizer, scheduled step-up of an ICS, and symptom-driven use of controller with reliever therapy, otherwise known as dynamic dosing or adjustable maintenance dosing (AMD). The regular scheduled use of SABA as the sole treatment for symptoms in the yellow zone is discouraged because it does not consistently prevent progression to the red zone and might increase the risk of progression.

Patients who are treated with daily ICS therapy can be advised to increase their total 24-hour ICS dose, for example, by 4-fold. Increase in the frequency of ICS administration over 24 hours also may result in improved efficacy. The EPR2 guidelines had recommended doubling the dose of ICS; however, EPR3 discouraged the use of doubling ICS doses and instead mentioned that preliminary evidence indicates that quadrupling the dose of an ICS for 7 days, starting at the first appearance of worsening symptoms, may prevent exacerbations requiring oral systemic corticosteroids. The key concept acknowledged in this practice parameter is that each yellow zone episode may require a different amount of supplemental ICS dose to prevent progression. For that reason, symptom-driven ICS use and dynamic dosing are attractive alternative options. In this model, patients receive a larger amount of ICS as they experience increasing loss of asthma control and a smaller amount of ICS as control is achieved. The evidence for dynamic dosing appears to be more consistent to that supporting the scheduled use of increased ICS dose in 24 hours.

Methods for administration of dynamic dosing include (1) separate use of reliever (ie, SABA) and controller inhalers in combination and (2) use of single inhalers that contain a reliever (SABA or quick-onset long-acting β agonists [LABA] such as formoterol) and a controller that is used for symptom relief (with accompanying escalation in controller therapy). Although the 2 approaches are effective, the use of a single inhaler with a reliever (ie, formoterol) and controller (ie, AMD) is more convenient and has been widely studied and used in other countries. A recent evidence-based review demonstrated that the AMD strategy can decrease exacerbations requiring oral corticosteroids (OCSs) compared with current best-practice strategies, although the authors do not recommend use of this approach in children and adolescents younger than 18 years because large-scale studies have not been conducted in this age group. Notably, although inhalers with the desired properties (ie, ICS with formoterol) are available in the United States, the FDA has not approved those inhalers for dynamic dosing or AMD therapy. In fact, the FDA specifically cautions against initiating use, or increasing the dose, of these inhalers during periods of acutely worsening asthma symptoms. As a result, these treatment options for yellow zone management of patients with asthma would be considered off-label in the United States, to be prescribed at the discretion and medical judgment of the individual provider, with additional extra caution to be exercised when using them in patients younger than 18 years.

The practice parameter concludes by briefly discussing additional approaches with limited or no evidence. Although these approaches may be beneficial for individual patients in special circumstances, they are not recommended for general use.

It is the hope of the Yellow Zone Workgroup that routine use of an effective yellow zone intervention for patients as part of an action plan will lead to decreased morbidity and improved quality of life for individuals with asthma. This document also highlights evidence gaps in yellow zone asthma management and strongly recommends conducting clinical trials to further validate the approaches explored in this document and to examine other effective options.

▶ The publication of this new practice parameter addressing management of acute loss of asthma control represented by patients' asthma entering the yellow zone (referring to the Asthma Action Plan) was developed by the Joint Task Force on Practice Parameters, representing the American Academy of Allergy, Asthma and Immunology; the American College of Allergy, Asthma and Immunology; and the Joint Council of Allergy, Asthma and Immunology. Eight summary statements, with defined strength of recommendation and graded evidence, are provided for the healthcare practitioner, along with an exhaustive review of the literature. This document is a must read for all who care for patients with asthma, because entry into the yellow zone represents acute loss of asthma control, and prompt and adequate intervention at this stage offers the opportunity to mitigate the need for entry into the red zone, the need for emergency department visits or hospitalization, and potentially the end result of reduced morbidity and mortality. Kudos to the working group for the labor put into this excellent work product; it is timely indeed and should be the topic of journal clubs in all academic settings, reiterated at all regional/national meetings and a required portion of online continuing medical education courses.

S. K. Willsie, DO, MA

A randomized trial of benralizumab, an antiinterleukin 5 receptor α monoclonal antibody, after acute asthma

Nowak RM, Parker JM, Silverman RA, et al (Henry Ford Health System, Detroit, MI; Clinical Development, Gaithersburg, MD; North Shore–Long Island Jewish Med Ctr, NY; et al)

Am J Emerg Med 33:14-20, 2015

Background.—Patients with frequent asthma exacerbations resulting in emergency department (ED) visits are at increased risk for future exacerbations. We examined the ability of 1 dose of benralizumab, an investigational antiinterleukin 5 receptor α monoclonal antibody, to reduce recurrence after acute asthma exacerbations.

Methods.—In this randomized, double-blind, placebo-controlled study, eligible subjects presented to the ED with an asthma exacerbation, had partial response to treatment, and greater than or equal to 1 additional exacerbation within the previous year. Subjects received 1 intravenous infusion of placebo (n = 38) or benralizumab (0.3 mg/kg, n = 36 or 1.0 mg/kg, n = 36) added to out patient management. The primary outcome was the

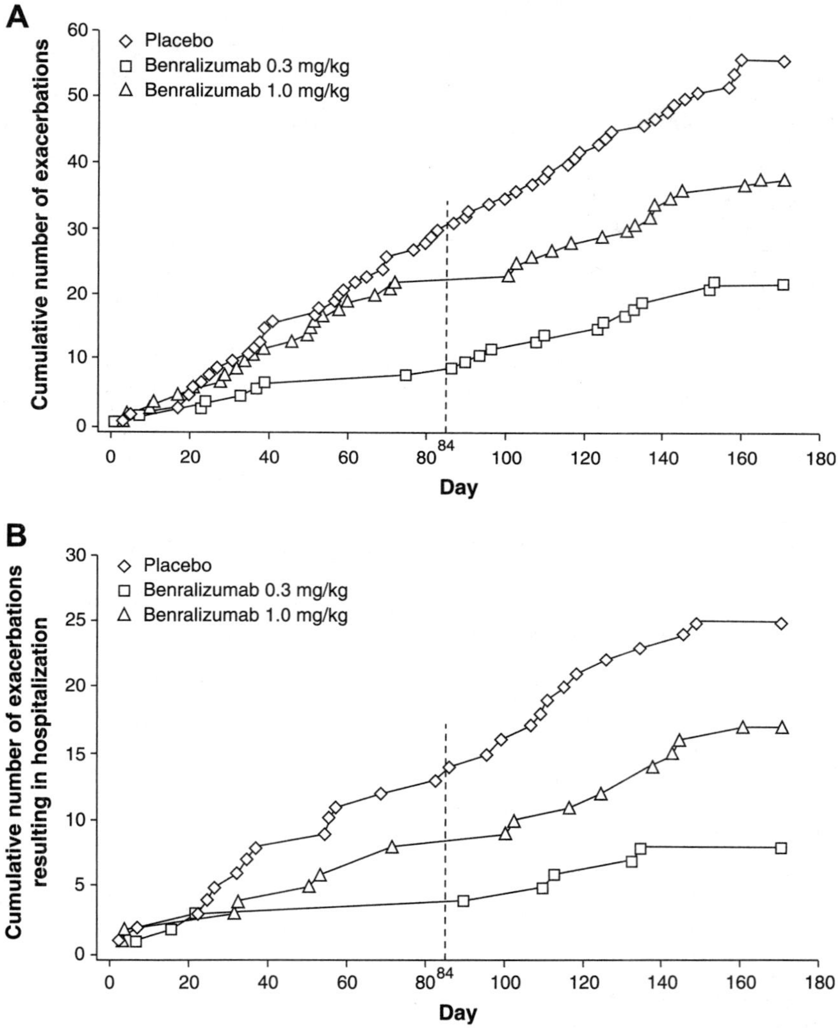

FIGURE 2.—Cumulative number of adjudicated asthma exacerbations. Analysis was performed on evaluable subjects. A, All exacerbations. B, Exacerbations requiring hospitalization. (Reprinted from the American Journal of Emergency Medicine. Nowak RM, Parker JM, Silverman RA, et al. A randomized trial of benralizumab, an antiinterleukin 5 receptor α monoclonal antibody, after acute asthma. *Am J Emerg Med*. 2015;33:14-20, Copyright 2015, with permission from Elsevier.)

proportion of subjects with greater than or equal to 1 exacerbation at 12 weeks in placebo vs the combined benralizumab groups. Other outcomes included the time-weighted rate of exacerbations at week 12, adverse events, blood eosinophil counts, asthma symptom changes, and healthcare resource utilization.

Results.—The proportion of subjects with greater than or equal to 1 asthma exacerbation at 12 weeks was not different between placebo and

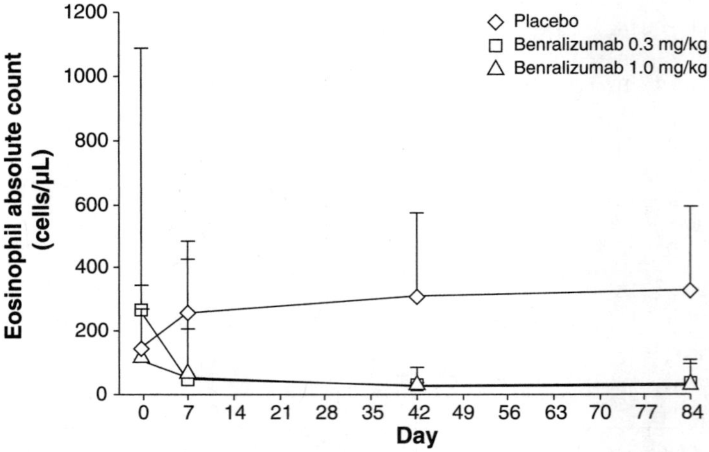

FIGURE 3.—Absolute eosinophil count by treatment group. (Reprinted from the American Journal of Emergency Medicine. Nowak RM, Parker JM, Silverman RA, et al. A randomized trial of benralizumab, an antiinterleukin 5 receptor α monoclonal antibody, after acute asthma. *Am J Emerg Med.* 2015;33:14-20, Copyright 2015, with permission from Elsevier.)

TABLE 2.—Outcome Measures (Evaluable Population)

Outcome Measure	Placebo n = 36	Benralizumab 0.3 mg/kg n = 36	Benralizumab 1.0 mg/kg n = 36	Benralizumab Total n = 72	*P*
Subjects with ≥1 asthma exacerbation, n (%)					
Wk 4	8 (22.2)	4 (11.1)	8 (22.2)	12 (16.7)	.60[b]
Wk 12[a]	14 (38.9)	9 (25.0)	15 (41.7)	24 (33.3)	.67[b]
Wk 24	17 (47.2)	13 (36.1)	18 (50.0)	31 (43.1)	.69[b]
Subjects with ≥1 exacerbation requiring hospitalization, n (%)					
Wk 4	4 (11.1)	3 (8.3)	2 (5.6)	5 (6.9)	.48[b]
Wk 12	7 (19.4)	3 (8.3)	5 (13.9)	8 (11.1)	.25[b]
Wk 24	10 (27.8)	6 (16.7)	7 (19.4)	13 (18.1)	.32[b]
Exacerbation rate through wk 12 (95% CI)[c]	3.59 (2.44, 5.10)	1.05 (0.48, 1.99)	2.61 (1.63, 3.95)	1.82 (1.24, 2.59)	.01[d]
Asthma hospitalization rate through wk 12 (95% CI)[c,e]	1.62 (0.89, 2.72)	0.35 (0.07, 1.02)	0.95 (0.41, 1.87)	0.65 (0.32, 1.16)	.02[f]

[a]Primary end point.
[b]*P* value by Fisher exact test comparing combined benralizumab groups with placebo.
[c]Time-weighted exacerbation rate = total number of exacerbations/total duration of person-year follow-up.
[d]*P* value by Poisson regression model without overdispersion comparing benralizumab combined group with placebo. *P* = .02 by Poisson regression model with overdispersion.
[e]Post hoc analysis.
[f]*P* value by Poisson regression model without overdispersion comparing benralizumab combined group with placebo. *P* = .02 by Poisson regression model with overdispersion.

Reprinted from the American Journal of Emergency Medicine. A randomized trial of benralizumab, an antiinterleukin 5 receptor a monoclonal antibody, after acute asthma. Am J Emerg Med. 2015;33:14-20. Copyright 2015, with permission from Elsevier.

TABLE 3.—Health Care Resource Utilization[a]

Health Care Resource	Placebo n = 36	Benralizumab 0.3 mg/kg n = 36	Benralizumab 1.0 mg/kg n = 36	Benralizumab Total n = 72
ED visits				
12 wk	4.40 (38)	3.73 (32)	2.96 (25)	3.35 (57)
24 wk	4.32 (65)	2.83 (42)	3.07 (44)	2.95 (86)[b]
Hospital admissions				
12 wk	1.51 (13)	0.82 (7)	0.95 (8)	0.88 (15)
24 wk	1.66 (25)	0.88 (13)	1.26 (18)	1.06 (31)
Total time spent in hospital at 24 wk, d	73	38	82	120
ICU admissions				
12 wk	0.12 (1)	0	0	0
24 wk	0.27 (4)	0.07 (1)	0.07 (1)	0.07 (2)
Total time spent in the ICU at 24 wk, d	14	2	8	10

[a]Values are expressed as rate (no. of events) for the evaluable population unless otherwise indicated. Rate for each group = total events/total duration of person-year follow-up.
[b]$P < .05$ between the combined treatment and placebo groups by Poisson regression.

the combined benralizumab groups (38.9% vs 33.3%; *P* =.67). However, compared with placebo, benralizumab reduced asthma exacerbation rates by 49% (3.59 vs 1.82; *P* =.01) and exacerbations resulting in hospitalization by 60% (1.62 vs 0.65; *P* =.02) in the combined groups. Benralizumab reduced blood eosinophil counts but did not affect other outcomes, while demonstrating an acceptable safety profile.

Conclusions.—When added to usual care, 1 dose of benralizumab reduced the rate and severity of exacerbations experienced over 12 weeks by subjects who presented to the ED with acute asthma (Figs 2 and 3, Tables 2 and 3).

▶ Phase II randomized double-blind placebo-controlled study of poorly controlled asthmatics with frequent emergency department visits who were randomized to receive a single intravenous infusion of placebo (P) or benralizumab (B) (0.3 mg/kg or 1.0 mg/kg), an anti-interleukin 5 receptor alpha monoclonal antibody (mAb), in addition to usual therapy. Subjects were followed to day 168, and a total of 103 and 80 subjects were followed for 12 and 24 weeks, respectively. Table 2 demonstrates a combined reduction in asthma exacerbations through week 12 for B groups of 49% (*P* = .01) and a combined reduction of 60% vs P through week 12 for subjects who required hospitalization for treatment of exacerbation (*P* = .02). Total eosinophil and basophil numbers were reduced (Fig 3) by B to a greater degree than by corticosteroids (systemic and airway levels), which the investigators hypothesize may be responsible for reduced events.[1-3] In addition, healthcare utilization (Table 3) demonstrated reduced emergency department visits at 24 weeks (combined B groups vs P, *P* = .05). Pharmacoeconomics of this therapy is not discussed, and additional, larger studies are needed. Is this another, more expensive Band-Aid treatment for asthmatics who choose to be noncompliant with treatment? Can the US healthcare system afford such therapies? These are questions that must be answered before we take such therapies mainstream to make up for noncompliant patients.

S. K. Willsie, DO, MA

References

1. Busse WW, Katial R, Gossage D, et al. Safety profile, pharmacokinetics and biologic activity of MEDI-563, an anti-IL-5 receptor alpha antibody, in a phase I subject with asthma. *J Allergy Clin Immunol.* 2010;125:1237-1244.
2. Kolbeck R, Kozhich A, Koike M, et al. MEDI-563, a humanized anti-IL-5 receptor alpha mAb with enhanced antibody-dependent cell-mediated cytotoxicity function. *J Allergy Clin Immunol.* 2010;125:1344-1353.
3. Laviolette M, Gossage DL, Gauvreau G, et al. Effects of benralizumab on airway eosinophils in asthmatic patients with sputum eosinophilia. *J Allergy Clin Immunol.* 2013;132:1086-1096.

The effect of fluticasone furoate/umeclidinium in adult patients with asthma: A randomized, dose-ranging study

Lee LA, Yang S, Kerwin E, et al (GlaxoSmithKline, Research Triangle Park, NC; GlaxoSmithKline, Uxbridge, Middlesex, UK; Clinical Res Inst of Southern Oregon, Medford, OR)

Respir Med 109:54-62, 2015

Background.—We evaluated the dose–response of umeclidinium (UMEC; a long-acting muscarinic antagonist) combined with fluticasone furoate (FF; an inhaled corticosteroid [ICS]) in patients with asthma.

Methods.—In a double-blind, three-period crossover study, 421 subjects (symptomatic on ICS), were randomized to a sequence of three of seven treatments: FF 100 mcg alone, FF 100 mcg combined with UMEC (15.6, 31.25, 62.5, 125, or 250 mcg), or vilanterol 25 mcg (a long-acting β-agonist), inhaled once-daily for 14 days (12–14-day washout). Trough forced expiratory volume in one second (FEV_1), peak expiratory flow (PEF), and safety were assessed.

Results.—Period baseline was a significant covariate, indicating a potential carryover effect between treatment periods. Across all treatment periods, trough FEV_1 improved with FF/UMEC 125 and 250 versus FF (treatment difference 0.055 L [both doses]; $p = 0.018$). FF/UMEC increased morning (15.9–22.9 L/min) and evening (16.2–28.8 L/min) PEF versus FF. As intended assessments were confounded, post hoc Period 1 data analyses were performed, demonstrating significant increases in trough FEV_1 with FF/UMEC 31.25, 62.5, and 250 versus FF. Trough FEV_1 improvements with FF/UMEC were greater in subjects with fixed (0.095–0.304 L) versus non-fixed (−0.084 to 0.041 L) obstruction. The incidence of on-treatment adverse events was 13–25% across groups. No treatment-related effects on laboratory parameters were reported.

Conclusion.—FF/UMEC may be a viable treatment for patients with asthma symptomatic on ICS; benefit may be most prominent in those

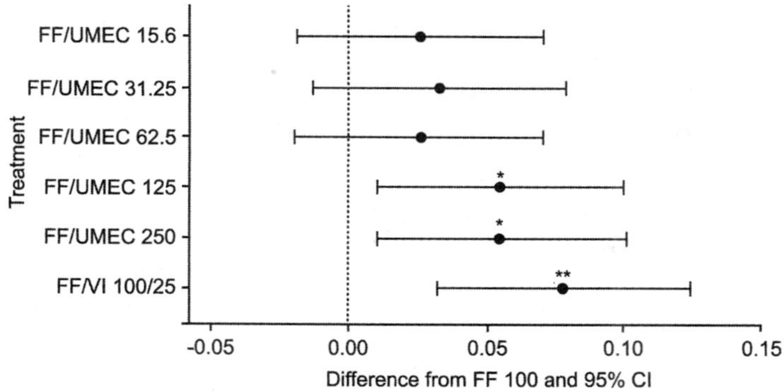

FIGURE 2.—Adjusted mean differences from FF 100 (95% CI) in change from baseline in trough FEV_1 (L) on Day 15 (ITT population). $^*p < 0.05$; $^{**}p < 0.001$. CI, confidence interval; FEV_1, forced expiratory volume in one second; FF, fluticasone furoate; ITT, intent-to-treat; UMEC, umeclidinium; VI, vilanterol. (Reprinted from Respiratory Medicine. Lee LA, Yang S, Kerwin E, et al. The effect of fluticasone furoate/umeclidinium in adult patients with asthma: a randomized, dose-ranging study. *Respir Med.* 2014;109:54-62, Copyright 2014, with permission from Elsevier.)

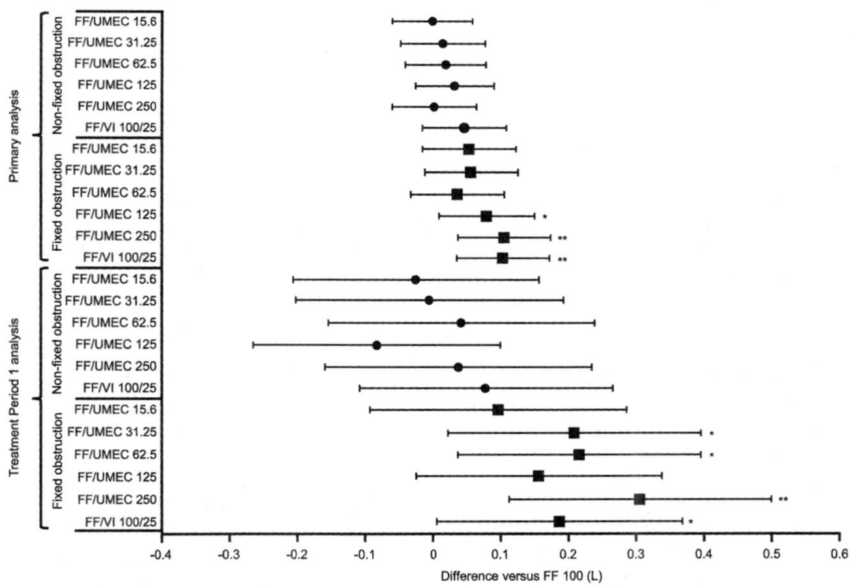

FIGURE 4.—Adjusted mean differences from FF 100 (95% CI) in change from baseline in trough FEV_1 on Day 15 in subjects with fixed obstruction versus non-fixed obstruction in the primary analysis (all treatment periods) and in Treatment Period 1. $p < 0.05$; $^{**}p < 0.001$. CI, confidence interval; FEV_1, forced expiratory volume in one second; FF, fluticasone furoate; UMEC, umeclidinium. (Reprinted from Respiratory Medicine. Lee LA, Yang S, Kerwin E, et al. The effect of fluticasone furoate/umeclidinium in adult patients with asthma: a randomized, dose-ranging study. *Respir Med.* 2014;109:54-62, Copyright 2014, with permission from Elsevier.)

with fixed obstruction. The carryover effect suggests future UMEC studies should use an alternative design.

ClinicalTrials.gov: NCT01573624 (Figs 2 and 4).

▶ Building on data from a randomized dose ranging study of umeclidinium (UME) in asthmatics,[1] this randomized double-blind, 3-period crossover study of 421 subjects who remained symptomatic on inhaled corticosteroids (ICS) was performed to compare fluticasone alone, 100 mcg (FF) to FF with UME (FF-UME) (varying doses) and FF combined with the long-acting beta-agonist (LABA) vilanterol 25 mcg (FF-LABA). Fig 2 demonstrates the mean differences in trough forced expiratory volume in 1 second (FEV_1) on day 15, with all FF-UME and FF-LABA achieving statistically significant improvement compared with FF alone ($P < .05$). Fig 4 depicts results of the mean differences in trough FEV_1 at day 15, with the subjects divided into those who had fixed obstruction and those without fixed obstruction. The trough FEV1 change at day 15 was greatest in the subjects who had fixed obstruction and was statistically significant in the FFMEC 125 mcg and 250 mcg groups ($P < .05$). The investigators suggest that the trough FEV_1 changes at day 15 may be the result of prolonged pulmonary effects of UME. The results of this investigation suggest that patients who remain symptomatic on ICS may benefit from the addition of UME, particularly the phenotype with fixed obstruction, as defined by this investigation (postalbuterol FEV_1/forced vital capacity ratio ≤ 0.70).

S. K. Willsie, DO, MA

Reference

1. Lee LA, Briggs A, Edwards LD, et al. A randomized, three-period crossover study of umeclidinium as monotherapy in adult patients with asthma. *Respir Med.* 2015; 109:63-73.

A randomized, three-period crossover study of umeclidinium as monotherapy in adult patients with asthma

Lee LA, Briggs A, Edwards LD, et al (GlaxoSmithKline, Research Triangle Park, NC; GlaxoSmithKline, Uxbridge, Middlesex, UK)

Respir Med 109:63-73, 2015

Background.—To our knowledge, no studies in patients with asthma have assessed a long-acting muscarinic antagonist in the absence of inhaled corticosteroids (ICS).

Objective.—Evaluate the dose–response, efficacy, and safety of umeclidinium (UMEC) in patients with asthma not receiving ICS.

Methods.—In this double-blind, three-period crossover study, 350 subjects were randomized to a sequence of three of eight inhaled treatments: UMEC 15.6, 31.25, 62.5, 125, or 250 mcg once daily (OD), UMEC 15.6 or 31.25 mcg twice daily (BID), or placebo, administered for 14 days (12–14-day washout). Trough forced expiratory volume in one second

(FEV_1), 0–24-h weighted mean (WM) FEV1, and safety were assessed. Serial spirometry and pharmacokinetic assessments were performed in a subgroup.

Results.—Subjects had a mean baseline pre- and post-bronchodilator FEV_1 of 71% and 88% predicted, respectively. Significant improvements in change from baseline trough FEV_1 were observed for UMEC 15.6 OD (0.066 L; $p = 0.036$) and UMEC 125 OD (0.088 L; $p = 0.005$) versus placebo, but not other OD or BID doses. UMEC increased 0–24-h WM FEV_1 versus placebo (0.068–0.121 L [$p \leq 0.017$] with no clear dose-response). Treatment differences were similar for corresponding OD and BID doses in serial assessments. UMEC was rapidly absorbed, with evidence of some accumulation. The incidence of on treatment adverse events was 9–21% for UMEC and 12% for placebo. There were no treatment-related effects on laboratory parameters.

Conclusion.—The modest trough FEV_1 improvements did not conclusively support a therapeutic benefit of UMEC in non-ICS treated patients with asthma.

ClinicalTrials.gov.—NCT01641692 (Figs 2 and 3, Tables 2 and 3).

▶ This randomized double-blind placebo-controlled, 3-period crossover study of mild adult asthmatics not receiving inhaled corticosteroids (ICS) was performed to evaluate efficacy and safety of monotherapy of a long-acting muscarinic agent (LAMA), umeclidinium (UME). LAMAs are included in guideline-directed care for chronic obstructive pulmonary disease (COPD), and some recently published studies have shown that the LAMA tiotropium has reduced asthmatic symptoms and improved pulmonary function when administered as add-on therapy with ICS[1,2] and has reduced the risk of severe asthma exacerbations when added to ICS and long-acting beta agonist therapy (LABA).[3] Studies in COPD patients have shown that UME has been well tolerated and has led to

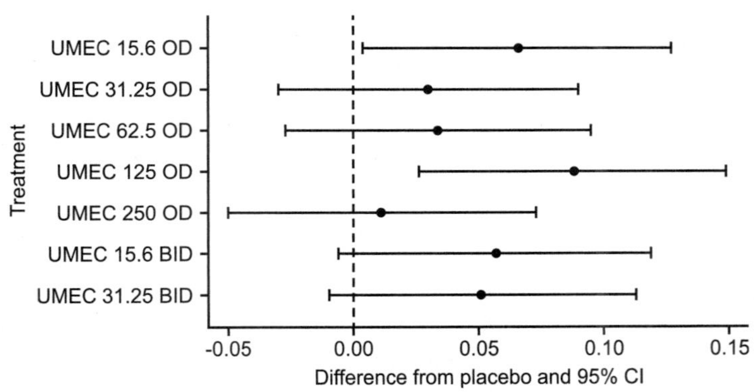

FIGURE 2.—Adjusted mean differences from placebo (95% CI) in change from baseline in trough FEV_1 (L) on Day 15. CI, confidence interval; BID, twice daily; FEV_1, forced expiratory volume in one second; OD, once daily; UMEC, umeclidinium. (Reprinted from Respiratory Medicine. Lee LA, Briggs A, Edwards LD, et al. A randomized, three-period crossover study of umeclidinium as monotherapy in adult patients with asthma. *Respir Med.* 2014;109:63-73, Copyright 2014, with permission from Elsevier.)

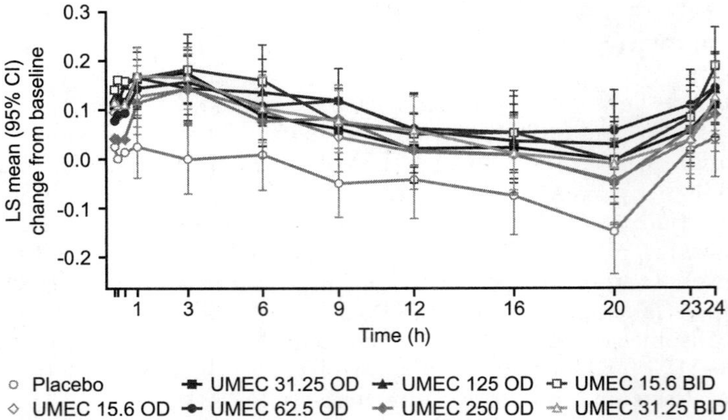

FIGURE 3.—Adjusted mean change from baseline (95% CI) in 0–24-h serial FEV_1 on Day 14. BID, twice daily; CI, confidence interval; FEV_1, forced expiratory volume in one second; LS, least squares; OD, once daily; UMEC, umeclidinium. (Reprinted from Respiratory Medicine. Lee LA, Briggs A, Edwards LD, et al. A randomized, three-period crossover study of umeclidinium as monotherapy in adult patients with asthma. *Respir Med.* 2014;109:63-73, Copyright 2014, with permission from Elsevier.)

TABLE 2.—Statistical Analysis of Change From Baseline in Trough FEV_1 (L) at Day 15

Trough FEV_1 (L)	Placebo	UMEC OD 15.6 mcg	UMEC OD 31.25 mcg	UMEC OD 62.5 mcg	UMEC OD 125 mcg	UMEC OD 250 mcg
n	110	120	124	122	113	117
LS mean (SE)	2.398 (0.0235)	2.464 (0.0226)	2.428 (0.0222)	2.432 (0.0224)	2.486 (0.0232)	2.409 (0.0228)
LS mean change (SE)	0.046 (0.0235)	0.112 (0.0226)	0.076 (0.0222)	0.080 (0.0224)	0.134 (0.0232)	0.057 (0.0228)
Treatment vs Placebo						
Difference		0.066	0.030	0.034	0.088	0.011
95% CI		0.004, 0.127	−0.030, 0.090	−0.027, 0.095	0.026, 0.149	−0.050, 0.073
p-value		0.036	0.331	0.272	0.005	0.722

Trough FEV_1 (L)	UMEC BID 15.6 mcg	UMEC BID 31.25 mcg
n	113	118
LS mean (SE)	2.455 (0.0232)	2.449 (0.0227)
LS mean change (SE)	0.103 (0.0232)	0.097 (0.0227)
Treatment vs Placebo		
Difference	0.057	0.051
95% CI	−0.006, 0.119	−0.010, 0.113
p-value	0.076	0.101

Analysis performed using a mixed model, including treatment, period, period baseline FEV_1 and mean baseline FEV_1 as fixed effects and subject as a random effect.

BID, twice daily; CI, confidence interval; FEV_1, forced expiratory volume in one second; L, liters; LS, least squares; OD, once daily; SE, standard error; UMEC, umeclidinium.

Reprinted from Respiratory Medicine. Lee LA, Briggs A, Edwards LD, et al. A randomized, three-period crossover study of umeclidinium as monotherapy in adult patients with asthma. Respir Med. 2014;109:63-73, Copyright 2014, with permission from Elsevier.

TABLE 3.—0–24-h WM FEV_1 at Day 14

WM FEV_1 (L)	Placebo	UMEC OD 15.6 mcg	UMEC OD 31.25 mcg	UMEC OD 62.5 mcg	UMEC OD 125 mcg	UMEC OD 250 mcg
n	33	35	49	42	45	38
LS mean (SE)	2.309 (0.0255)	2.394 (0.0249)	2.410 (0.0222)	2.426 (0.0232)	2.427 (0.0229)	2.382 (0.0243)
LS mean change (SE)	−0.025 (0.0255)	0.060 (0.0249)	0.077 (0.0222)	0.092 (0.0232)	0.094 (0.0229)	0.048 (0.0243)
Treatment vs placebo						
Difference		0.085	0.101	0.117	0.119	0.073
95% CI		0.025, 0.145	0.047, 0.156	0.061, 0.173	0.064, 0.174	0.015, 0.131
p-value		0.006	<0.001	<0.001	<0.001	0.014

WM FEV_1 (L)	UMEC BID 15.6 mcg	UMEC BID 31.25 mcg
n	35	43
LS mean (SE)	2.430 (0.0252)	2.377 (0.0231)
LS mean change (SE)	0.097 (0.0252)	0.043 (0.0231)
Treatment vs placebo		
Difference	0.121	0.068
95% CI	0.061, 0.182	0.012, 0.124
p-value	<0.001	0.017

Note: Analysis performed using a mixed model, including treatment, period, period baseline FEV_1 and mean baseline FEV_1 as fixed effects and subject as a random effect.

BID, twice daily; CI, confidence interval; FEV_1, forced expiratory volume in one second; L, liters; LS, least squares; OD, once daily; SE, standard error; UMEC, umeclidinium; WM, weighted mean.

Reprinted from Respiratory Medicine. Lee LA, Briggs A, Edwards LD, et al. A randomized, three-period crossover study of umeclidinium as monotherapy in adult patients with asthma. Respir Med. 2014;109:63-73, Copyright 2014, with permission from Elsevier.

significantly improved lung function, reduced dyspnea, and improved overall health status versus placebo (P).[4-7] All consented subjects entered a 9- to 14-day run-in period, after which reversibility testing with ipratropium bromide was performed. Eligible subjects were stratified by age in a 1:2:2 ratio (18–29, 30–49, ≥50 years) and were randomized at visit 3 to a sequence of 3 of 8 potential treatments. Treatments included UME at 5 different concentrations once daily, UME at 2 concentrations twice daily, or placebo. Each treatment period was 14 days in duration and separated by a 12- to 14-day washout period. The final follow-up visit occurred 5 to 9 days following the last treatment period. All treatments were delivered by dry powder inhaler via metered dose inhaler (MDI). Fig 2 and Table 2 together demonstrate that the trough forced expiratory volume at 1 second (FEV_1) increased for all UME doses vs P; however, only the 15.6 and 125 once-daily doses of UME reached statistical significance vs P ($P < .05$). Table 3 and Fig 3 depict results from the subgroup of subjects who underwent serial spirometry; significant statistical improvement was seen in the 0- to 24-hour weighted mean FEV_1 vs P, with the largest increase ($P \leq .005$) noted 3 hours after dosing. Results of bid dosing were similar to once-daily dosing. Although all doses of UME produced statistically significant increases in the 0- to 6-hour weighted mean FEV_1 vs P on Day 1 with the exception of UME administered 31.25 once and twice daily, there was no clear dose response evident in any of the serial spirometry measurements. Additional studies are indicated, particularly in asthmatics who are known to exhibit elevated cholinergic tone, and, in those subjects particularly, as adjunctive to ICS therapy.

S. K. Willsie, DO, MA

References

1. Peters SP, Kunselman SJ, Icitovic N, et al. Tiotropium bromide step-up therapy for adults with uncontrolled asthma. *N Engl J Med.* 2010;363:1715-1726.
2. Beeh KM, Moroni-Zentgraf P, Ablinger O, et al. Tiotropium in asthma: a dose-finding study in adult patients with moderate persistent asthma. *Respir Res.* 2013;187:A1283.
3. Kerstjens HA, Engel M, Dahl R, et al. Tiotropium in asthma poorly controlled with standard combination therapy. *N Engl J Med.* 2012;367:1198-1207.
4. Decramer M, Maltais F, Feldman G, et al. Bronchodilatation of umeclidinium, a new long-acting muscarininc antagonist, in COPD patients. *Respir Physiol Neurobiol.* 2013;185:393-399.
5. Tal-Singer R, Cahn A, Mehta R, et al. Initial assessment of single and repeat dose of inhaled umeclidinium in patients with COPD: two randomized studies. *Eur J Pharmacol.* 2013;701:40-48.
6. Trivedi R, Richard N, Mehta R, Church A. Umeclidinium in patients with COPD: a randomised, placebo controlled study. *Eur Respir J.* 2014;43:72-81.
7. Donohue JF, Anzueto A, Brooks J, Mehta R, Kalberg C, Crater G. A randomized, double-blind dose-ranging study of the novel LAMA GSK573719 in patients with COPD. *Respir Med.* 2012;106:970-979.

Cluster Analysis and Characterization of Response to Mepolizumab: A Step Closer to Personalized Medicine for Patients with Severe Asthma

Ortega H, Li H, Suruki R, et al (GlaxoSmithKline, Research Triangle Park, NC; et al)

Ann Am Thorac Soc 11:1011-1017, 2014

Rationale.—Detailed characterization of asthma phenotypes is essential for identification of responder populations to allow directed personalized medical intervention.

Objectives.—The aim of this study was to identify distinctive patient characteristics within subgroups of a well-characterized severe asthma population at risk for exacerbations and to determine the treatment response within each subgroup.

Methods.—A supervised cluster analysis with recursive partitioning approach was applied to data from the Dose Ranging Efficacy And safety with Mepolizumab (DREAM) study to identify characteristics that maximized the differences across subgroups. Exacerbation rate ratios were calculated for each cluster comparing mepolizumab versus placebo.

Measurements and Main Results.—Three predictors were identified in four primary clusters: blood eosinophils, airway reversibility, and body mass index. The reduction in exacerbations was significantly greater in patients who received mepolizumab (clusters 2, 3, and 4) with raised eosinophils (responder population). Cluster 2 with low airway reversibility

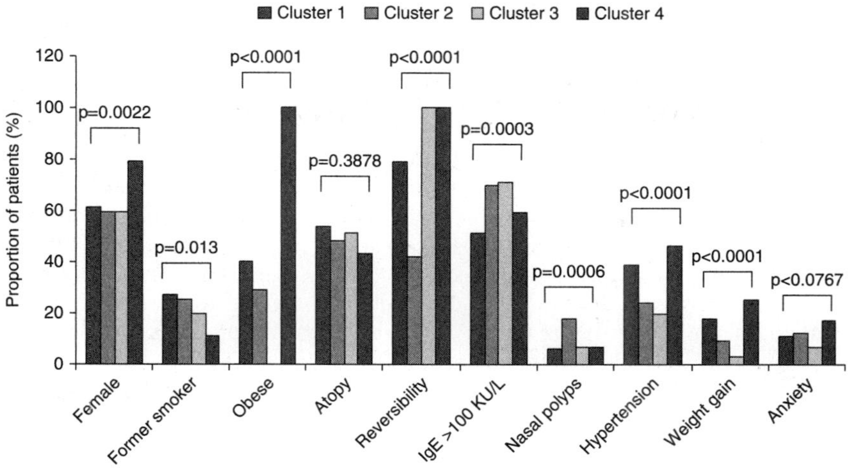

FIGURE 3.—Proportion of patients with key clinical characteristics by cluster. *P* value represents any difference across the clusters. (Reprinted from Ortega H, Li H, Suruki R, et al. Cluster analysis and characterization of response to mepolizumab: a step closer to personalized medicine for patients with severe asthma. *Ann Am Thorac Soc.* 2014;11:1011-1017, with permission from the American Thoracic Society.)

(mean, 11%) had a 53% reduction in exacerbations. These patients more frequently reported sinusitis and nasal polyposis. Those with higher airway reversibility (mean, 28%) were further split by body mass index. The non-obese versus obese (clusters 3 and 4) had a 35 and 67% reduction in exacerbations, respectively. Cluster 4 also had patients with more comorbidities, including hypertension, weight gain, and anxiety.

Conclusions.—Using supervised cluster analysis helped identify specific patient characteristics related to disease and therapeutic response. Patients with eosinophilic inflammation received significant therapeutic benefit with mepolizumab, and responses differed within clusters. Clinical trial registered with www.clinicaltrials.gov (NCT01000506) (Fig 3).

▶ This is a post-hoc analysis of the DREAM study (Dose Ranging Efficacy and Safety with Mepolizumab [M]) with the aim to determine whether specific characteristics might predict increased efficacy with M. The DREAM study evaluated the exacerbation rate of 616 severe asthmatics administering 3 dose levels of M (75 mg, 250 mg, 750 mg intravenously every 4 weeks) compared with placebo (P) for 12 months. Several clusters of subjects were developed based on specific criteria: Cluster 1: mean age of 51 years, 62.7% female; relative low level of eosinophils; lower total immunoglobulin E, elevated fractional excretion of nitric oxide (FENO), and > 50% with atopy; 12% reduction of asthma exacerbations (AE) with M; Cluster 2: mean age 48 years; low airway reversibility of 11%; high proportion of sinusitis and polyposis; 53% reduction of AE with M. Cluster 3: mean age 49 years; 28.7% airway reversibility; body mass index (BMI) 25.3; 36% reduction of AE with M; Cluster 4: 96 subjects with mean age of 50; majority were female; high airway reversibility 28.3%; obese,

BMI 33.9; 43.1% atopic; 67% reduction of AE with M; lowest mean post-bronchodilator forced expiratory volume in 1 second of 66% (most severe cluster). Fig 3 represents the key features by cluster. The investigators summarize their response data to advise that the severe asthmatic subjects with phenotypes showing higher blood eosinophilia (>150 cell/μ) and obesity were the subjects most likely to have the greatest reduction in AEs when treated with M. What does this mean? So-called personalized asthma treatment options may be possible by predetermining which asthma phenotype your patient has and then applying the therapy most likely to lead to the best response. Although we might not be there with all asthma therapies, the past few years have brought us closer to that goal. It just might not be that much longer before we are able to plan optimal treatment for our asthmatics just as we plan best antihypertensive therapy from the get-go for certain populations. Exciting? Yes!

S. K. Willsie, DO, MA

Comprehensive efficacy of omalizumab for severe refractory asthma: a time-series observational study

Tajiri T, Niimi A, Matsumoto H, et al (Kyoto Univ, Japan)

Ann Allergy Asthma Immunol 113:470-475, 2014

Background.—Omalizumab, a humanized anti-IgE monoclonal antibody, is reportedly an effective treatment for severe allergic asthma. However, there have been few comprehensive analyses of its efficacy, including assessments of small airways or airway remodeling.

Objective.—To comprehensively evaluate the efficacy of omalizumab, including its effects on small airways and airway remodeling, in adult patients with severe refractory asthma.

Methods.—In this prospective, time-series, single-arm observational study, 31 adult patients with severe refractory asthma despite the use of multiple controller medications, including high-dose inhaled corticosteroids (1,432 ± 581 μg/d of fluticasone propionate equivalent), were enrolled. Clinical variables, including Asthma Quality of Life Questionnaire, asthma exacerbations, exhaled nitric oxide, pulmonary function, methacholine airway responsiveness, induced sputum, and chest computed tomogram, were assessed at baseline and after 16 and 48 weeks of treatment with omalizumab.

Results.—Twenty-six of the 31 patients completed 48 weeks of treatment. For these patients, Asthma Quality of Life Questionnaire scores and peak expiratory flow values significantly and continuously improved throughout the 48 weeks ($P < .001$ for all comparisons). Unscheduled physician visits, asthma exacerbations requiring systemic corticosteroids, fractional exhaled nitric oxide at 50 mL/s and alveolar nitric oxide levels, sputum eosinophil proportions, and airway-wall thickness as assessed by computed tomography significantly decreased at 48 weeks ($P < .05$ for all comparisons).

Conclusion.—Omalizumab was effective for adult patients with severe refractory asthma. Omalizumab may have anti-inflammatory effects on small airways and reverse airway remodeling.

Trial Registration.—UMIN000002389 (Figs 2-4, Tables 2-4).

▶ Omalizumab, an anti-immunoglobulin E (IgE) monoclonal antibody approved for adjunctive treatment of severe allergic asthma, was prospectively administered every 2 to 4 weeks in addition to stable inhaled corticosteroid doses and other asthma therapy for 48 weeks to 31 subjects with severe refractory asthma. Twenty-six subjects complete the study, which included frequent detailed assessments throughout the study, including pulmonary function: Asthma Quality of Life Questionnaires (AQLQ), asthma exacerbations, exhaled nitric oxide (ENO), methacholine (MC) airway responsiveness, serum IgE levels, induced sputum, and chest computed tomography (CT). Table 2 depicts changes at baseline, 16 weeks, and 48 weeks in the AQLQ, which demonstrated statistically significant and maintained improvement over the 48-week period ($P < .05$). Figs 2-4 depict changes in the rate of unscheduled clinic visits and asthma exacerbations requiring systemic steroids for at least 3 days; changes in fractional ENO vs alveolar NO over time, all statistically significant; and changes across time in peak expiratory flow showing significant improvement ($P < .001$), respectively. Table 3 depicts the results of pulmonary function that did not significantly

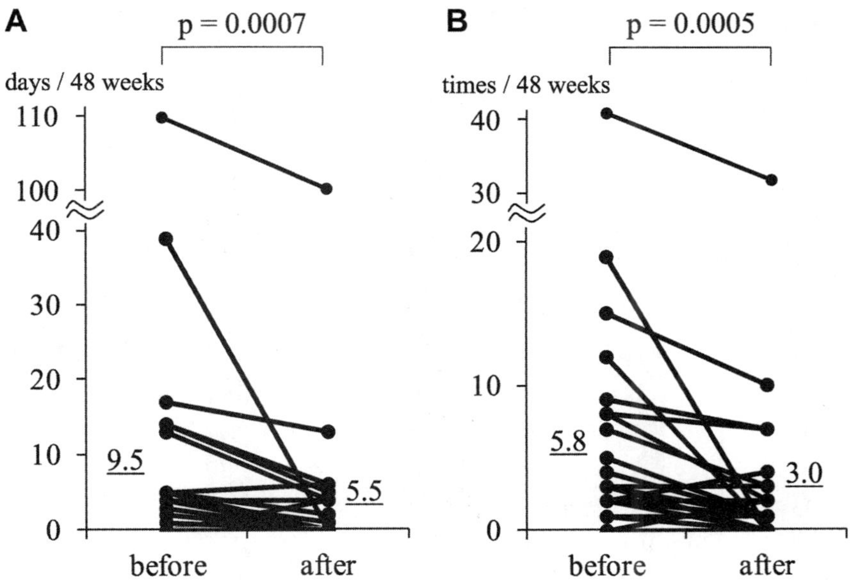

FIGURE 2.—Changes from 48 weeks before treatment to 48 weeks after treatment in *(A)* the rate of unscheduled physician visits and *(B)* the rate of asthma exacerbations that required systemic corticosteroids for at least 3 days. Each point represents a single patient and values indicate means. (Reprinted from Annals of Allergy, Asthma and Immunology. Tajiri T, Niimi A, Matsumoto H, et al. Comprehensive efficacy of omalizumab for severe refractory asthma: a time-series observational study. *Ann Allergy Asthma Immunol.* 2014;113:470-475, Copyright 2014, with permission from American College of Annals of Allergy, Asthma & Immunology.)

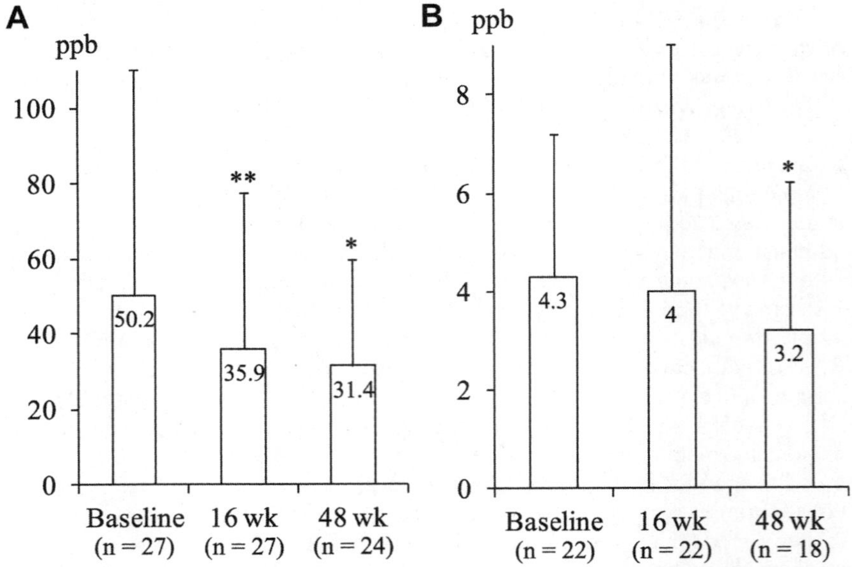

FIGURE 3.—Changes from baseline to 48 weeks of treatment in *(A)* fractional exhaled nitric oxide at 50-mL/s levels and *(B)* alveolar nitric oxide levels. *$P < .05$, **$P < .01$ compared with baseline values. Values and bars indicate means and SDs. (Reprinted from Annals of Allergy, Asthma and Immunology. Tajiri T, Niimi A, Matsumoto H, et al. Comprehensive efficacy of omalizumab for severe refractory asthma: a time-series observational study. *Ann Allergy Asthma Immunol.* 2014;113:470-475, Copyright 2014, with permission from American College of Annals of Allergy, Asthma & Immunology.)

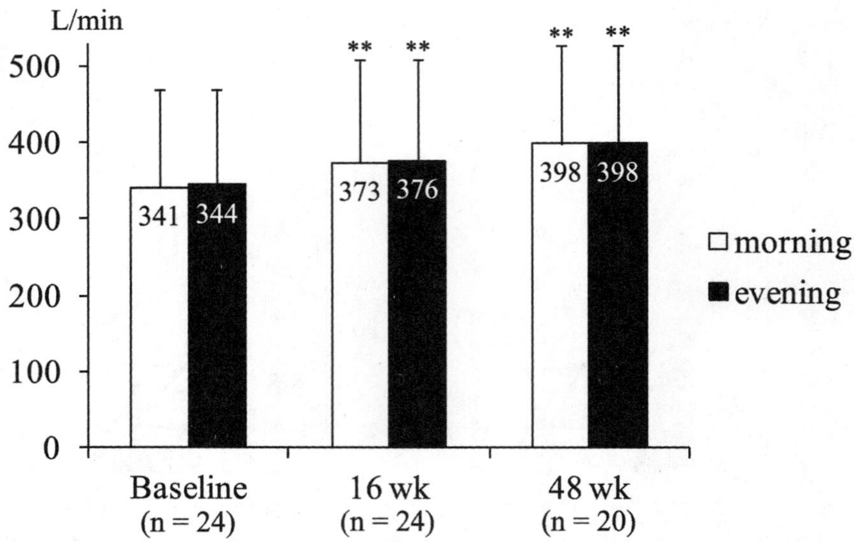

FIGURE 4.—Changes from baseline to 48 weeks of treatment in peak expiratory flow values in the morning and evening. **$P < .001$ compared with baseline values. Values and bars indicate means and SDs. (Reprinted from Annals of Allergy, Asthma and Immunology. Tajiri T, Niimi A, Matsumoto H, et al. Comprehensive efficacy of omalizumab for severe refractory asthma: a time-series observational study. *Ann Allergy Asthma Immunol.* 2014;113:470-475, Copyright 2014, with permission from American College of Annals of Allergy, Asthma & Immunology.)

TABLE 2.—Changes From Baseline and 16 Weeks in SGRQ, AQLQ, and ACQ Scores[a]

Questionnaire and Domain	Baseline (n = 31)	Baseline vs 16 wk (n = 31)	16 vs 48 wk (n = 26)	Baseline vs 48 wk (n = 26)
SGRQ				
Symptoms	65.7 ± 24.1	−10.08[b]	−12.45[c]	−22.49[d]
Activities	51.6 ± 27.8	−4.31	−12.04[b]	−14.41[d]
Impact	40.6 ± 23.4	−9.81[c]	−9.70[c]	−19.08[d]
Total	48.1 ± 23.1	−4.88[b]	−14.81[c]	−18.24[d]
AQLQ				
Symptoms	4.3 ± 1.6	0.97[d]	0.66[c]	1.74[d]
Activities	4.1 ± 1.4	0.59[b]	0.48[c]	1.07[d]
Emotions	4.4 ± 1.6	0.86[c]	0.42[b]	1.29[d]
Environment	4.5 ± 1.7	0.62[b]	0.47[b]	1.09[d]
Overall	4.2 ± 1.4	0.81[c]	0.50[b]	1.36[d]
ACQ				
Total	2.0 ± 1.0	−0.62[c]	−0.37[b]	−1.11[d]

Abbreviations: ACQ, Asthma Control Questionnaire; AQLQ, Asthma Quality of Life Questionnaire; SGRQ, St George's Respiratory Questionnaire.

[a]Values at baseline are presented as mean ± SD. Values at 16 and 48 weeks are average changes in score from baseline values.

[b]$P < .05$ compared with baseline by paired t test.

[c]$P < .01$ compared with baseline by paired t test.

[d]$P < .001$ compared with baseline by paired t test.

TABLE 3.—Effects of Omalizumab on Pulmonary Function[a]

Variables	Baseline (n = 29)	Time Points 16 wk (n = 29)	48 wk (n = 25)	*P* Value[b]
Pulmonary function				
VC (L)	3.02 ± 0.73	3.13 ± 0.75[c]	3.05 ± 0.61	.07
FVC (L)	2.93 ± 0.68	3.02 ± 0.71	2.96 ± 0.61	.41
FEV_1 (L/s)	2.17 ± 0.53	2.25 ± 0.56	2.24 ± 0.55	.09
$FEF_{25\text{-}75}$ (L/s)	1.86 ± 1.01	1.85 ± 1.03	1.89 ± 1.13	.09
RV/TLC (%)	32.1 ± 8.1	31.2 ± 5.6	30.7 ± 6.3	.61
ΔN2	2.52 ± 2.85	2.17 ± 1.95	1.78 ± 1.37	.06
Impulse oscillometry				
R5 (kPa/L/s)	0.41 ± 0.23	0.40 ± 0.22	0.36 ± 0.20	.06
R20 (kPa/L/s)	0.30 ± 0.10	0.29 ± 0.09	0.28 ± 0.10	.07
R5−R20 (kPa/L/s)	0.11 ± 0.15	0.11 ± 0.15	0.08 ± 0.12	.16
AX (kPa/L)	1.13 ± 1.96	1.19 ± 2.09	0.91 ± 1.68	.47

Abbreviations: AX, integrated area of low-frequency reactance; ΔN_2, slope of phase 3 of nitrogen single-breath washout curve; $FEF_{25\text{-}75}$, forced expiratory flow at 25% to 75%; FEV_1, forced expiratory volume in 1 second; FVC, forced vital capacity; R20, respiratory resistance at 20 Hz; R5, respiratory resistance at 5 Hz; R5−R20, difference in respiratory resistance between 5 and 20 Hz; RV, residual volume; TLC, total lung capacity; VC, vital capacity.

[a]Values are presented as mean ± SD.

[b]P values for baseline vs 48 weeks by paired t test.

[c]$P < .05$ compared with baseline by paired t test.

TABLE 4.—Effects of Omalizumab on Computed Tomographic Indices[a]

	Time Points			
	Baseline	16 wk[b]	48 wk	*P* Value[c]
Airway dimensions	21	21	14	
WA (mm^2)	30.3 ± 12.6	29.5 ± 12.5	26.0 ± 7.6	.09
WA/BSA (mm^2/m^2)	18.6 ± 8.2	18.1 ± 7.9	11.0 ± 3.3	.09
WA%	62.0 ± 7.2	60.6 ± 7.3	57.1 ± 6.2	.002
Ao (mm^2)	49.7 ± 21.7	48.9 ± 21.5	45.6 ± 13.1	.51
Ao/BSA (mm^2/m^2)	30.6 ± 13.8	30.1 ± 13.5	27.9 ± 7.2	.54
Ai (mm^2)	19.5 ± 9.8	19.4 ± 9.9	19.6 ± 6.6	.024
Ai/BSA (mm^2/m^2)	12.0 ± 6.1	12.0 ± 6.2	12.1 ± 4.0	.025
Lung density	24	24	17	
LAA% of inspiratory scans	22.2 ± 7.6	22.4 ± 6.5	24.8 ± 5.1	.07
LAA% of expiratory scans	9.8 ± 4.9	10.4 ± 6.6	9.9 ± 4.6	.43
E/I ratio of LAA%	0.51 ± 0.51	0.46 ± 0.27	0.39 ± 0.15	.89
MLD of inspiratory scans (HU)	−859.7 ± 35.6	−863.4 ± 28.4	−874.0 ± 16.9	.10
MLD of expiratory scans (HU)	−761.6 ± 58.9	−762.6 ± 62.6	−764.8 ± 50.3	.71
E/I ratio of MLD	0.89 ± 0.06	0.88 ± 0.06	0.87 ± 0.05	.78

Abbreviations: Ai, luminal area; Ao, outer area of bronchus; BSA, body surface area; E/I ratio, percentage of low-attenuation area to lung area and mean lung density on inspiratory and expiratory computed tomographic scans and the ratios of these values at expiration to the respective values at inspiration; LAA%, percentage of low-attenuation area to lung area; MLD, mean lung density; WA%, percentage of wall area equal to wall area divided by outer area of bronchus multiplied by 100; WA, wall area.

[a]Values are presented as number of patients or mean ± SD.

[b]$P > .05$ for all indices compared with baseline by paired *t* test.

[c]*P* value for baseline vs 48 weeks by paired *t* test.

improve over time, and Table 4 demonstrates the results of chest CT, which showed evidence of statistically significant increase in luminal area and wall area/outer area of bronchus (%WA) at 48 weeks but not at 16 weeks. The reduced %WA seen at 48 weeks was associated with a reduced ENO and sputum eosinophil numbers. These same type of CT changes have been suggested to be associated with possible reversal in airway remodeling.[1] These results add to the body of knowledge related to using this drug in severe refractory asthma. The data regarding the potential for reversal of airway remodeling, albeit in limited numbers of subjects, holds potential promise for the future, pending confirmation by larger prospective, randomized studies.

S. K. Willsie, DO, MA

Reference

1. Niimi A, Matsumoto H, Amitani R, et al. Effect of short-term treatment with inhaled corticosteroid on airway wall thickening in asthma. *Am J Med.* 2004; 116:725-731.

Tiotropium in asthmatic adolescents symptomatic despite inhaled corticosteroids: A randomised dose-ranging study

Vogelberg C, Engel M, Moroni-Zentgraf P, et al (Univ Hosp Carl Gustav Carus, Dresden, Germany; Boehringer Ingelheim Pharma GmbH & Co. KG, Ingelheim am Rhein, Germany; et al)

Respir Med 108:1268-1276, 2014

Introduction.—Tiotropium, a once-daily long-acting anticholinergic agent, has been shown to be an efficacious and safe add-on treatment for adults with symptomatic asthma, despite treatment with inhaled corticosteroids (ICS). A large proportion of asthmatic adolescents have symptomatic disease despite a wide range of therapeutic options. We investigated the efficacy and safety of three doses of tiotropium, administered in the evening (via Respimat® SoftMist™ inhaler), versus placebo in asthmatic adolescents symptomatic despite ICS treatment.

Methods.—This randomised, double-blind, placebo-controlled, incomplete crossover study evaluated once-daily tiotropium 5 μg, 2.5 μg and 1.25 μg versus placebo in three 4-week treatment periods. Primary efficacy end point was change in peak forced expiratory volume in 1 s within 3 h post-dose from baseline (peak $FEV_{1(0-3h)}$).

Results.—From 139 enrolled patients, 105 were randomised to receive one of four treatment sequences. Peak $FEV_{1(0-3h)}$ response for tiotropium 5 μg was significantly greater versus placebo ($p = 0.0043$). Trough FEV_1 responses were significantly greater for tiotropium 5 μg ($p < 0.00001$) and 1.25 μg ($p = 0.0134$) versus placebo, but not for 2.5 μg ($p = 0.0975$), while FEV_1 area under the $\text{curve}_{(0-3h)}$ responses were significant for all doses ($p = 0.00001-0.0398$). Overall incidence of adverse events was balanced across treatment groups, with no dosedependent observations. The majority of adverse events were mild to moderate in intensity.

Conclusion.—This first study of tiotropium in adolescents with symptomatic asthma demonstrates that tiotropium is well tolerated and efficacious as add-on to maintenance treatment with ICS.

ClinicalTrials.gov identifier; NCT01122680 (Figs 1-3 and 5).

► This dose-ranging randomized double-blind placebo-controlled incomplete-crossover study evaluated 3 doses (5, 2.5, and 1.25 μg) of tiotropium (T) in adolescent asthmatics who remained symptomatic despite receiving medium-doses of inhaled corticosteroids (ICS). Global asthma guidelines have recommended the addition of short-acting anticholinergic agents to short-acting beta agonists as reliever medications.[1] Following a 4-week run-in period, moderate persistent asthmatics on medium-dose ICS were randomized in a 1:1:1:1 ratio to receive once-daily placebo (P) or T 5, 2.5, or 1.25 μg, all delivered via a SoftMist (superscript TM) inhaler, every evening for each of the three 4-week treatment periods. A final follow-up visit occurred 3 weeks after the final treatment period. All subjects continued baseline treatment, which included medium doses of ICS and rescue short-acting beta agonists, with or without leukotriene modifiers. Fig 1 depicts the study design and outcome assessments performed; Fig 2 demonstrates a

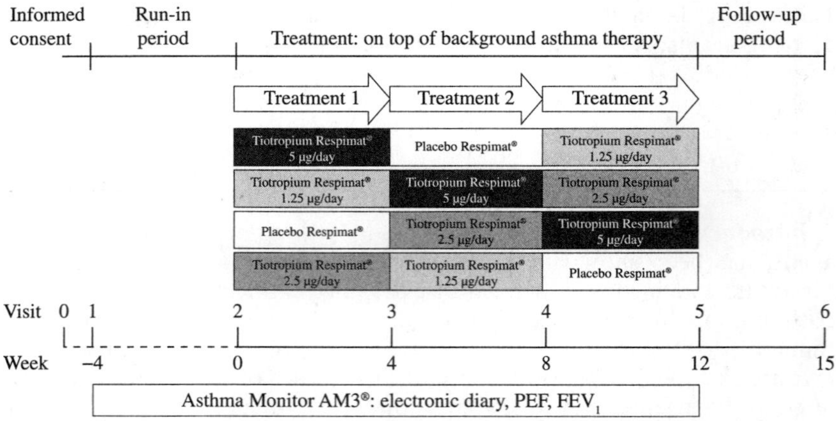

FIGURE 1.—Study design. FEV_1, forced expiratory volume in 1 s; PEF, peak expiratory flow. (Reprinted from Respiratory Medicine. Vogelberg C, Engel M, Moroni-Zentgraf P, et al. Tiotropium in asthmatic adolescents symptomatic despite inhaled corticosteroids: a randomised dose-ranging study. *Respir Med.* 2014;108:1268-1276, Copyright 2014, with permission from Elsevier.)

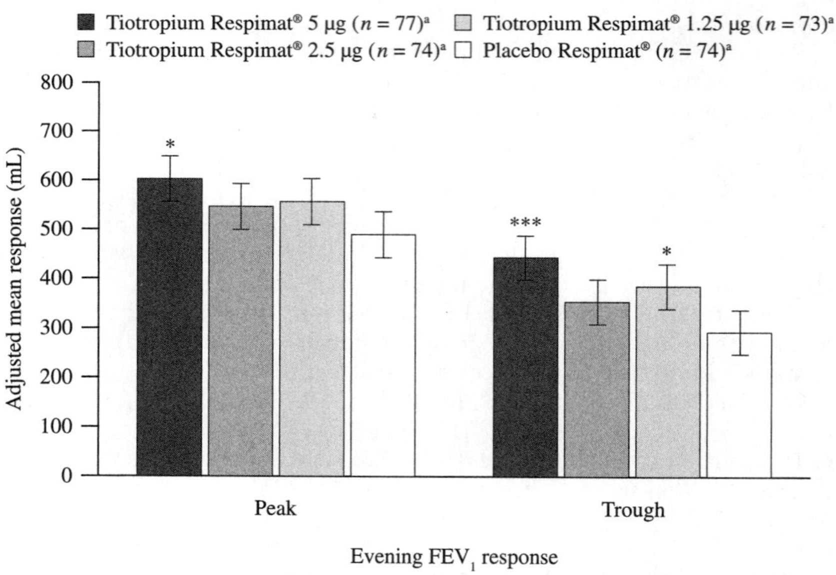

FIGURE 2.—Evening peak FEV_1 within 3 h post-dose from baseline and trough FEV_1 responses to tiotropium Respimat® and placebo Respimat® (full analysis set). $*p < 0.05$; $***p < 0.001$ versus placebo Respimat®. [a]The number of patients within the full analysis set for whom the end point measurement is available. FEV_1, forced expiratory volume in 1 s. (Reprinted from Respiratory Medicine. Vogelberg C, Engel M, Moroni-Zentgraf P, et al. Tiotropium in asthmatic adolescents symptomatic despite inhaled corticosteroids: a randomised dose-ranging study. *Respir Med.* 2014;108:1268-1276, Copyright 2014, with permission from Elsevier.)

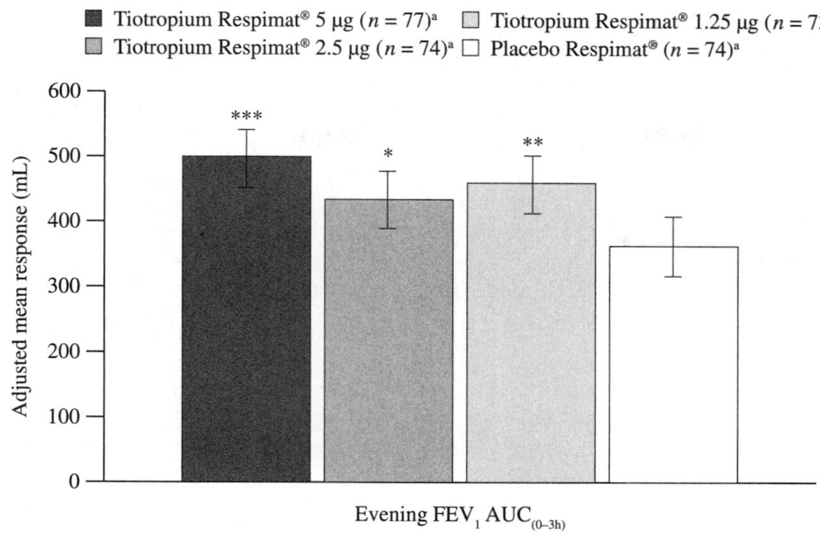

FIGURE 3.—Evening FEV_1 AUC responses to tiotropium Respimat® and placebo Respimat® (full analysis set). $*p < 0.05$; $**p < 0.01$; $***p < 0.001$ versus placebo Respimat®. [a]The number of patients within the full analysis set for whom the end point measurement is available. AUC, area under the curve; FEV_1, forced expiratory volume in 1 s. (Reprinted from Respiratory Medicine. Vogelberg C, Engel M, Moroni-Zentgraf P, et al. Tiotropium in asthmatic adolescents symptomatic despite inhaled corticosteroids: a randomised dose-ranging study. *Respir Med.* 2014;108:1268-1276, Copyright 2014, with permission from Elsevier.)

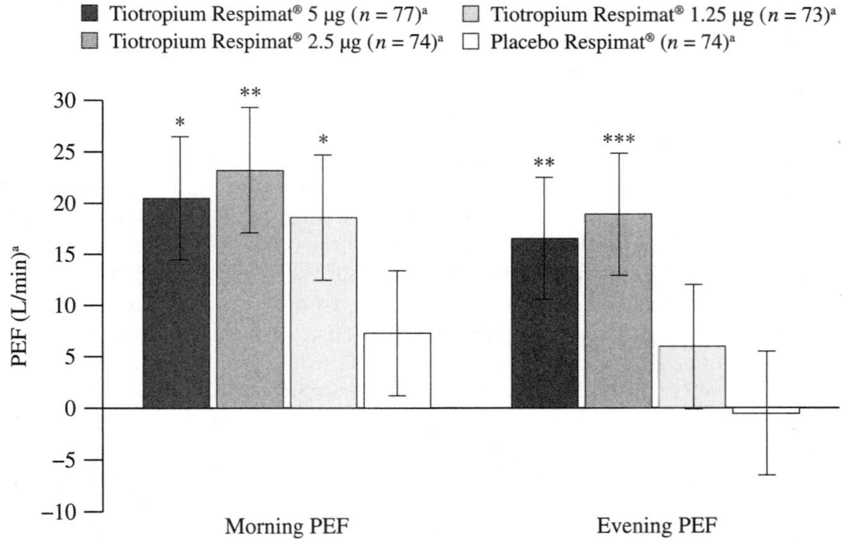

FIGURE 5.—Morning and evening PEF response to tiotropium Respimat® and placebo Respimat® (full analysis set). $*p < 0.05$; $**p < 0.01$; $***p < 0.001$ versus placebo Respimat®. [a]Determined as a response from baseline on the weekly mean of the last week of treatment for each treatment period. [b]The number of patients within the full analysis set for whom the end point measurement is available. PEF, peak expiratory flow. (Reprinted from Respiratory Medicine. Vogelberg C, Engel M, Moroni-Zentgraf P, et al. Tiotropium in asthmatic adolescents symptomatic despite inhaled corticosteroids: a randomised dose-ranging study. *Respir Med.* 2014;108:1268-1276, Copyright 2014, with permission from Elsevier.)

statistically significant increase in evening peak forced expiratory volume in 1 second (FEV_1) observed only with the 5-μg dose vs P ($P < .05$). The adjusted FEV_1 area under the curve was statistically significant for all doses vs P (Fig 3). Fig 5 displays morning and evening peak expiratory flow response to T and P, demonstrating statistically significant changes for all doses of T vs P. A dose of 5 μg was suggested by the investigators as the target dose for adolescents, and more studies are indicated before generalizing adolescent data for T to children <12 years of age. Additional tolerability data will be forthcoming: A 1-year study is underway for a randomized double-blind placebo-controlled, parallel-group Phase III study in adolescents with moderate persistent asthma. In other words, stay tuned.

S. K. Willsie, DO, MA

Reference

1. Global Initiative for Asthma. Global strategy for asthma management and prevention. Updated 2012. http://www.ginasthma.org/local/uploads/files/GINA_Report_2012Feb13.pdf. Accessed January 28, 2015.

Inhaled corticosteroid beliefs, complementary and alternative medicine, and uncontrolled asthma in urban minority adults

George M, Topaz M, Rand C, et al (Univ of Pennsylvania School of Nursing, Philadelphia; Univ of Pennsylvania, Philadelphia; et al)

J Allergy Clin Immunol 134:1252-1259, 2014

Background.—Many factors contribute to uncontrolled asthma; negative inhaled corticosteroid (ICS) beliefs and complementary and alternative medicine (CAM) endorsement are 2 that are more prevalent in black compared with white adults.

Objectives.—This mixed-methods study (1) developed and psychometrically tested a brief self-administered tool with low literacy demands to identify negative ICS beliefs and CAM endorsement and (2) evaluated the clinical utility of the tool as a communication prompt in primary care.

Methods.—Comprehensive literature reviews and content experts identified candidate items for our instrument that were distributed to 304 subjects for psychometric testing. In the second phase content analysis of 33 audio-recorded primary care visits provided a preliminary evaluation of the instrument's clinical utility.

Results.—Psychometric testing of the instrument identified 17 items representing ICS beliefs ($\alpha = .59$) and CAM endorsement ($\alpha = .68$). Test-retest analysis demonstrated a high level of reliability (intraclass correlation coefficient 5 0.77 for CAM items and 0.79 for ICS items). We found high rates of CAM endorsement (93%), negative ICS beliefs (68%), and uncontrolled asthma (69%). CAM endorsement was significantly associated with uncontrolled asthma ($P = .04$). Qualitative data analysis provided preliminary evidence for the instrument's clinical utility in that knowledge of ICS beliefs and CAM endorsement prompted providers to initiate discussions with patients.

TABLE 2.—CAM-A* Instrument Items (n = 304)

Item	Item Domain	Positive Response, no. (%)
(Insert BRAND NAME ICS) controls my asthma	Positive ICS belief	250 (82)
Having air movement from a fan, air conditioner or open window helps my asthma	CAM endorsement	202 (66)
I need my (insert BRAND NAME ICS) every day	Positive ICS belief	227 (75)
It is important to me that I find a natural way to treat my asthma	CAM endorsement	128 (42)
Drinking water helps my asthma	CAM endorsement	128 (42)
I am the best judge of whether I need to take my (Insert BRAND NAME ICS)	Negative ICS belief	127 (42)
Steam or warm things on my chest helps my asthma	CAM endorsement	116 (38)
Praying, or having someone pray for me, helps my asthma	CAM endorsement	114 (37)
My asthma can get worse if I go out with a wet head	CAM endorsement	109 (36)
I make decisions about whether I need my (Insert BRAND NAME ICS) on a day-by-day dose-by-dose basis	Negative ICS belief	106 (35)
Drinking tea (herbal or regular) helps my asthma	CAM endorsement	99 (32)
I am afraid that I will build up a tolerance to (Insert BRAND NAME ICS)	Negative ICS belief	71 (23)
Drinking coffee helps my asthma	CAM endorsement	61 (20)
Using Vicks VapoRub helps my asthma	CAM endorsement	53 (17)
Doctors compensated for writing ICS prescriptions	Negative ICS belief	39 (13)
ICS causes cancer or organ damage	Negative ICS belief	35 (11)
ICS causes side effects	Negative ICS belief	33 (11)

Conclusion.—Negative ICS beliefs and CAM endorsement were common and associated with uncontrolled asthma. A brief self-administered instrument that identifies beliefs and behaviors that likely undermine ICS adherence might be a leveraging tool to change the content of communications during clinic visits (Tables 2 and 3).

▶ This interesting study showed high correlation between poorly controlled asthma and negative belief endorsement by urban subjects (more black than white participants). The results of this questionnaire study point out what many medical schools have been trying to teach their students for years: The great majority of practicing physicians are not comfortable with and/or do not condone complementary and alternative medicine (CAM) and therefore do not ask about and do not encourage their patients to discuss whether or not they are using any type of CAM. Worrisome factors related to the results of this study include that uncontrolled asthmatics thought there was a possibility they might develop bad side effects from inhaled corticosteroid (ICS) and that they were in the best position to know how to treat their asthma and make the decision about whether they would use the ICS on a daily basis. CAM methods (Table 2) used instead by subjects for their asthma included praying or having someone else pray for them,

TABLE 3.—Bivariate Comparisons and Multivariate Logistic Regression of Factors Associated with Asthma Control

Characteristics	Bivariate Comparison Controlled Asthma (n = 97)	Bivariate Comparison Uncontrolled Asthma (n = 207)	*P* Value	Logistic Regression† OR (95% CI), *P* Value
Level of CAM endorsement, mean (SD)	2.9 (2.1)	3.5 (0.15)	**.032**	1.41 (1.1-2.31), **.04**
Level of ICS negative belief endorsement, mean (SD)	1.12 (1.19)	1.5 (1.33)	**.035**	1.4 (0.94-2.1), .099
Age (y), mean (SD)	48.1 (1.53)	50.5 (0.87)	.15	
Sex			.29	
Male	26 (27%)	44 (21%)		
Female	71 (73%)	163 (79%)		
Race			**.001**	.56
White	28 (29%)	20 (10%)		Referent
Black/African American	63 (65%)	174 (84%)		1.6 (0.55-4.63), .39
Other*	6 (6%)	13 (6%)		2.37 (0.43-12.9), .32
Marital status				.33
Single	36 (37%)	99 (49%)		
Married	32 (34%)	50 (25%)		
Divorced/separated	19 (21%)	43 (21%)		
Widowed	8 (8%)	11 (5%)		
Occupation			.06	
Unemployed	30 (31%)	99 (49%)		
Manual/service	11 (11%)	27 (13%)		
Skilled professional	35 (36%)	36 (18%)		
Student	4 (4%)	6 (3%)		
Retired	12 (13%)	22 (11%)		
Other (chef, EMS, on disability)	5 (5%)	11 (6%)		
Highest educational level			**.001**	.011
Some high school	7 (7%)	46 (22%)		Referent
Completed high school/obtained GED/vocational training	31 (32%)	87 (42%)		0.44 (0.15-1.34), .17
Some college	23 (24%)	52 (25%)		0.32 (0.1-1.1), .07
College graduate/postgraduate	36 (37%)	22 (11%)		0.09 (0.02-0.38), **.048**
Insurance			**.002**	.77
Medicaid	27 (27%)	91 (45%)		Referent
Medicare/SSI	15 (16%)	46 (22%)		1.57 (0.61-4.03), .35
Commercial	48 (50%)	53 (26%)		1.11 (0.46-2.7), .81
Other	7 (7%)	15 (7%)		0.83 (0.22-3.04), .78
Income			.08	
$0-$9,999	23 (24%)	91 (44%)		
$10,000-$19,999	16 (17%)	40 (20%)		
$20,000-$29,999	12 (12%)	24 (12%)		
$30,000-$39,999	12 (12%)	14 (7%)		
$40,000-$40,999	10 (10%)	11 (5%)		
≥$50,000	17 (18%)	11 (5%)		
Refused to disclose	7 (7%)	14 (7%)		
Age when first given a diagnosis of asthma (y), mean (SD)	22.4 (18.1)	23.6 (18.6)	.588	

Values shown in boldface are statistically significant.

EMS, Emergency medical services; *SSI*, Social Security Income.

*Including American Indian/Alaskan Native, Asian, and Native Hawaiian/Pacific Islander.

†For the logistic regression, 0 indicated controlled asthma and 1 indicated uncontrolled asthma.

fresh-air breathing (including use of fans, open windows), breathing steam, drinking coffee, drinking plenty of water, using Vicks VapoRub, and drinking tea/herbal tea. Many subjects thought doctors got paid for writing ICS prescriptions for patients and worried that they would build up a tolerance to ICS therapy. Table 3 depicts the results of a multivariate analysis of study data, showing a statistically significant difference between controlled and uncontrolled asthmatics related to level of CAM endorsement and negative ICS beliefs. The bottom line is that it's the 21st century; patients are using CAM in large numbers, and we all need to accept that and get on the same page; we do not have to encourage them to use CAM for their asthma (although some CAM methods can be helpful in some disease settings, such as massage in fibromyalgia). However, we can at least take a few minutes or ask our office assistants to have the opening conversation so that we know what patients are taking; we can recognize patients do not trust all medical providers and all medications; and we can understand where patients are coming from and what their misgivings might be. Only then we will be able to educate them on what ICS and other life-sustaining and changing therapies can do for their asthma.

S. K. Willsie, DO, MA

Impact of exhaled nitric oxide measurements on treatment decisions in an asthma specialty clinic

LaForce C, Brooks E, Herje N, et al (North Carolina Clinical Res, Raleigh; Reimbursement Principles, Littleton, CO; Aerocrine, Inc, Morrisville, NC; et al)
Ann Allergy Asthma Immunol 113:619-623, 2014

Background.—Asthma management in an outpatient setting is best accomplished by clinical evaluation coupled with spirometry and symptom evaluation, but these assessments do not provide information about airway inflammation. Exhaled nitric oxide (fraction of exhaled nitric oxide [FeNO]) measures T-helper cell type 2–mediated airway inflammation and may be a useful adjunct in asthma management.

Objective.—To determine whether the use of FeNO in the specialist management of asthma results in more effective and cost-effective treatment decisions.

Methods.—Fifty subjects 7 to 60 years old with established asthma participated in this observational study. Subjects were evaluated by clinical examination, spirometry, and symptom assessment using the Asthma Control Test, and clinicians estimated airway inflammation and made treatment decisions based on these assessments. Then, FeNO was measured, and changes in therapy based on FeNO levels were documented. The estimated cost impact of using FeNO was calculated presuming ongoing FeNO use in patient management.

Results.—Without FeNO, the clinician's assessment of airway inflammation was incorrectly classified in 50% of subjects. FeNO results substantially altered treatment decisions in more than one third of subjects, notably medication augmentation in 10 (20%) and medication decreases

TABLE 2.—Airway Inflammation: Subjects Categorized by Clinical Appraisal vs Observed FeNO Levels

Observed FeNO Level of Airway Inflammation	Clinical Appraisal of Airway Inflammation Low	Intermediate	High	Total
Low	21 (42%)	7 (14%)	1 (2%)	29 (58%)
Intermediate	7 (14%)	3 (6%)	0	10 (20%)
High	6 (12%)	4 (8%)	1 (2%)	11 (22%)
Total	34 (68%)	14 (28%)	2 (4%)	

Abbreviation: FeNO, fraction of exhaled nitric oxide.

TABLE 4.—Asthma Medication Changes Based on FeNO Results

	Overall (N = 50)
Overall	
No change	32 (64%)
Added medication or increased medication dose	10 (20%)
Subtracted medication or decreased medication dose	8 (16%)
OCS	
No change	50 (100%)
Added or increased dose	0
Subtracted or decreased dose	0
ICS-LABA	
No change	46 (92%)
Added or increased dose	3 (6%)
Subtracted or decreased dose	1 (2%)
ICS	
No change	35 (70%)
Added or increased dose	8 (16%)
Subtracted or decreased dose	7 (14%)
LTRA	
No change	47 (94%)
Added or increased dose	2 (4%)
Subtracted or decreased dose	1 (2%)

Abbreviations: ICS, inhaled corticosteroid; ICS-LABA, inhaled corticosteroid plus long-acting β agonist; LTRA, leukotriene receptor antagonist; OCS, oral corticosteroid.

in 8 (16%). Use of FeNO in addition to standard of care was estimated to save $629 per subject per year.

Conclusion.—Measurement of FeNO augments routine clinical assessment of asthma by measuring airway inflammation. Knowledge of FeNO affects medication treatment decisions to augment or decrease pharmacotherapy, which has important long-term asthma management implications, most notably the potential to lower the costs and morbidity associated with asthma exacerbation.

TABLE 6.—Estimated Annual Asthma Management Costs (per Subject)

	Maintenance Medications (US$)	Exacerbations (US$)[a]	Scheduled Physician Office Visits (US$)[b]	All Asthma-Related Care (US$)
Standard guidelines	1,601.16	864.37	281.68	2,747.21
FeNO in addition to standard guidelines	1,376.30	410.90	331.48	2,118.38

Abbreviation: FeNO, fraction of exhaled nitric oxide.

[a]Includes direct payer costs of unscheduled physician office visits, outpatient visits, hospital emergency department visits, inpatient hospitalizations, FeNO testing, spirometry, and rescue medications.

[b]Includes level III physician office visits, FeNO testing, and spirometry.

Trial Registration.—ClinicalTrials.gov identifier NCT01729247 (Tables 2, 4 and 6).

▶ Previous investigations have indicated that high levels of exhaled nitric oxide (ENO) portend uncontrolled asthma and increased risk of deterioration and potential for future deterioration.[1-3] This interesting single-center, single-observation study of children and adults with asthma measured ENO after completion of clinician assessment of asthma stability. The clinician was not provided with the results of the ENO levels until all medical decision making had been completed. Table 2 compares and depicts measured ENO vs clinician appraisal of inflammatory status and expected ENO level in each subject. In more than 50% of the cases, the level of severity/inflammation was underestimated based on spirometry, Asthmas Control Test questionnaire, and clinician assessment. Table 4 details medication changes made by the clinician after being provided with the measured ENO levels for each asthmatic. Thirty-six percent of subjects had a medication change made by the clinician following review of the ENO level review: 20% of subjects had their inhaled corticosteroid (ICS) dose increased; 2 subjects who were on moderate to high doses of ICS had leukotriene modifiers added to their medication regimen. Table 6 provides estimated annual asthma management costs per subjects in the case of using ENO levels at each visit; note that the overall asthma cost saves shows that utilization of ENO would actually lead to significant cost savings related to reduced exacerbation costs, increase in scheduled office visits, and overall reduction in all asthma-related care. Unstated in the table's depiction is the overall reduction of asthma morbidity due to fewer cases of emergency department visits and hospitalizations related to underestimation of asthma severity. It's time that point-of-care testing for ENO becomes routine in the care of asthma.

S. K. Willsie, DO, MA

References

1. Agache I, Ciobanu C. Predictive value of lung function trend and FENO for difficult asthma in children. *J Investig Allergol Clin Immunol.* 2012;22:419-426.

2. Dweik RA, Sorkness RL, Wenzel S, et al. Use of exhaled nitric oxide measurement to identify a reactive, at risk phenotype among patients with asthma. *Am J Respir Crit Care Med.* 2010;181:1033-1041.
3. van Veen IH, Ten Brinke A, Sterk PJ, et al. Exhaled nitric oxide predicts lung function decline in difficult to treat asthma. *Eur Resp J.* 2008;32:344-349.

Linking Patient-Centered Medical Home and Asthma Measures Reduces Hospital Readmission Rates

Bergert L, Patel SJ, Kimata C, et al (Univ of Hawaii John A. Burns School of Medicine, Honolulu; Hawaii Pacific Health, Honolulu)
Pediatrics 134:e249-e256, 2014

Objective.—We sought to achieve 100% compliance with all 3 Children's Asthma Care (CAC; CAC-1, CAC-2, CAC-3) measures and track attendance at follow-up appointments with the patient-centered medical home. The impact of these measures on readmission and emergency department utilization rates was evaluated.

Methods.—This quality improvement study evaluated compliance with CAC measures in pediatric patients aged 2 to 18 years old hospitalized with a primary diagnosis of asthma from January 1, 2008, through June 30, 2012. A multidisciplinary Asthma Task Force was assembled to develop interventions. Attendance at the follow-up appointment was tracked monthly from January 1, 2009. Readmission and emergency department utilization rates were compared between the preimplementation period (January 1, 2006, through December 31, 2007) and the postimplementation period (January 1, 2008, through June 30, 2012).

Results.—The preimplementation period included 231 subjects and the postimplementation period included 532 subjects. Compliance with CAC-3 was 95% from October 1, 2009, through June 30, 2012. Compliance with the postdischarge follow-up appointment was 69% from January 1, 2009 through September 30, 2009, increasing significantly to 90% from October 1, 2009, through June 30, 2012 ($P < .001$). Postimplementation readmission rates significantly decreased in the 91- to 180-day postdischarge interval (odds ratio: 0.29; 95% confidence interval: 0.11−0.78).

Conclusions.—In children hospitalized with asthma, compliance with the asthma core measures and the postdischarge follow-up appointment with the primary care provider was associated with reduced readmission rates at 91 to 180 days after discharge. We attribute our results to a comprehensive set of interventions designed by our multidisciplinary Asthma Task Force.

► This article describes a successful quality improvement project incorporating all 3 Children's Asthma Care (CAC) measures (1-bronchodilator/reliever use, 2-systemic corticosteroid use, 3-completion of home management plan of care). An institution-wide task force, consisting of the usual parties involved in care delivery to children with asthma, worked together to design a process-oriented approach to the identification of weaknesses within their system. Statistically significant improvement with sustainment of improvement over nearly 3 years was demonstrated. The most difficult of the CACs to comply with, CAC-3, was successfully managed by this group with an improvement from 74% compliance (22% SD) before implementation of the process changes vs 95% sustained compliance (7% SD) after implementation (Fig 1 in the original article). Table 1 in the original article shows compliance and follow-up rates with medical home appointments (CAC-3). The successful process improvements that resulted from this group's work, particularly the sustained improvements for CAC-3, may serve as a model for other institutions hoping to improve outcomes.

S. K. Willsie, DO, MA

Evolution of occupational asthma: Does cessation of exposure really improve prognosis?

Munoz X, Viladrich M, Manso L, et al (Hosp Vall d'Hebron, Barcelona, Spain; Ciber Enfermedades Respiratorias (CibeRes), Spain; et al)
Respir Med 108:1363-1370, 2014

Aim.—To assess the evolution of occupational asthma (OA) depending on whether the patient avoids or continues with exposure to the offending agent.

Methods.—Study in patients diagnosed with OA using a specific inhalation challenge. Patients underwent the following examinations on the same day: clinical interview, physical examination, forced spirometry, methacholine test and determination of total IgE. Clinical improvement, deterioration or no change were defined according to the changes seen on the GINA severity scale at the time of diagnosis.

Results.—Of the 73 patients finally included, 55 had totally ended exposure and 18 continued to be exposed at work. Clinical improvement was observed in 47% of those who had terminated exposure and in 22% of those who remained exposed; clinical deterioration was observed in 14% and 17% respectively ($p = 0.805$). Logistical regression analysis, including the type of agent and the persistence or avoidance of exposure among the variables, did not show any predictive factors of clinical evolution. Similarly, the changes in FEV_1 and in bronchial hyperresponsiveness were not associated with the avoidance or continuation of exposure to the causative agent.

Conclusions.—Avoiding exposure to the causative agent in patients with OA does not seem to improve prognosis in this disease. Despite these findings, there is insufficient evidence to recommend a change in current management guidelines (Table 2).

▶ This is an interesting study from 2 centers treating a mixed group of occupational asthma (OA) patients, some of whom were promptly removed from the place of their OA exposure and some who had remained in their place of work but were provided with appropriate exposure-limiting technology or avoidance

TABLE 2.—Baseline and Follow-up Characteristics of Patients Finally Included (Divided According to Exposure/Non-exposure to the Causative Agent)

	Non-exposed $n = 55$			Exposed $n = 18$		
	Baseline	Follow-up	p	Baseline	Follow-up	p
Age, yrs	41 (18–65)	–	–	44 (25–57)	–	–
Sex, M/F	35/20	–	–	7/11	–	–
Smoking habit S/NS/ExS	11/36/8			4/12/2		
Pack/year	15 (5–60)			14.5 (7–21)		
Time from exposure to diagnosis, months	120 (6–710)	–	–	242 (12–539)	–	–
Time from symptom onset to diagnosis, months	48 (2–377)	–	–	41 (1–430)	–	–
Time from diagnosis to avoidance, months	–	1.5 (0–224)	–	–	30 (6–120)	–
Agent, LMW/HMW	38/17	–	–	12/6	–	–
Atopy, yes/no (% yes)	23/21 (52%)	–	–	8/10 (44%)	–	–
Rhinitis, yes/no (% yes)	39/16 (71%)	22/32 (41%)	0.001	14/4 (78%)	14/4 (78%)	0.182
Conjunctivitis, yes/no (% yes)	25/30 (45%)	13/41 (24%)	0.027	8/10 (44%)	9/9 (50%)	0.149
Dermatitis, yes/no (% yes)	13/42 (31%)	6/48 (11%)	0.065	6/12 (33%)	4/14 (22%)	0.125
Total IgE; kU/L	118 (5–2393)	101 (5.9–1611)	0.858	75 (10–696)	105.5 (18–1212)	0.362
% Blood eosinophils	4.5 (0–29.9)	3.0 (0.9–29.2)	0.006	5 (0–25)	2.6 (0.8–4.8)	0.028
FEV_1; % predicted	93 (60–130)	90 (52–131)	0.072	89.5 (64–113)	93 (60–131)	0.554
FVC; % predicted	95.5 (71–148)	91.5 (49–138)	0.011	93 (74–123)	90 (70–120)	0.434
FEV_1/FVC%	78 (58–99.2)	77 (50–97)	0.150	76 (52–92)	78.3 (58.4–89.7)	0.777
Methacholine, % +	89%	78%	0.0001	67%	51%	0.006
PC_{20}, mg/ml	2 (0.06–16)	1.6 (0.06–16)	0.780	1.2 (0.13–8)	1.3 (0.4–8.5)	0.925
Response to SIC (E/L/D/O)	17/24/12/2	–	–	6/5/4/3	–	–
% fall SIC	25 (12–50)	–	–	22 (8–41)	–	–
GINA NA/I/MiP/ModP/SP	0/16/6/20/13	1/30/6/8/10	0.001	0/7/5/5/1	0/8/4/4/2	0.861
Better/worse/same*	–	26/8/21 47%/14%/38%		–	4/3/11 22%/17%/61%	
ACQ: Control/Parcial Control/no control**	–	34/14/7 62%/25%/13%		–	13/2/3 72%/15%/23%	

LMW – low molecular weight; HMW – high molecular weight; SIC – specific inhalation challenge; NA – no asthma; , I – intermittent; MiP – mild persistent; ModP – moderate persistent; , SP – severe persistent; E – early; L – late; D – dual; O – others.

*$p = 0.805$.

**$p = 0.437$.

Reprinted from Munoz X, Viladrich M, Manso L, et al. Evolution of occupational asthma: Does cessation of exposure really improve prognosis? Respir Med. 2014;108:1363-1370.

measures. Table 2 depicts subjects no longer exposed (n = 55) and those who continue in the exposure environment (n = 18), allowing comparison of baseline and follow-up data (*P* values shown). Statistically significant changes from baseline to follow-up within the no-longer-exposed group were seen for rhinitis, conjunctivitis, blood eosinophilia, % predicted forced vital capacity; % positivity on methacholine challenge, and GINA classification. Statistically significant changes for the continually exposed group of subjects were seen only for % blood eosinophils, % positivity on methacholine challenge. The group who avoided exposure to the causative agent (OA) did not have an overall improved prognosis. The investigators state that avoiding exposure is independent of both the type of agent and whether the agent is subsequently and promptly avoided. In addition, the group of subjects who did not leave the work site failed to have significant reductions in airway obstruction or airway hyperresponsiveness. Despite these findings, because of the small numbers of subjects, the authors caution against changing the current guidelines, which suggest that removal from exposure for patients with OA is recommended in all cases until further research is performed.[1,2]

S. K. Willsie, DO, MA

References

1. Tarlo SM, Balmes J, Balkissoon R, et al. Diagnosis and management of work-related asthma: American College of Chest Physicians consensus statement. *Chest*. 2008;134:1S-41S.
2. Perfetti L, Cartier A, Ghezzo H, Gautrin D, Malo JL. Follow-up of occupational asthma after removal from or diminution of exposure to the responsible agent: relevance of the length of the interval from cessation of exposure. *Chest*. 1998; 114:398-403.

Comparison of US emergency department acute asthma care quality: 1997-2001 and 2011-2012

Hasegawa K, on behalf of the MARC-36 Investigators (Massachusetts General Hosp, Boston; et al)

J Allergy Clin Immunol 135:73-80, 2015

Background.—It remains unclear whether the quality of acute asthma care in US emergency departments (EDs) has improved over time.

Objectives.—We investigated changes in concordance of ED asthma care with 2007 National Institutes of Health guidelines, identified ED characteristics predictive of concordance, and tested whether higher concordance was associated with lower risk of hospitalization.

Methods.—We performed chart reviews in ED patients aged 18 to 54 years with asthma exacerbations in 48 EDs during 2 time periods: 1997-2001 (2 prior studies) and 2011-2012 (new study). Concordance with guideline recommendations was evaluated by using item-by-item quality measures and composite concordance scores at the patient and ED levels; these scores ranged from 0 to 100.

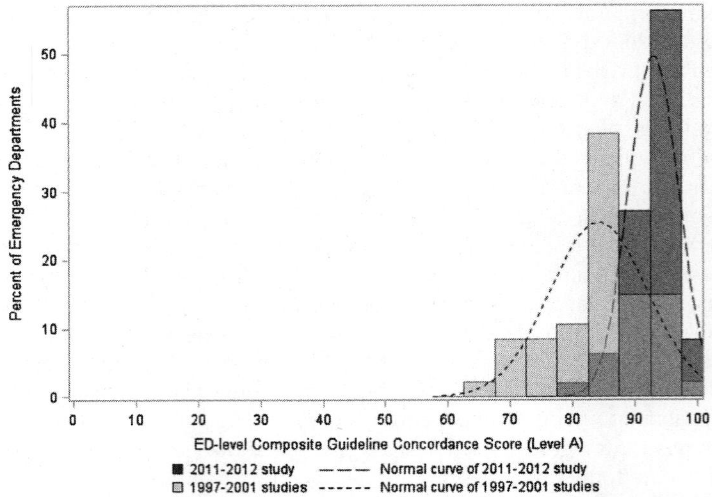

FIGURE 2.—Distribution of composite guideline concordance with level A recommendations at the ED level according to time period. Compared with the 1997-2001 period, concordance with the level A recommendations was significantly higher in the 2011-2012 period (mean composite score, 84 vs 93; $P < .001$), with a smaller variation in concordance (SD, 8 vs 4). The *superimposed curves* represent the normal curve based on each sample mean and SD. (Reprinted from The Journal of Allergy and Clinical Immunology. Hasegawa K, on behalf of the MARC-36 Investigators. Comparison of US emergency department acute asthma care quality: 1997-2001 and 2011-2012. *J Allergy Clin Immunol.* 2015;135:73-80, Copyright 2015, with permission from Elsevier.)

Results.—The analytic cohort comprised 4039 patients (2119 from 1997-2001 vs 1920 from 2011-2012). Over these 16 years, emergency asthma care became more concordant with level A recommendations at both the patient and ED levels (both $P < .001$). By contrast, concordance with non–level A recommendations (peak expiratory flow measurement and timeliness) decreased at both the patient (median score, 75 [interquartile range, 50-100] to 50 [interquartile range, 33-75], $P < .001$) and ED (mean score, 67 [SD, 7] to 50 [SD, 16], $P < .001$) levels. Multivariable analysis demonstrated ED concordance was lower in Southern and Western EDs compared with Midwestern EDs. After adjusting for severity, guidelineconcordant care was associated with lower risk of hospitalization (odds ratio, 0.37; 95% CI, 0.26-0.53).

Conclusions.—Between 1997 and 2012, we observed changes in the quality of emergency asthma care that differed by level of guideline recommendation and substantial interhospital and geographic variations. Greater concordance with guidelinerecommended management might reduce unnecessary hospitalizations (Fig 2).

▶ Prospective, multicenter, observational study of asthmatics receiving care at emergency departments (ED); subjects were recruited and provided with routine ED care for asthma exacerbations. Chart reviews were conducted by trained observers without interference with treatment or disposition of subject.

Subjects were enrolled and followed during 2 time periods—1997–2001 and 2011–2012—to allow for comparison of quality of care. Forty-eight participating EDs enrolled subjects during both time periods; all participating EDs recorded a decrease in the number of asthma ED visits from the first to second time period ($P < .01$). The percent of EDs that were affiliated with a university-associated ED residency program increased from the first to second observational period ($P < .001$). Fig 2 depicts composite guideline concordance with level A recommendations for the 2011–2012 time period ($P < .001$ vs 1997–2001 period). Of note is that more than 30% of subjects were not on ICS at the time of admission, and more than 10% of subjects left the ED without an ICS prescription. The results of this study show that even though overall compliance with guideline care has improved from the time of the original observation, there is still great room for improvement of asthma care administered during ED visits. The investigators hypothesize that focusing on guideline adherence during ED visits would lessen the number of unnecessary hospitalizations related to asthma exacerbation and/or relapse. Such a study needs to be conducted on a large-scale particularly given the roll out of major health care reform and looming attendant costs; pay for performance will be even more important given the overall incidence of asthma and the still too frequent use of the ED as the primary care office by many patients.

S. K. Willsie, DO, MA

EAACI position paper: irritant-induced asthma

Vandenplas O, Wiszniewska M, Raulf M, et al (Université Catholique de Louvain, Yvoir, Belgium; Nofer Inst of Occupational Medicine, Lodz, Poland; Inst of the Ruhr-Universität Bochum, Germany; et al)
Allergy 69:1141-1153, 2014

The term irritant-induced (occupational) asthma (IIA) has been used to denote various clinical forms of asthma related to irritant exposure at work. The causal relationship between irritant exposure(s) and the development of asthma can be substantiated by the temporal association between the onset of asthma symptoms and a single or multiple high-level exposure(s) to irritants, whereas this relationship can only be inferred from epidemiological data for workers chronically exposed to moderate levels of irritants. Accordingly, the following clinical phenotypes should be distinguished within the wide spectrum of irritant-related asthma: (i) definite IIA, that is acute-onset IIA characterized by the rapid onset of asthma within a few hours after a single exposure to very high levels of irritant substances; (ii) probable IIA, that is asthma that develops in workers with multiple symptomatic high-level exposures to irritants; and (iii) possible IIA, that is asthma occurring with a delayed-onset after chronic exposure to moderate levels of irritants. This document prepared by a panel of experts summarizes our current knowledge on the diagnostic approach, epidemiology, pathophysiology, and management of the various phenotypes of IIA.

▶ This European Academy of Allergy and Clinical Immunology position paper on Irritant-Induced Asthma (IIA) offers an expert panels' opinion, based on currently available information and published literature, on what was once referred to as occupational asthma. Occupational asthma's acute form was originally referred to as Reactive Airways Dysfunction Syndrome, or RADS, by Stuart Brooks who coined the term in 1985,[1] to refer to acute asthmatic symptoms following a single exposure to an irritant in the workplace. Table 1 in the original article lists current diagnostic criteria for IIA, adapted from those originally suggested by Brooks and *Chest*.[1-3] The position paper defines definite, probable, and possible phenotypes of IIA, and Table 2 in the original article provides a listing of common exposures leading to IIA. Fig 6 in the original article provides a useful algorithm by which to diagnose and manage these forms of IIA.

S. K. Willsie, DO, MA

References

1. Brooks SM, Weiss MA, Bernstein IL. Reactive airways dysfunction syndrome (RADS). Persistent asthma syndrome after high level irritant exposures. *Chest*. 1985;88:376-384.
2. Brooks SM, Bernstein IL. Irritant-induced airway disorders. *Immunol Allergy Clin North Am*. 2011;31:747-768.
3. Tarlo SM, Balmes J, Balkissoon R, et al. Diagnosis and management of work-related asthma: American College Of Chest Physicians Consensus Statement. *Chest*. 2008;134:1S-41S.

Rates and Correlates of Relapse Following ED Discharge for Acute Asthma: A Canadian 20-Site Prospective Cohort Study

Rowe BH, for the AIR Investigators (Univ of Alberta, Edmonton, Canada; et al)
Chest 147:140-149, 2015

Background.—Acute asthma is a common ED presentation. In a prospective, multicenter cohort study, we determined the frequency and factors associated with asthma relapse following discharge from the ED.

Methods.—Adults aged 18 to 55 years who were treated for acute asthma and discharged from 20 Canadian EDs underwent a structured ED interview and a follow-up telephone interview 4 weeks later. Standardized anti-inflammatory treatment was offered at discharge. Multivariable analyses were performed.

Results.—Of 807 enrolled patients, 58% were women, and the median age was 30 years. Relapse occurred in 144 patients (18%) within 4 weeks of ED discharge. Factors independently associated with relapse occurrence were female sex (women, 22% vs men, 12%; adjusted OR [aOR], 1.9; 95% CI, 1.2-3.0); symptom duration of ≥24 h prior to ED visit (long duration, 19% vs short duration, 13%; aOR, 1.7; 95% CI, 1.3-2.3); ever using oral corticosteroids (ever use, 21% vs never use, 12%; aOR, 1.5; 95% CI, 1.1-2.0); current use of an inhaled corticosteroid [ICS]/long-acting β-agonist combination product (combination product, 25% vs ICS monotherapy, 15%; aOR, 1.9; 95% CI, 1.1-3.2); and owning a spacer device (owning one, 24% vs not owning one, 15%; aOR, 1.6; 95% CI, 1.3-1.9).

Conclusions.—Despite receiving guideline-concordant antiinflammatory treatments at ED discharge, almost one in five patients relapsed within 4 weeks. Female sex, prolonged symptoms, treatment-related factors, and markers of prior asthma severity were significantly associated with relapse. These results may help physicians target more aggressive interventions for patients at high risk of relapse.

▶ This study was a prospective multicenter cohort study of patients with acute exacerbations of asthma presenting to 20 emergency departments (ED) in Canada (universal healthcare access system) to evaluate the incidence of relapse in this setting. A structured ED interview took place, and a telephone call was made to subjects 4 weeks after the ED visit. The study attempted to control for aftercare, aiming to provide evidence-based anti-inflammatory treatment to all subjects on discharge from the ED. A total of 807 subjects were enrolled, 57% of which were women. Before the ED visit, 25% of the subjects were steroid naive, 29% were using inhaled corticosteroid (ICS) monotherapy, and 46% using ICS/long-acting beta-agonist (LABA) treatment. A total of 144 subjects (18%) relapsed within 4 weeks (86 at 1 week, 112 total by 2 weeks); 16% of all relapses led to hospitalization for asthma. Tables 1-3 in the original article demonstrate that the following factors were independently associated with increased risk of relapse: Females were more likely to relapse than males (adjusted odds ratio [aOR] 1.9; 95% confidence interval [CI], 1.2–3.0); having previously taken corticosteroids vs never having taken corticosteroids (aOR 1.5; 95% CI, 1.1–2.0); using ICS monotherapy on admission to ED (aOR 1.9; 95% CI, 1.1–3.2); owning a spacer device vs not owning a spacer device (aOR 1.6; 95% CI, 1.2–1.9); having an action plan; having influence immunization ever taken oral corticosteroids for asthma. Table 2 in the original article shows only the following lines: duration of symptoms (the 3 lines < 24 h, > 24 hr, and not documented); respiratory rate. Fig 2 in the original article depicts medication at entrance to ED (those that relapsed vs no relapse), and Fig 3 in the original article depicts medications at presentation vs discharge. Note that even though the study called for all subjects to receive anti-inflammatory therapy at discharge, approximately 10% did not receive anti-inflammatory therapy. Fig 4 in the original article depicts incidence of relapse over 30 days, males vs females. What this study shows us is that in a universal healthcare system, even with the best of intentions, evidence-based guidelines may not be followed; in addition, the study has identified specific factors that portend relapse, which are listed above. With this information, healthcare providers can scrutinize patients a little bit closer when evaluating them in the ED, perhaps hold females who meet the high-risk relapse criteria a little longer, have a lower threshold to admit them earlier, and/or to refer them for earlier follow-up (eg, next day or within a few days).

Taking this approach could result in significant savings for the healthcare system and less morbidity for patients.

S. K. Willsie, DO, MA

Vitamin D, asthma prevalence and asthma exacerbations: a large adult population-based study

Confino-Cohen R, Brufman I, Goldberg A, et al (Meir Med Ctr, Kfar Saba, Israel; Clalit Health Services, Tel Aviv, Israel)
Allergy 69:1673-1680, 2014

Background.—The impact of low vitamin D status on asthma, asthma morbidity and control is unclear. We aimed to investigate in adults the associations between serum 25-hydroxyvitamin D level and prevalent asthma as well as asthma exacerbations.

Methods.—A cohort of Israeli adults aged 22–50 years with documented vitamin D status were extracted from Clalit Health Services (HMO) between July 1, 2008 and July 1, 2012. Among this population, those with physician-diagnosed asthma and asthma exacerbations were identified. Asthma exacerbations were defined as any of the following: prescription for oral corticosteroids, >5 prescriptions for short acting beta agonists and more than four visits to a physician for asthma. Logistic regression models assessed the associations between vitamin D and both asthma and asthma exacerbations.

Results.—Approximately 308 000 members with at least one vitamin D measurement were included in the cohort. Among them, 6.9% (21 237) had physician-diagnosed asthma *vs* 5.7% in the general population. Serum 25-OHD levels across both groups were similar. However, among those with vitamin D deficiency, the odds of having an exacerbation were 25% greater compared to those with levels in the normal range. This association remained significant after controlling for known confounders.

Conclusion.—While there was no significant association between vitamin D status and physician-diagnosed asthma, there was a strong association with asthma exacerbations. The presented evidence supports vitamin D screening in the subgroup of asthmatics that are uncontrolled and experience recurrent exacerbations.

▶ This is an interesting health maintenance organization study in which the records of 308 000 members between the ages of 22 and 50 years of age with at least 1 vitamin D level were reviewed. Of this group, 6.9%, or 21 237 people, carried a physician diagnosis of asthma. No correlation existed between vitamin D deficiency and physician-diagnosed asthma; however, asthmatics with vitamin D deficiency (≤50 nmol/L) were more likely to have uncontrolled asthma (1 or more exacerbation within the past year). Table 1 in the original article depicts that 66.1% of the asthmatics with 1 or more exacerbation in the previous year had vitamin D levels ≤50 (nmol/L, equated with vitamin D deficiency). Table 3 in the original article demonstrates that 2.584 of all asthmatics (12.3%)

had more than 1 exacerbation during the previous year. Fig 1 in the original article depicts asthma exacerbation in the year before the vitamin D level, by type of exacerbation and vitamin D level group. In summary, this large-scale investigation clearly demonstrates an inverse linear association between the proportion of asthmatics with exacerbations and vitamin D levels ($P < .001$). For those caring for asthmatics, if you are not yet sold on the relationship between vitamin D and asthma, might this data perhaps cause you now to consider, as the investigators recommend, to at the least check vitamin D levels in your uncontrolled asthmatics? Given the high incidence of vitamin D deficiency in the American population, I am certainly checking all my patients and have been for some time.

S. K. Willsie, DO, MA

Risk of congenital malformations for asthmatic pregnant women using a long-acting β₂-agonist and inhaled corticosteroid combination versus higher-dose inhaled corticosteroid monotherapy

Eltonsy S, Forget A, Beauchesne MF, et al (Université de Montréal, Quebec, Canada)

J Allergy Clin Immunol 135:123-130, 2014

Background.—Current recommendations for managing persistent asthma during pregnancy when low-dose inhaled corticosteroids (ICSs) are insufficient include adding a long-acting β_2-agonist (LABA) or increasing the ICS dose. However, there are no data to help clinicians evaluate the safest regimen during pregnancy.

Objective.—We sought to compare the risk of major congenital malformations in asthmatic women exposed to a LABA plus ICS combination and those exposed to ICS monotherapy at higher doses during the first trimester.

Methods.—A cohort of asthmatic pregnant women exposed to ICSs during the first trimester who delivered between January 1990 and March 2009 was established. The primary outcome was major malformation recorded at birth or during the first year of life. Two subcohorts were established as follows: (1) users of a LABA plus low-dose ICS combination or users of a medium-dose ICS and (2) users of a LABA plus medium-dose ICS combination or users of a high-dose ICS. Generalized estimating equations were used to compare the risk of major malformations between the groups.

Results.—In one subcohort there were 643 women who used a LABA plus low-dose ICS and 305 who used a medium-dose ICS; the other subcohort included 198 users of a LABA plus medium-dose ICS and 156 users of a high-dose ICS. The prevalence of major malformations was 6.9% and 7.2%, respectively. The adjusted odds ratio for major malformations was 1.1 (95% CI, 0.6-1.9) when a LABA plus low-dose ICS was used compared with a medium-dose ICS and 1.2 (95% CI, 0.5-2.7) when a LABA plus medium-dose ICS was used compared with a high-dose ICS.

Conclusion.—The risk of major malformations was similar with a LABA plus ICS combination and ICS monotherapy at higher doses, suggesting that both therapeutic options can be considered during pregnancy (Tables 1 and E2).

▶ The issue of whether to control asthma during pregnancy (when required) with higher doses of inhaled corticosteroids (ICS) vs medium-dose ICS with long-acting beta-agonists (LABA) is one that has been discussed among healthcare providers for decades. The answer to this question is that it has never been prospectively answered! This group of investigators aimed to answer this question by reviewing data from 1302 pregnancies in 1249 women who were all exposed to ICS during the first trimester of pregnancy. This population-based safety study uses a database from Quebec: 948 pregnancies with moderate asthma and 354 pregnancies with severe asthma. Ninety-six (7.4%) of these pregnancies resulted in major malformations diagnosed within the first year of life. Table 1 demonstrates the differences between the moderate and severe asthma cohorts. Women in the severe asthma cohort were more likely to have experienced exacerbated asthma ($P < .001$) and have used more than 3 doses of short-acting beta-agonists (SABA) per week in the 3 months preceding conception ($P < .001$). In the severe asthma cohort, 14 cases (7.1%) of major congenital malformations were detected in women receiving combination therapy (medium-dose ICS and LABA), whereas 15 cases (9.6%) of major malformations occurred in the cohort

TABLE 1.—Distribution of Maternal Characteristics According to Exposure to ICSs and LABAs During the First Trimester of Pregnancy in Each Subcohort of Asthmatic Women

	Moderate Asthma Subcohort			Severe Asthma Subcohort		
	LABA Plus Low-dose ICS	Medium-dose ICS	*P* Value	LABA Plus Medium-dose ICS	High-dose ICS	*P* Value
Total no. of pregnancies in subcohort (%)	305 (32.2)	643 (67.8)		198 (55.9)	156 (44.1)	
No. (%) of pregnancies						
Maternal age at beginning of pregnancy						
18-34 y	268 (87.9)	544 (84.6)	.180	171 (86.4)	119 (76.3)	.014
<18 or ≥35 y	37 (12.1)	99 (15.4)		27 (13.6)	37 (23.7)	
Receipt of social assistance during pregnancy	130 (42.6)	374 (58.2)	<.001	89 (45.0)	116 (74.4)	<.001
Urban area of residence at delivery	243 (79.7)	497 (77.3)	.409	152 (76.8)	125 (80.1)	.447
Chronic hypertension	7 (2.3)	16 (2.5)	.857	8 (4.0)	6 (3.9)	.926
Diabetes mellitus	12 (3.9)	33 (5.1)	.418	8 (4.0)	12 (7.7)	.139
Exacerbation of asthma 3 mo before pregnancy	46 (15.1)	75 (11.7)	.141	35 (17.7)	33 (21.2)	.410
SABA doses/wk 3 mo before pregnancy						
0-3	144 (47.2)	249 (38.7)	.013	59 (29.8)	21 (13.5)	<.001
>3	161 (52.8)	394 (61.3)		139 (70.2)	135 (86.5)	

TABLE E2.—Distribution of Major Congenital Malformations in the Moderate and Severe Asthma Subcohorts

	Moderate Asthma Subcohort				Severe Asthma subcohort			
	LABA Plus Low-dose ICS		Medium-dose ICS		LABA Plus Medium-Dose ICS		High-dose ICS	
	No.	Percent	No.	Percent	No.	Percent	No.	Percent
≥1 Major malformation*	21	6.9	46	7.2	14	7.1	15	9.6
Specific major malformations								
Nervous system	4	1.3	4	0.6	2	1.0	2	1.3
Cardiac	8	2.6	15	2.3	4	2.0	5	3.2
Circulatory system	1	0.3	2	0.3	2	1.0	2	1.3
Respiratory system	3	1.0	4	0.6	1	0.5	0	0.0
Eye	0	0.0	1	0.2	0	0.0	0	0.0
Ear, face, and neck	0	0.0	0	0.0	0	0.0	0	0.0
Cleft palate and cleft lip	1	0.3	3	0.5	0	0.0	0	0.0
Digestive system	0	0.0	11	1.7	1	0.5	2	1.3
Genital organs	1	0.3	2	0.3	1	0.5	1	0.6
Urinary system	0	0.0	3	0.5	3	1.5	6	3.9
Limbs	0	0.0	1	0.2	0	0.0	2	1.3
Musculoskeletal†	2	0.7	6	0.9	1	0.5	3	1.9
Integument	4	1.3	2	0.3	2	1.0	2	1.3
Chromosomal	1	0.3	3	0.5	2	1.0	1	0.6
Other congenital anomalies	2	0.7	2	0.3	0	0.0	2	1.3

*The total sum of all major specific malformations exceeded the number of cases (96 infants with major malformations) because an infant could have more than 1 malformation.

†Including all musculoskeletal malformations, except limb malformations.

Reprinted from The Journal of Allergy and Clinical Immunology. Eltonsy S, Forget A, Beauchesne MF, et al. Risk of congenital malformations for asthmatic pregnant women using a long-acting β_2-agonist and inhaled corticosteroid combination versus higher-dose inhaled corticosteroid monotherapy. J Allergy Clin Immunol. 2014;135:123-130, Copyright 2014, with permission from Elsevier.

of women receiving high doses of ICS only. The difference between the incidence of major malformation between the severe asthmatic groups, by treatment, did not reach statistical significance: odds ratio 1.0, 95% confidence interval 0.5–2.7. Although these data were not prospectively obtained, they were based on high-quality data and suggest overall fetal safety of combination therapy with LABA/ICS during pregnancy. The results of this investigation may lend encouragement to providers who wish to maintain prepregnancy combination asthma therapy for a controlled asthmatic or, alternatively, choose to use one of several available types of combination therapy as opposed to monotherapy with ICS alone during pregnancy or following exacerbation.

S. K. Willsie, DO, MA

PRAM Score as Predictor of Pediatric Asthma Hospitalization

Alnaji F, Zemek R, Barrowman N, et al (Univ of Ottawa, Ontario, Canada; Children's Hosp of Eastern Ontario Res Inst, Ottawa, Ontario, Canada)

Acad Emerg Med 21:872-878, 2014

Objectives.—The objective was to determine the association between asthma severity as measured by the Pediatric Respiratory Assessment Measure (PRAM) score and the likelihood of admission for pediatric

TABLE 3.—PRAM Score Predictability Odds Ratios

Time	Odds Ratio (95% CI)	Test of Goodness-of-Fit* p-Value
PRAM as a predictor of admission		
Triage	1.82 (1.42–2.35)	0.15
2-hour	1.84 (1.47–2.29)	0.88
3-hour	2.05 (1.57–2.68)	0.87
4-hour	1.85 (1.46–2.35)	0.37
PRAM as a predictor of long ED stay > 8 hours		
Triage	1.26 (1.03–1.55)	0.79
2-hour	1.41 (1.14–1.74)	0.29
3-hour	1.49 (1.20–1.86)	0.25
4-hour	1.50 (1.20–1.88)	0.16

PRAM = Pediatric Respiratory Assessment Measure.
*le Cessie-van Houwelingen test for goodness of fit.
Reprinted from Alnaji F, Zemek R, Barrowman N, et al. PRAM Score as Predictor of Pediatric Asthma Hospitalization. Acad Emerg Med. 2014;21:872-878, with permission from Academy of Emergency Medicine and John Wiley and Sons, www.interscience.wiley.com.

patients who present to the emergency department (ED) with moderate-to-severe asthma exacerbations and who receive intensive asthma therapy.

Methods.—This was a secondary analysis of a prospective study of triage nurse-initiated steroid therapy in pediatric asthma. Children aged 2 to 17 years inclusive, presenting with moderate-to-severe acute asthma exacerbations (defined as PRAM ≥ 4), were included. To be eligible for inclusion in the study, children must have received "intensive asthma therapy," defined as nurse-initiated initial bronchodilator and oral steroid therapy at arrival to triage. PRAM scores were measured hourly as per ED protocol. The primary outcome was inpatient hospitalization; secondary outcome was ED stay greater than 8 hours. Logistic regression models were used to predict admission based on PRAM score at triage and then hourly thereafter. The area under the receiver operating characteristic curve (AUC) was calculated for each hour.

Results.—A total of 297 patients were included in the analysis, with an admission rate of 11.4% for patients receiving intensive therapy. The 3-hour PRAM (AUC = 0.85) significantly improved prediction of admission compared to PRAM at triage ($p = 0.04$).

Conclusions.—The 3-hour PRAM scores best predicts the need for hospitalization. These results may be applied in clinical settings to facilitate the decision to admit or initiate more aggressive adjunctive therapy to decrease the need for hospitalization (Table 3).

▶ This retrospective study of emergency department (ED) visits for moderate and severe pediatric asthmatics evaluated the use of the Pediatric Respiratory Assessment Measure (PRAM) to determine its utility at different time points versus triage with regard to efficacy in decision making about need for hospitalization. Table 3 demonstrates the utility of the PRAM score for decision making regarding admission and predicting the need for prolonged ED visits. This table shows that although the triage and hourly PRAMs were of use in determining the need to admission, only the 3-hour PRAM outperformed the triage PRAM for this purpose. The investigators suggest that the 3-hour PRAM score might be used to improve ED flow and better apply triage and maximization of therapy for asthmatics who appear to require admission.

S. K. Willsie, DO, MA

Comparing the Asthma APGAR System and the Asthma Control Test™ in a Multicenter Primary Care Sample

Rank MA, Bertram S, Wollan P, et al (Mayo Clinic, Scottsdale, AZ; Olmsted Med Ctr Res, Rochester, MN)
Mayo Clin Proc 89:917-925, 2014

Objective.—To compare asthma control assessment using the Asthma APGAR system, a tool developed by primary care clinicians, in a multicenter primary care sample with the Asthma Control Test (ACT™)/Childhood Asthma Control Test (CACT™), a tool developed by asthma specialists.

Patients and Methods.—This is a substudy of a multicenter, randomized, controlled pragmatic trial that tests the effectiveness of the Asthma APGAR system in primary care practices. As part of the study, enrolled patients completed both the ACT™/CACT™ and the Asthma APGAR system between March 1, 2011, and December 31, 2011. Kappa and McNemar statistics were used to compare the results of questionnaires.

Results.—Of the 468 patients in our sample, 306 (65%) were classified as not controlled by the ACT™/CACT™ or the Asthma APGAR system. The overall agreement was 84.4%, with a kappa value of .68 (substantial agreement) and a McNemar test P value of .35 (suggesting no significant difference in the direction of disagreement). Of those with poor control as defined by the Asthma APGAR system, 23.8% (73) had no controller medications and 76.5% (234) were seldom or sometimes able to avoid identified triggers for their asthma. Of those who stated that they had been prescribed controller medications, 116 of 332 (35%) stated that they did not use the controller medication on a daily basis.

Conclusion.—The Asthma APGAR system and the ACT™/CACT™ similarly assess asthma control in a multicenter primary care–based sample. The Asthma APGAR system identified an "actionable item" in more than 75% (234) of the individuals with poor asthma control, thus linking an assessment of poor asthma control with a management strategy (Figs 1-4).

▶ Remember when the term "APGAR" brought forth images of a delivery room where a score is given to each newborn infant reflecting his or her well-being at 1 and 5 minutes after birth?[1] Well, the Asthma APGAR Score (AAS) tool represents a whole new ballgame, developed by primary care clinicians to bridge the gap in the primary care management of asthma. Fig 1 is representative of the patient completed AAS form. Fig 2 depicts the AAS algorithm that is used by the

A

Name **APGAR PLUS** *Date* ____________

Asthma Tools

A = Activities
P = Persistent
G = triGGers
A = Asthma medications
R = Response to therapy

P = Asthma Plan
L = Lung function
U= Use of inhaler
S = Steroids

Please circle your answers:

A **1. In the past 2 weeks, how many times did any breathing problems (such as asthma) interfere with your ACTIVITIES or activities you wanted to do?**

Never 1-2 times 3 or more times

P **2. How many DAYS in the past 2 weeks did you have shortness of breath, wheezing, chest tightness, cough or felt you should use your rescue inhaler?**

None 1-2 DAYS 3 or more DAYS

3. How many NIGHTS in the past 2 weeks did you wake up or have trouble sleeping due to coughing, shortness of breath, wheezing, chest tightness or get up to use your rescue medication?

None 1-2 NIGHTS 3 or more NIGHTS

G **4. Do you know what makes your breathing problems or asthma worse?**

Yes No Unsure

- **Please circle things that make your breathing problems or asthma worse:**

Cigarettes Smoke Cold Air Colds Exercise Dust Dust Mites
Trees Flowers Cats Dogs Mold Other: ____________

- **Can you avoid the things that make your breathing problems or asthma worse?**

Seldom Sometimes Most of the time

A **5. List or describe medications you've taken for breathing problems or asthma in the past 2 weeks: Remember you may use Nasal, Oral, or Inhaler medications.**

Breathing or Asthma Medication	When taken?		Reasons for taking medication:	Reasons for not taking medication:
	☐ Daily	☐ As needed		
	☐ Daily	☐ As needed		
	☐ Daily	☐ As needed		
	☐ Daily	☐ As needed		

R **6. When I use my breathing or asthma medicines I feel:**

Worse No Different A Little Better A Lot Better

FIGURE 1.—Patient Asthma APGAR system form. (Reproduced with permission from Mayo Clinic Proceedings. Rank MA, Bertram S, Wollan P, et al. Comparing the asthma APGAR system and the asthma control Test™ in a multicenter primary care sample. *Mayo Clin Proc.* 2014;89:917-925, Copyright 2014, Dowden Health Media.)

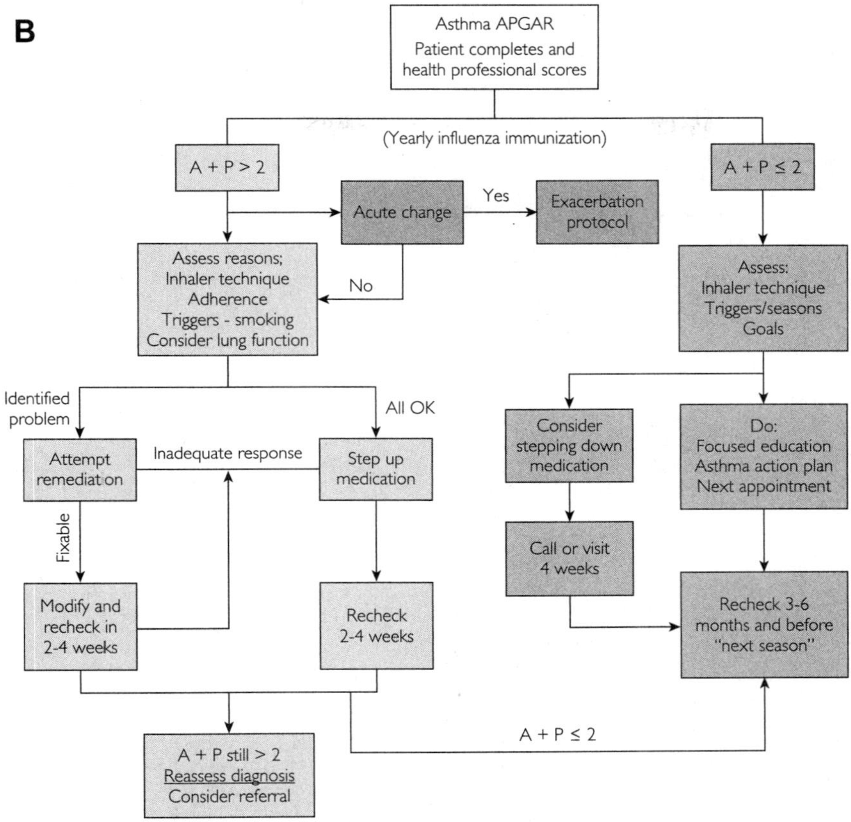

FIGURE 2.—Asthma APGAR system algorithm. (Reproduced with permission from Mayo Clinic Proceedings. Rank MA, Bertram S, Wollan P, et al. Comparing the asthma APGAR system and the asthma control Test™ in a multicenter primary care sample. *Mayo Clin Proc.* 2014;89:917-925, Copyright 2014, Dowden Health Media.)

clinician scoring the patient's answers on the questionnaire to determine next steps in the patient's asthma care. The profile of patients who are identified using the AAS as having uncontrolled asthma includes the following categories: age 19 years or older, female, black, smokers, and exposed to secondhand smoke. Patients most likely to be in control are those in the highest income group (≥$75 000 annual household income). Comparison between the AAS and the Asthma Control Test (ACT) or Asthma Control Questionnaire (ACQ) showed that overall agreement existed in this study (controlled vs not controlled); 15.6% of subjects were classified differently by the 2 systems. Results on the AAS for more than 70% of subjects with uncontrolled asthma detailed 1 or more actionable items according to the Asthma APGAR algorithm. The overall benefit of the AAS is that these interventions (eg, identifying and removing triggers; adherence to medications; teaching appropriate inhaler technique) can be undertaken at the time of the healthcare provider visit to improve control. Of

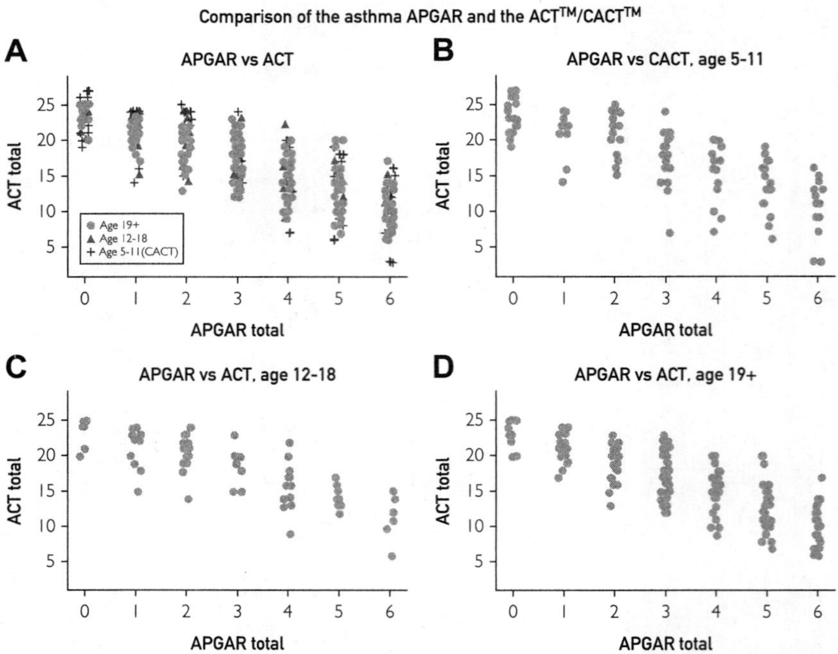

FIGURE 3.—A, Agreement on the degree of asthma control by ACT™/CACT™ and Asthma APGAR system scores for the study group (N = 468). The left upper and the right lower quadrants represent the patients for whom the 2 scores agree. The right upper quadrant represents patients for whom the Asthma APGAR system indicates not controlled and the ACT™/CACT™ indicates controlled; and the left lower quadrant shows those for whom the Asthma APGAR system indicates in control and the ACT™/CACT™ not controlled. B, Agreement on the degree of asthma control by ACT™ and Asthma APGAR system scores for those aged 5 to 11 years. C, Agreement on the degree of asthma control by ACT™ and Asthma APGAR system scores for those aged 12 to 18 years. D, Agreement on the degree of asthma control by ACT™ and Asthma APGAR system scores for those older than 19 years. (Reproduced with permission from Mayo Clinic Proceedings. Rank MA, Bertram S, Wollan P, et al. Comparing the asthma APGAR system and the asthma control Test™ in a multicenter primary care sample. *Mayo Clin Proc.* 2014;89:917-925, Copyright 2014, Dowden Health Media.)

those who scored as not controlled by the AAS, 23.8% had no daily medications, and 76.5% reported being seldom or only sometimes able to avoid identified triggers for their asthma. Thirty-five percent stated that they did not use prescribed daily controller medications, instead using the controller medication on an as-needed basis. Fig 4 depicts recommended approaches after use of the ACT/ACQ versus the AAS, suggesting ways in which primary care providers can take actionable intervention steps to improve overall patient compliance and control. More studies are underway, but the message is clear: Better educate yourself and get used to the term APGAR in the asthma clinic, and soon.

S. K. Willsie, DO, MA

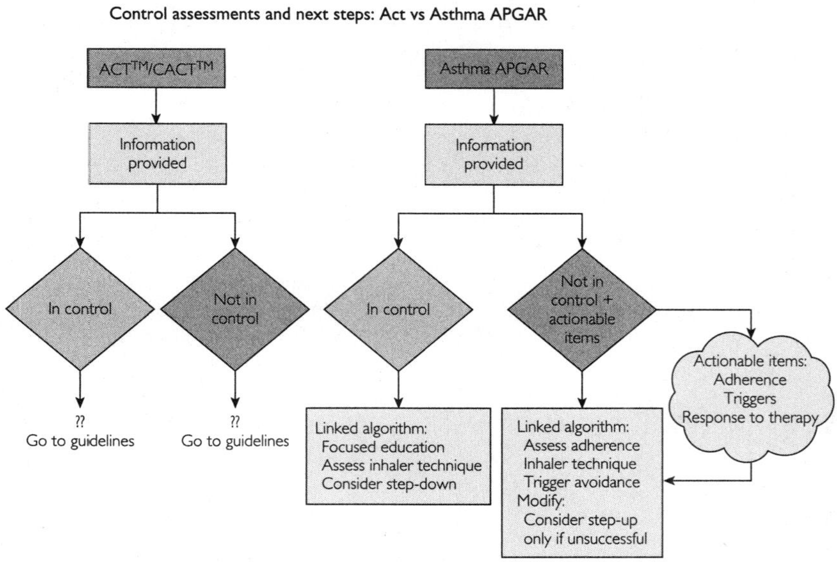

FIGURE 4.—Control assessments and next steps: The ACT™ vs the Asthma APGAR system. (Reproduced with permission from Mayo Clinic Proceedings. Rank MA, Bertram S, Wollan P, et al. Comparing the asthma APGAR system and the asthma control Test™ in a multicenter primary care sample. *Mayo Clin Proc*. 2014;89:917-925, Copyright 2014, Dowden Health Media.)

Reference

1. Yawn BP, Bertram S, Wollan P. Introduction of Asthma APGAR tools to improve asthma management in primary care practices. *J Asthma Allergy*. 2008;1:1-10.

Cystic Fibrosis

Gene therapy in cystic fibrosis

Armstrong DK, Cunningham S, Davies JC, et al (UK CF Gene Therapy Consortium)
Arch Dis Child 99:465-468, 2014

The principal cause of morbidity and mortality in cystic fibrosis (CF) is pulmonary disease, so the focus of new treatments in this condition is primarily targeted at the lungs. Since the cloning of the *Cystic Fibrosis.*
Transmembrane Conductance Regulator (CFTR) gene in 1989, there has been significant interest in the possibility of gene therapy as a treatment for CF. Early studies using viral vectors carrying a healthy CFTR plasmid highlighted the difficulties with overcoming the body's host defences. This article reviews the work on gene therapy in CF to date and describes the ongoing

work of the UK CF Gene Therapy Consortium in investigating the potential of gene therapy as a treatment for patients with CF.

▶ This article is a must read for all healthcare providers caring for patients with cystic fibrosis (CF) and educators preparing the next generation of healthcare providers! It provides an excellent review of the status of gene therapy for CF, the most common lethal autosomal recessive genetic defect in European Caucasians.[1,2] Describing major efforts since the gene's discovery in 1989 to successfully implant and cure CF with gene therapy and the attendant failures, the authors describe current investigations, the results of which should be published soon and sound promising for CF patients and their families. Numerous cohorts receiving different routes of small molecule delivery have been studied long term, and the results of these investigations stand to offer groundbreaking and life-changing therapies, potentially prolonging life for those with this deadly disease. At last .... But we must wait for the results.

S. K. Willsie, DO, MA

References

1. Farrell PM. The prevalence of cystic fibrosis in the European Union. *J Cyst Fibros.* 2008;7:450-453.
2. Dodge JA, Morison S, Lewis PA, et al. Incidence, population, and survival of cystic fibrosis in the UK, 1968–95. UK Cystic Fibrosis Survey Management Committee. *Arch Dis Child.* 1997;77:493-496.

Cystic Fibrosis Foundation Pulmonary Guideline: Pharmacologic Approaches to Prevention and Eradication of Initial *Pseudomonas aeruginosa* Infection

Mogayzel PJ Jr, the Cystic Fibrosis Foundation Pulmonary Clinical Practice Guidelines Committee (The Johns Hopkins Med Institutions, Baltimore, MD; et al)

Ann Am Thorac Soc 11:1640-1650, 2014

Description.—The Cystic Fibrosis (CF) Foundation developed clinical care guidelines for the prevention of *Pseudomonas aeruginosa* infection, the treatment of initial *P. aeruginosa* infection, and the use of bronchoscopy to obtain routine airway cultures in individuals with CF.

Methods.—A multidisciplinary committee developed questions about the prevention and treatment of initial *P. aeruginosa* infection and the use of bronchoscopy to obtain routine airway cultures. The outcome measure of interest was cultures without *P. aeruginosa* growth. Systematic reviews of PubMed, EMBASE, and the Cochrane Central Register of Controlled Trials were conducted in May 2012 and August 2013. Searches combined controlled vocabulary terms and text words for CF and terms relevant to each question. The entire committee reviewed the evidence, and final recommendation statements were graded using the U.S. Preventive Services Task Force system.

Recommendation 1.—The CF Foundation strongly recommends inhaled antibiotic therapy for the treatment of initial or new growth of *P. aeruginosa* from an airway culture (certainty of net benefit, high; estimate of net benefit, substantial; grade of recommendation, A). The favored antibiotic regimen is inhaled tobramycin (300 mg twice daily) for 28 days.

Recommendation 2.—The CF Foundation recommends against the use of prophylactic antipseudomonal antibiotics to prevent the acquisition *P. aeruginosa* (certainty of net benefit, moderate; estimate of net benefit, zero; grade of recommendation, D).

Recommendation 3.—The CF Foundation recommends routine oropharyngeal cultures rather than bronchoalveolar lavage cultures obtained by bronchoscopy in individuals with CF who cannot expectorate sputum to determine if they are infected with *P. aeruginosa* (certainty of net benefit, moderate; estimate of net benefit, moderate; grade of recommendation, B).

▶ Hot off the presses is the must-read Pulmonary Guideline for Cystic Fibrosis (CF) published by the Cystic Fibrosis Foundation. The methodologies used by the Clinical Practice Guideline committee are detailed extensively in the clinical practice guideline and will not be reiterated here. The US Preventive Services Task Force system was used for grading recommendations, which assesses net benefit and certainty of net benefit.[1] Key Recommendations from the Clinical Practice Guideline Committee are listed in the abstract of this article. With regard to the recommendation of 28 days of twice-daily inhaled tobramycin 80 mg for a newly acquired infection with *Pseudomonas aeruginosa*, the committee noted that the recently convened European CF Society has adopted the same recommendation. In finding no benefit of preventive antibiotic therapy to stave off *P aeruginosa* infection, the committee notes that not only is there no benefit in doing so, but prolonged use of such antibiotics may increase the risk of acquiring other potential pathogenic microorganisms. Oropharyngeal cultures are the preferred alternative to bronchoalveolar lavage to evaluate for the absence of *P aeruginosa*. The remaining question posed at the end of the guideline is how best to treat the *P aeruginosa* initial infection, which does not respond to the recommended therapy.

S. K. Willsie, DO, MA

Reference

1. Sawaya GF, Guirguis-Blake J, LeFevre M, Harris R, Petitti D, US Preventive Health Services Task Force. Update on the methods of the U.S. Preventive Services Task Force: estimating certainty and magnitude of net benefit. *Ann Intern Med.* 2007;147:871-875.

Viability of *Pseudomonas aeruginosa* in cough aerosols generated by persons with cystic fibrosis

Knibbs LD, Johnson GR, Kidd TJ, et al (Queensland Univ of Technology, Brisbane, Australia; The Univ of Queensland, Herston, Australia; et al)
Thorax 69:740-745, 2014

Background.—Person-to-person transmission of respiratory pathogens, including *Pseudomonas aeruginosa,* is a challenge facing many cystic fibrosis (CF) centres. Viable *P aeruginosa* are contained in aerosols produced during coughing, raising the possibility of airborne transmission.

Methods.—Using purpose-built equipment, we measured viable *P aeruginosa* in cough aerosols at 1, 2 and 4 m from the subject (distance) and after allowing aerosols to age for 5, 15 and 45 min in a slowly rotating drum to minimise gravitational settling and inertial impaction (duration). Aerosol particles were captured and sized employing an Anderson Impactor and cultured using conventional microbiology. Sputum was also cultured and lung function and respiratory muscle strength measured.

Results.—Nineteen patients with CF, mean age 25.8 (SD 9.2) years, chronically infected with *P aeruginosa*, and 10 healthy controls, 26.5 (8.7) years, participated. Viable *P aeruginosa* were detected in cough aerosols from all patients with CF, but not from controls; travelling 4 m in 17/18 (94%) and persisting for 45 min in 14/18 (78%) of the CF group. Marked inter-subject heterogeneity of *P aeruginosa* aerosol colony counts was seen and correlated strongly ($r = 0.73 - 0.90$) with sputum bacterial loads. Modelling decay of viable *P aeruginosa* in a clinic room suggested that at the recommended ventilation rate of two air changes per hour almost 50 min were required for 90% to be removed after an infected patient left the room.

Conclusions.—Viable *P aeruginosa* in cough aerosols travel further and last longer than recognised previously, providing additional evidence of airborne transmission between patients with CF.

▶ This is an important investigation documenting that person-to-person transmission of *Pseudomonas aeruginosa* is possible and that current room air exchanges and distance between beds required by standard infection controls may be inadequate to prevent person-to-person transmission of this pathogenic organism, which is responsible for much of the morbidity and lung parenchymal damage in patients with cystic fibrosis. It's time for hospital and infectious control experts to revisit the current infection control guidelines.

S. K. Willsie, DO, MA

Longevity of Patients With Cystic Fibrosis in 2000 to 2010 and Beyond: Survival Analysis of the Cystic Fibrosis Foundation Patient Registry

MacKenzie T, Gifford AH, Sabadosa KA, et al (Geisel School of Medicine at Dartmouth and Dartmouth Inst for Health Policy and Clinical Practice, Hanover, NH; Dartmouth—Hitchcock Med Ctr, Lebanon, NH; Cystic Fibrosis Foundation, Bethesda, MD; et al)

Ann Intern Med 161:233-241, 2014

Background.—Advances in treatments for cystic fibrosis (CF) continue to extend survival. An updated estimate of survival is needed for better prognostication and to anticipate evolving adult care needs.

Objective.—To characterize trends in CF survival between 2000 and 2010 and to project survival for children born and diagnosed with the disease in 2010.

Design.—Registry-based study.

Setting.—110 Cystic Fibrosis Foundation-accredited care centers in the United States.

Patients.—All patients represented in the Cystic Fibrosis Foundation Patient Registry (CFFPR) between 2000 and 2010.

Measurements.—Survival was modeled with respect to age, age at diagnosis, gender, race or ethnicity, F508del mutation status, and symptoms at diagnosis.

Results.—Between 2000 and 2010, the number of patients in the CFFPR increased from 21 000 to 26 000, median age increased from 14.3 to 16.7 years, and adjusted mortality decreased by 1.8% per year (95% CI, 0.5% to 2.7%). Males had a 19% (CI, 13% to 24%) lower adjusted risk for death than females. Median survival of children born and diagnosed with CF in 2010 is projected to be 37 years (CI, 35 to 39 years) for females and 40 years (CI, 39 to 42 years) for males if mortality remains at 2010 levels and more than 50 years if mortality continues to decrease at the rate observed between 2000 and 2010.

Limitations.—The CFFPR does not include all patients with CF in the United States, and loss to follow-up and missing data were observed. Additional analyses to address these limitations suggest that the survival projections are conservative.

Conclusion.—Children born and diagnosed with CF in the United States in 2010 are expected to live longer than those born earlier. This has important implications for prognostic discussions and suggests that the health care system should anticipate greater numbers of adults with CF.

▶ This selection reports survival analysis from the Cystic Fibrosis (CF) National Registry, 2000—2010 that, although rich with data, has several key points that are of great importance to the entire healthcare community and patients with CF. Males had a 19% lower risk of death than females from 2000 to 2010, and overall, there was a 1.8% reduction in mortality per year from 2000 to 2010 for all CF patients. For patients born with CF in 2010 will be diagnosed earlier in life in large part because of newborn screening for CF. Table 3 in the original article depicts CF mortality as a function of gender and genotype. It is known that chronic renal insufficiency, hypertriglyceridemia, and colon cancer affect CF patients more commonly than non-CF patients. Thirty percent of adults with CF have depression, which can affect adherence to medication regimens and follow-up visits to healthcare providers. Table 3 in the original article depicts "what if" ages of survival for CF patients based on predicted improvement survival and genotype. For example, given what was seen from 2000 to 2010, that is, a 1.8% increase in survival per year, what would that mean to survival of a CF patient? He or she could survive between 53 and 67 years of age, dependent on genotype and presuming that no life-changing event occurs in medical care between now and his or her death. This represents a startling increase in longevity for CF patients, and if this trend continues, this will be a game changer for healthcare providers, patients, and families as they prognosticate and plan for the future. Healthcare providers will have to be educated about the aging CF patient and more centers that specialize in treating CF will need to be established, or else these patients will have to be redistributed to primary care providers, who require additional education on their specialized health care needs. Stay tuned—we've come a long way with CF, the most common fatal autosomal recessive genetically transmitted disease in primarily Caucasians of European descent.

S. K. Willsie, DO, MA

Medical and obstetric complications among pregnant women with cystic fibrosis

Patel EM, Swamy GK, Heine RP, et al (Duke Univ School of Medicine, Durham, NC; et al)

Am J Obstet Gynecol 212:98.e1-98.e9, 2015

Objective.—The objective of this study was to estimate the nationwide prevalence of cystic fibrosis (CF) in pregnancy and determine what medical complications exist at delivery among pregnant women with CF.

Study Design.—The Nationwide Inpatient Sample (NIS) was queried for all delivery-related discharges. Women with CF were identified by *International Classification of Diseases, 9th revision, Clinical Modifications* codes and compared with women without CF. The prevalence of selected severe medical complications was compared between the 2 groups (NIS years 2008-2010) using multivariable logistic regression and the linear change in prevalence of CF at delivery determined (NIS years 2000-2010).

Results.—From 2000 to 2010, there was a significant linear increase in the prevalence of CF at delivery from 3.0 to 9.8 per 100,000 deliveries, in 2000 and 2010, respectively ($R^2 = 0.92$, $P < .0001$). From 2008-2010, there were 1119 deliveries to women with CF and 12,627,627 to women without CF. Women with CF were more likely to be white ($P < .0001$) and have diabetes (odds ratio [OR], 14.0; 95% confidence interval [CI], 11.8–16.7) or asthma (OR, 5.1; 95% CI, 4.3–6.1).

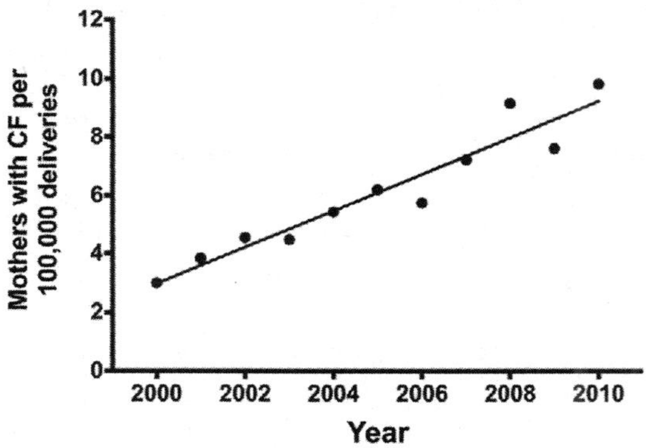

FIGURE 1.—Trend in the number of pregnant women with cystic fibrosis per 100,000 deliveries. There was a significant linear increase in the number of women with cystic fibrosis at delivery from 2.99 per 100,000 deliveries in 2000 to 9.84 per 100,000 in 2010 ($P < .0001$, $R^2 = 0.91$). (Reprinted from American Journal of Obstretics & Gynecology. Patel EM, Swamy GK, Heine RP, et al. Medical and obstetric complications among pregnant women with cystic fibrosis. *Am J Obstet Gynecol.* 2015;212:98.e1-98.e9, Copyright 2015, with permission from Elsevier.)

TABLE 2.—Medical Conditions Present at Time of Delivery Among Women with CF

Condition, n (%)[a]	CF n = 1119	No CF n = 12,627,627	OR (95% CI)	*P* Value
Cardiac conduction disorders	39 (3.5)	83,146 (0.7)	5.5 (4.0–7.6)	< .0001
Asthma	165 (14.7)	411,451 (3.3)	5.1 (4.3–6.1)	< .0001
Diabetes (nongestational)	147 (13.1)	134,209 (1.1)	14.0 (11.8–16.7)	< .0001
Thyroid disorder	33 (2.9)	299,896 (2.4)	1.2 (0.9–1.7)	.24
Thrombophilia/APS	36 (3.2)	71,418 (0.6)	5.7 (2.7–12.1)	< .0001
Anemia	154 (13.8)	1,363,611 (10.8)	1.3 (1.1–1.6)	.001
Thrombocytopenia	11 (1.0)	114,686 (0.9)	1.1 (0.6–1.9)	.85
Drug use	14 (1.2)	165,626 (1.3)	0.9 (0.5–1.6)	.80
Tobacco	90 (8.0)	794,831 (6.3)	1.3 (1.04–1.6)	.02

APS, antiphospholipid antibody syndrome; *CF*, cystic fibrosis; *CI*, confidence interval; *NIS*, Nationwide Inpatient Sample; *OR*, odds ratio.

[a]The NIS does not allow reporting the number of cases when the cell frequency is less than or equal to 10. There were 10 or fewer cases of chronic hypertension, systemic lupus erythematosus, rheumatoid arthritis, human immunodeficiency virus, alcohol use, and chronic renal failure among women with CF.

Reprinted from American Journal of Obstretics & Gynecology. Patel EM, Swamy GK, Heine RP, et al. Medical and obstetric complications among pregnant women with cystic fibrosis. Am J Obstet Gynecol. 2015;212:98.e1-98.e9. Copyright 2015, with permission from Elsevier.

Multivariable logistic regression demonstrated that women with CF were more likely to die (adjusted OR [aOR], 76.0; 95% CI, 31.6–183), require mechanical ventilation (aOR, 18.3; 95% CI, 10.8–31.2), or have pneumonia (aOR, 56.5; 95% CI, 43.2–74.1), acute renal failure (aOR, 17.3; 95% CI, 9.1–32.6), preterm labor (aOR, 2.2; 95% CI, 1.9–2.6), or an adverse composite CF outcome (aOR, 28.1; 95% CI, 21.8–36.3).

Conclusion.—Pregnant women with CF are more likely to die, require mechanical ventilation, and have infectious complications compared

TABLE 3.—Medical Events Present at Time of Delivery Among Women with CF

Condition, n (%)[a]	CF n = 1119	No CF n = 12,627,627	OR (95% CI)	*P* Value
Death	11 (1.0)	921 (0.007)	125 (67–233)	< .0001
Mechanical ventilation	25 (2.2)	9003 (0.07)	31.9 (21.4–47.5)	< .0001
Transfusion	20 (1.8)	131,684 (1.0)	1.7 (1.1–2.7)	.01
Pneumonia	75 (6.7)	13,150 (0.1)	68.7 (54.3–86.9)	< .0001
Acute respiratory failure	14 (1.2)	5450 (0.04)	29.6 (16.7–48.0)	< .0001
Acute renal failure	11 (1.0)	7075 (0.06)	16.4 (8.9–30.4)	< .0001
Composite CF outcome[b]	95 (8.5)	33,275 (0.26)	35.3 (28.6–43.5)	< .0001

CF, cystic fibrosis; *CI*, confidence interval; *NIS*, Nationwide Inpatient Sample; *OR*, odds ratio.

[a]The NIS does not allow reporting the number of cases when the cell frequency is less than or equal to 10. There were 10 or fewer cases of myocardial infarction, cardiac arrest, acute heart failure, pulmonary edema, acute respiratory distress syndrome, pulmonary embolism, deep vein thrombosis, stroke/cerebral vascular accident, sepsis, pyelonephritis and influenza among women with CF.

[b]Composite CF outcome includes any of the following: death, mechanical ventilation, sepsis, pneumonia, acute respiratory failure, acute respiratory distress syndrome, or acute renal failure.

TABLE 4.—Obstetric Events Present at time of Delivery Among Women with CF

Condition, n (%)[a]	CF n = 1119	No CF n = 12,627,627	OR (95% CI)	*P* Value
Cesarean delivery	351 (31.4)	4,041,005 (32.0)	1.0 (0.9–1.1)	.67
Operative vaginal delivery	100 (8.9)	792,143 (6.3)	1.5 (1.2–1.8)	.0002
Multiple gestation	39 (3.5)	267,193 (2.1)	1.7 (1.2–2.3)	.0013
GDM	148 (13.2)	714,940 (5.7)	2.5 (2.1–3.0)	< .0001
Preeclampsia, eclampsia, gest HTN	76 (6.8)	931,154 (7.4)	0.9 (0.7–1.1)	.48
Preterm labor	209 (18.7)	1,051,494 (8.3)	2.5 (2.2–2.9)	< .0001
Abruption	16 (1.4)	136,053 (1.1)	1.3 (0.8–2.2)	.22
Fetal growth restriction	29 (2.6)	271,882 (2.2)	1.2 (0.8–1.8)	.26
Postpartum hemorrhage	15 (1.3)	321,959 (2.5)	0.5 (0.3–0.9)	.012
Chorioamnionitis	36 (3.2)	323,531 (2.6)	1.3 (0.9–1.8)	.17

CF, cystic fibrosis, *CI*, confidence interval; *GDM*, gestational diabetes; gest *HTN*, gestational hypertension; *NIS*, Nationwide Inpatient Sample; *OR*, odds ratio.

[a]The NIS does not allow reporting the number of cases when the cell frequency is less than or equal to 10. There were 10 or fewer cases of fetal demise and placenta previa among women with CF.

with women without CF, although the absolute risks are low and these events are relatively rare (Fig 1, and Tables 2-5).

▶ This investigation used the Nationwide Inpatient Sample (NIS) from the Healthcare Cost and Utilization Project of the Agency for Healthcare Research and Quality to gain information related to pregnancy related discharges from 2008 to 2010 and specifically evaluated pregnancies of women with cystic fibrosis (CF) compared with pregnancies of women without CF. Between 2000 and 2010, a statistically significant increase in women with CF at delivery was documented as noted in Fig 1, rising from 2.99 per 100 000 deliveries in 2000

TABLE 5.—Multivariable Logistic Regression Model for Complications Among Women with CF

Maternal Condition	Adjusted OR (95% CI)	*P* Value
Death	76.0 (31.6–183)	< .0001
Mechanical ventilation	18.3 (10.8–31.2)	< .0001
Transfusion	1.68 (1.01–2.81)	.045
Pneumonia	56.5 (43.2–74.1)	< .0001
Acute respiratory failure	20.3 (10.5–39.0)	< .0001
Acute renal failure	17.3 (9.1–32.6)	< .0001
Composite CF outcome	28.1 (21.8–36.3)	< .0001
Preterm labor	2.2 (1.9–2.6)	< .0001

Multivariable logistic regression analysis for the listed outcomes among women with CF at delivery while controlling for age, race/ethnicity, diabetes, hypertension, gestational diabetes, preeclampsia, multiple gestation, and mode of delivery.

CF, cystic fibrosis; *CI*, confidence interval; *OR*, odds ratio.

to 9.84 per 100 000 ($P < .0001$; $R^2 = 0.91$). Women with CF at delivery were more likely to be white and younger compared with women at delivery without CF. Preexisting conditions in women at delivery are displayed in Table 2, showing that women with CF were more likely to have significant medical comorbidities, including asthma (odds ratio 5.1; 95% confidence interval 4.3–6.1; $P < .0001$) and diabetes mellitus (odds ratio 14.0; 95% confidence interval, 11.8–16.7; $P < .0001$). In addition, women with CF were more likely to have cardiac conduction disorders and thrombophilia ($P < .0001$). Medical conditions occurring at delivery (Table 3) show that women with CF at delivery were statistically significantly more likely to die, develop acute respiratory failure, require mechanical ventilation, have pneumonia, or experience acute renal failure. Table 4 demonstrates that obstetric events more common in women with CF at delivery include operative vaginal delivery, multiple gestation, and preterm labor. Despite these findings, the incidence of these events remain low and women with CF are generally considered good candidates for pregnancy, provided that they have intermediate to good pulmonary function (forced expiratory volume at 1 second 50%–75%), which is considered the strongest predictor of maternal morbidity and mortality.[1-4]

S. K. Willsie, DO, MA

References

1. Gilljam M, Antoniou M, Shin J, Dupuis A, Corey M, Tullis De. Pregnancy in cystic fibrosis: fetal and maternal outcome. *Chest*. 2000;118:85-91.
2. Lau EM, Barnes DJ, MOriarty C, et al. Pregnancy outcomes in the current era of cystic fibrosis care: a 15 year experience. *Aust N Z J Obstet Gynaecol*. 2011;51: 220-224.
3. Thorpe-Geeston JG, Madge S, Gyi K, Hodson M, Bilton D. The outcome of pregnancies in women with cystic fibrosis-single centre experience. 1998–2011. *BJOG*. 2013;120:354-361.
4. Cheng EY, Goss CH, McKone EF, et al. Aggressive prenatal care results in successful fetal outcomes in CF women. *J Cyst Fibros*. 2006;5:85-91.

Miscellaneous

Scientific Foundations of Allergen-Specific Immunotherapy for Allergic Disease

Soyka MB, van de Veen W, Holzmann D, et al (Univ of Zurich, Davos, Switzerland; Univ Hosp Zurich, Switzerland)

Chest 146:1347-1357, 2014

Allergen-specific immunotherapy (AIT) was described as a therapeutic option for the treatment of allergies > 100 years ago. It is based on administration of allergen extracts and leads to the development of clinical allergen tolerance in selected patients. According to current knowledge, AIT results in the restoration of immune tolerance toward the allergen of interest. It is mainly accompanied by the induction of regulatory and suppressive subsets of T and B cells, the production of IgG4 isotype allergen-specific blocking antibodies, and decreased inflammatory responses to allergens by effector cells in inflamed tissues. Currently, AIT is mainly applied subcutaneously or sublingually and is suitable for both children and adults for pollen, pet dander, house dust mite, and venom allergies. It not only affects rhinoconjunctival symptoms but also has documented short- and long-term benefits in asthma treatment. Clinically, a fast onset of tolerance is achieved during desensitization, with a tolerable amount of side effects. The disease modification effect leads to decreased disease severity, less drug usage, prevention of future allergen sensitizations, and a long-term curative effect. Increasing safety while maintaining or even augmenting efficiency is the main goal of research for novel vaccine development and improvement of treatment schemes in AIT. This article reviews the principles of allergen-specific immune tolerance development and the effects of AIT in the clinical context.

► This is a solid review of the state-of-the-art of allergen-specific immunotherapy for allergic disease. Fig 2 in the original article depicts induction of tolerance by allergen-specific immunotherapy, and Table 1 in the original article identifies cellular sources for a variety of important cytokines, their main targets, general mechanisms, and potential roles in allergen immunotherapy. The review focuses on selection of candidates for immunotherapy, and schedules for same, including defining rush, ultra-rush, and short-course regimens. Sublingual and subcutaneous routes are compared with regard to efficacy and tolerance. Contraindications for allergen immunotherapy and long-term effects are discussed. Table 2 in the original article provides the results of large-scale clinical trials and systemic reviews, including efficacy of various therapies and associated side effects. Future research areas defined include discovery of biomarkers that signal clinical response to immunotherapy.

S. K. Willsie, DO, MA

2 Chronic Obstructive Pulmonary Disease

Introduction

The topic areas covered in the Chronic Obstructive Pulmonary Disease (COPD) chapter in this YEAR BOOK include research in risk factors for development of the disease and related complications, new or new uses of existing assessment tools for disease severity, prognosis and outcomes, and medications and their use in COPD.

The relationship between childhood asthma and adult COPD is often assumed and has been documented in other studies, but the actual correlation is still vague. Tai et al followed children over 40 years and found that those with severe asthma were much more likely to develop COPD. Risk factors for a common complication of COPD, pneumothorax, were identified and reported by Hobbs et al from a population of more than 9000 patients with and without in the COPD Genetic Epidemiology Study. This is the largest population that has been used to look at pneumothorax risk.

New uses of existing COPD severity/measurement/prognosis/outcome tools were reported in several studies. A rather unusual "tool" is the microbiome of the lung. Garcia-Nunez et al reported changes in the microbiome related to the severity of disease. The clinical utility of this finding is not yet defined. The BODE Index representing measures of weight, flow obstruction, dyspnea, and exercise capacity has been widely adopted as a prognostic tool in COPD. de Torres et al published a study in which they added a co-morbidity index (called COTE) to the BODE Index and showed a much-improved ability to determine patient prognosis. Thabut et al applied the BODE Index measure to a national population of alpha-1 antitrypsin deficient COPD patients; the results were less sensitive than in the original cohorts of COPD patients tested.

The COPD Assessment Test (CAT) is a relatively recently developed health-related, quality-of-life tool designed with the help of COPD patients that is designed to be more sensitive and accurate than traditional tools. Gupta et al report on a systematic review of studies using CAT to determine its reliability, validity, responsiveness, and minimal clinically important difference.

Of the multiple predictive and outcome tools available for COPD, there is little focus on readmission to hospital, which is currently a very important issue in Medicare reimbursement. Chawla et al identified physical activity—and especially decreasing physical activity levels—as a sensitive predictor of all cause readmission. One area that remains relatively unexplored is the role of co-morbidity in COPD. Few tools assess the overall prognostic impact on common co-morbidities such as coronary disease. Williams et al used coronary calcium scores to identify coronary disease in COPD patients and were able to correlate higher scores with outcomes.

COPD medication management was the focus of many studies this past year. Rodrigo et al reported a systematic review of the first combination inhaler with both long-acting beta agonist and long-acting anticholinergic drug, both recommended for management of COPD but currently available only as individual inhalers. Gershon et al examined the use of long-acting beta agonists and inhaled corticosteroids in older patients with COPD and found that older patients tended not to be prescribed inhaled corticosteroids even though they might meet published guidelines. In a another study, Magnusson et al report a prospective, randomized trial in which inhaled corticosteroids were removed (or not) from a regimen, including long-acting bronchodilators and inhaled steroids; the withdrawal of corticosteroids resulted in worse lung function and quality of life, but no significant increase in exacerbations. Han et al reanalyzed a previously reported trial from the COPD Clinical Research Network to try to determine patients that are most likely to exacerbate if removed from Azithromycin treatment. Tse et al, also concerned with reducing COPD exacerbations, reported a post-hoc analysis of a study originally reported in 2013 showing modest benefit of an old drug, n-acetyl cysteine, in patients with more severe disease.

Another study addresses the needs of palliative care in patients with advanced chronic lung disease and lung cancer. The last study included is a systematic review of management of stable bronchiectasis with inhaled antibiotics.

Janet R. Mauer, MD, MBA

The association between childhood asthma and adult chronic obstructive pulmonary disease

Tai A, Tran H, Roberts M, et al (Women's and Children's Hosp, Adelaide, South Australia, Australia; Murdoch Children's Res Inst, Melbourne, Victoria, Australia; Royal Children's Hosp Melbourne, Victoria, Australia; et al)

Thorax 69:805-810, 2014

Introduction.—There is epidemiological evidence to suggest that events in childhood influence lung growth and constitute a significant risk for adult COPD. The aim of the study is to evaluate for an association between childhood asthma and adult COPD.

Methods.—This longitudinal, prospective study of 6–7-year-old children with asthma has been regularly reviewed every 7 years to the current analysis at 50 years of age. Participants completed respiratory questionnaires and lung function spirometry with postbronchodilator response. At the age of 50, subjects were classified to the following subgroups: non-asthmatics, asthma remission, current asthma and COPD which was defined by FEV_1 to FVC ratio postbronchodilator of less than 0.7.

Results.—Of the remaining survivors, 346 participated in the current study (participation rate of 76%) of whom 197 completed both questionnaire and lung function testing. As compared with children without symptoms of wheeze to the age of 7, (non-asthmatics) children with severe asthma had an adjusted 32 times higher risk for developing COPD (95% CI 3.4 to 269). In this cohort, 43% of the COPD group had never smoked. There was no evidence of a difference in the rate of decline in FEV_1 (mL/year, 95th CI) between the COPD group (17, 10 to 23) and the other groups: non-asthmatics (16, 12 to 21), asthma remission (20, 16 to 24) and current asthma (19, 13 to 25).

Conclusions.—Children with severe asthma are at increased risk of developing COPD.

► Adult chronic obstructive pulmonary disorder (COPD) is an amalgam of many diseases, the most common of which are tobacco-related, inhalation of toxic materials, and genetic mutations. It has long been suggested that another determinant of adult lung obstruction is airway disease as a child. In a large cohort of adults older than 20 years and followed for 20 years from the American Southwest, the presence of childhood asthma had a large impact on the development of subsequent obstructive disease in adulthood.[1] This report is of a study of children started more than 40 years ago. The cohort of asthmatic children has been reviewed every 7 years until age 50. At age 50, of the 34 patients with severe asthma as children, nearly half had a diagnosis of COPD. This represented a far greater percentage of patients progressing to COPD than any other group with lesser degrees of asthma or wheezing. In fact, children with these lesser degrees of airway disease did not appear to be at increased risk of adult obstructive disease. Forty plus years ago, of course, the medications available for managing asthma and the general approach to management were much less effective than today's antiinflammatory/bronchodilator approach. Hopefully, current management with good control will reduce the impact of childhood on adult lung health.

J. R. Maurer, MD

Reference

1. Silva GE, Sherrill DL, Guerra S, Barbee RA. Asthma as a risk factor for COPD in a longitudinal study. *Chest.* 2004;126:59-65.

Pneumothorax Risk Factors in Smokers with and without Chronic Obstructive Pulmonary Disease

Hobbs BD, the COPDGene Investigators (Brigham and Women's Hosp and Harvard Med School, Boston, MA; et al)

Ann Am Thorac Soc 11:1387-1394, 2014

Rationale.—The demographic, physiological, and computed tomography (CT) features associated with pneumothorax in smokers with and without chronic obstructive pulmonary disease (COPD) are not clearly defined.

Objectives.—We evaluated the hypothesis that pneumothorax in smokers is associated with male sex, tall and thin stature, airflow obstruction, and increased total and subpleural emphysema.

Methods.—The study included smokers with and without COPD from the COPDGene Study, with quantitative chest CT analysis. Pleural-based emphysema was assessed on the basis of local histogram measures of emphysema. Pneumothorax history was defined by subject self-report.

Measurements and Main Results.—Pneumothorax was reported in 286 (3.2%) of 9,062 participants. In all participants, risk of prior pneumothorax was significantly higher in men (odds ratio [OR], 1.55; 95% confidence interval [CI], 1.08–2.22) and non-Hispanic white subjects (OR, 1.90; 95% CI, 1.34–2.69). Risk of prior pneumothorax was associated with increased percent CT emphysema in all participants and participants with COPD (OR, 1.04 for each 1% increase in emphysema; 95% CI, 1.03–1.06). Increased pleural-based emphysema was independently associated with risk of past pneumothorax in all participants (OR, 1.05 for each 1% increase; 95% CI, 1.01–1.10). In smokers with normal spirometry, risk of past pneumothorax was associated with non-Hispanic white race and lifetime smoking intensity (OR, 1.20 for every 10 pack-years; 95% CI, 1.09–1.33).

Conclusions.—Among smokers, pneumothorax is associated with male sex, non-Hispanic white race, and increased percentage of total and subpleural CT emphysema. Pneumothorax was not independently associated with height or lung function, even in participants with COPD.

Clinical trial registered with www.clinicaltrials.gov (NCT00608764).

▶ Pulmonary lore surrounding the occurrence of primary spontaneous pneumothoraces (not those occurring in the context of diseases that predispose to pneumothorax, such as lymphangioleiomyomatosis or chronic obstructive pulmonary disease [COPD]) is that they occur in tall, thin males; smokers; and in the presence of atmospheric pressure changes. Studies have identified subpleural blebs as well as decreased lung density on computed tomography (CT) in many of the patients who develop spontaneous pneumothoraces.[1,2] Secondary spontaneous pneumothoraces occur in the context of known disease, most commonly COPD. In COPD, severe disease has been reported to be associated with more pneumothoraces, which can be a devastating complication.[3] However, these anecdotal risk factors have not previously been verified by a large, population-based study. In this report, the investigators looked at a population of more than 9000 patients in the COPD Genetic Epidemiology (COPDGene) Study to get a more complete and accurate view of the demographics of pneumothorax and the associated risk factors. This included a large population of smokers with a broad range of lung function values. The authors were particularly interested in the difference in risk factors for pneumothorax in patients with COPD compared with those with normal spirometry. Their hypothesis was to test the traditionally held beliefs about the demographics of patients who develop pneumothorax in this large population. In addition, they hypothesized that quantitative CT measures of pleural-based emphysema would be associated with histories of pneumothorax. The results were mixed. To start, the entire population smoked, so these are risk factors within smokers. Risk factors included male sex and increased percentage of total and subpleural emphysematous changes. However, neither height nor lung function were supported as risk factors, the latter contradicting previous cohort studies. In smokers with normal spirometry, risk of pneumothorax increased with increased pack-years of smoking. Of particular interest was the finding that non-Hispanic white patients had a greater risk than African-Americans in that two-thirds of the population was non-Hispanic white, but 80% of the pneumothoraces occurred in that group. This latter finding was noted both in patients with normal and abnormal spirometry and deserves more investigation.

J. R. Maurer, MD

References

1. Casali C, Stefani A, Ligabue G, et al. Role of blebs and bullae detected by high-resolution computed tomography and recurrent spontaneous pneumothorax. *Ann Thorac Surg*. 2013;95:249-255.
2. Lesur O, Delorme N, Fromaget JM, Bernadac P, Polu JM. Computed tomography in the etiologic assessment of idiopathic spontaneous pneumothorax. *Chest*. 1990; 98:341-347.
3. Sahn SA, Heffner JE. Spontaneous pneumothorax. *N Engl J Med*. 2000;342: 868-874.

Severity-Related Changes of Bronchial Microbiome in Chronic Obstructive Pulmonary Disease

Garcia-Nuñez M, Millares L, Pomares X, et al (Fundació Parc Taulí, Sabadell/Badalona, Spain; Universitat Autonoma de Barcelona, Esfera (UAB), Barcelona, Spain; et al)
J Clin Microbiol 52:4217-4223, 2014

Bronchial colonization by potentially pathogenic microorganisms (PPMs) is often demonstrated in chronic obstructive pulmonary disease (COPD), but culture-based techniques identify only a portion of the bacteria in mucosal surfaces. The aim of the study was to determine changes in the bronchial microbiome of COPD associated with the severity of the disease. The bronchial microbiome of COPD patients was analyzed by 16S rRNA gene amplification and pyrosequencing in sputum samples obtained during stable disease. Seventeen COPD patients were studied (forced expiratory volume in the first second expressed as a percentage of the forced vital capacity [FEV_1%] median, 35.0%; interquartile range [IQR], 31.5 to 52.0), providing a mean of 4,493 (standard deviation [SD], 2,598) sequences corresponding to 47 operational taxonomic units (OTUs) (SD, 17) at a 97% identity level. Patients were dichotomized according to their lung function as moderate to severe when their FEV_1% values were over the median and as advanced when FEV_1% values were lower. The most prevalent phyla in sputum were *Proteobacteria* (44%) and *Firmicutes* (16%), followed by *Actinobacteria* (13%). A greater microbial diversity was found in patients with moderate-to-severe disease, and alpha diversity showed a statistically significant decrease in patients with advanced disease when assessed by Shannon ($\rho = 0.528$; $P = 0.029$, Spearman correlation coefficient) and Chao1 ($\rho = 0.53$; $P = 0.028$, Spearman correlation coefficient) alpha-diversity indexes. The higher severity that characterizes advanced COPD is paralleled by a decrease in the diversity of the bronchial microbiome, with a loss of part of the resident flora that is replaced by a more restricted microbiota that includes PPMs.

▶ Ever since a much more diverse set of microbiota than we have ever cultured in the lung as well as in other organs was found by using molecular techniques, we have been trying to determine the role of these microbes. Naturally, in pulmonary medicine, we would like to identify a "normal" microbiome of the pulmonary system, then see if it changes in disease states and, if so, what these changes mean. In 2014, several groups published reports on the microbiome in chronic obstructive pulmonary disease (COPD). Garcia-Nunez et al described changes in the microbiome that appear to occur at different levels of severity of disease. The most interesting finding by this group was that the diversity of the microorganisms decreases with disease severity, a finding that differs from a previous study by Pragman et al, who did not find a restricted microbiome in more severe cases.[1] The authors speculate that this may be due to differences in patient samples. More data are clearly needed to reach any definitive conclusions. Huang et al and his investigators studied the microbiome in patients with COPD exacerbations.[2] They identified various changes in the microbiome depending on the type of treatment the patient received; for example, systemic steroids led to enrichment of members of the microbiota. Many bacterial groups were identified in the microbiota that are not typical COPD exacerbation pathogens but were involved in the compositional changes. During an exacerbation, proteobacteria were primarily increased and use of antibiotic treatment alone suppressed these and the other groups of microorganisms. Changes in function of some of the microbiota members appeared to reverse as the patient recovered. The changes were variable among patients. Because of the heterogenicity of changes in microbiota and the variable amount of changes, the authors of this study suggest that a much larger data set is needed to better understand how the microbiota functions in COPD exacerbations and what clinical implications these changes might have. The microbiome in general is fascinating and undoubtedly will stimulate research, leading to a sea change in the way we think about and manage pulmonary disease.

J. R. Maurer, MD

References

1. Pragman AA, Kim HB, Reilly CS, Wendt C, Isaacson RE. The lung microbiome in moderate and severe chronic obstructive pulmonary disease. *PLoS One*. 2012;7: e47305.
2. Huang YJ, Sethi S, Murphy T, Nariya S, Boushey HA, Lynch SV. Airway microbiome dynamics in exacerbations of chronic obstructive pulmonary disease. *J Clin Microbiol*. 2014;52:2813-2823.

Prognostic evaluation of COPD patients: GOLD 2011 versus BODE and the COPD comorbidity index COTE

de Torres JP, Casanova C, Marín JM, et al (Clínica Universidad de Navarra, Pamplona, Spain; Hospital Ntra Sra de Candelaria, Tenerife, Spain; Hospital Universitario Miguel Servet, Zaragoza, Spain; et al)
Thorax 69:799-804, 2014

Background.—The Global Obstructive Lung Disease (GOLD) 2011 revision recommends the multidimensional assessment of COPD including comorbidities and has developed a disease categories system (ABCD) attempting to implement this strategy. The added value provided by quantifying comorbidities and integrating them to multidimensional indices has not been explored.

Objective.—Compare the prognostic value of the GOLD ABCD categories versus the BMI, Obstruction, Dyspnea, Exercise (BODE) index, and explore the added prognostic value of comorbidities evaluation to this multidimensional assessment.

Methods.—From the patients who have been enrolled in the BODE study, we selected the most recent ones who had the available information needed to classify them by the ABCD GOLD categories. Cox proportional hazards ratios for all-cause mortality were performed for GOLD categories and BODE index. The added value of the comorbidity Copd cOmorbidity TEst (COTE) index was also explored using receiver operating curves (ROC) values.

Results.—707 patients were followed for 50 ± 30 months including all degrees of airway limitation and BODE index severity. ABCD GOLD predicted global mortality (HR: 1.47; 95% CI 1.28 to 1.70) as did the BODE index (HR: 2.02; 95% CI 1.76 to 2.31). Area under the curve (AUC) of ROC for ABCD GOLD was 0.68; (95% CI 0.64 to 0.73) while for the BODE index was 0.71 (95% CI 0.67 to 0.76). The C statistics value was significantly higher for the observed difference. Adding the COTE index to the BODE index improved its AUC to 0.81 (95% CI 0.77 to 0.85), ($\chi^2 = 40.28$, $p < 0.001$).

Conclusions.—In this population of COPD patients, the BODE index had a better survival prediction than the ABCD GOLD categories. Adding the COTE to the BODE index was complimentary and significantly improved outcome prediction.

▶ De Torres and colleagues present an interesting study in which they used chronic obstructive pulmonary disease (COPD) patients from the BODE (body mass index, obstruction, dyspnea, and exercise capacity) cohort to compare prognostic value of the GOLD 2011 guidelines to the BODE index.[1,2] In 2011, the Global Obstructive Lung Disease guidelines were changed to include not only degree of airway obstruction but also the phenotype or clinical components of the disease in the individual patient. Four groupings reflected a combination of either more or less airway obstruction in conjunction with more or fewer symptoms/hospitalizations. Although this change in the GOLD guidelines was designed to assist in appropriate management of COPD and not to serve as a prognostic tool, a number of studies have tried to compare the prognostic value (in terms of survival) of this enhanced model with the traditional approach that classified patients only by degree of airway obstruction. The traditional approach was notoriously poor at predicting survivals. However, the multifactorial BODE mode has been much better at this. De Torres et al assess the prognostic value of the GOLD model against the prognostic value of BODE and find the BODE index to be slightly better across the severity classifications of COPD in predicting survival. The most interesting part of this study is not the comparison of BODE versus GOLD, but rather the addition of patient medical comorbidities into the predictive model. The investigators used a comorbidity index called COTE (COPD Comorbidity Test Index) developed by many of this same group of investigators and published by Divo et al.[3] The COTE index includes 12 comorbidities that were shown previously in the BODE cohort of COPD patients to be associated with increased mortality. A scoring system was developed to incorporate these comorbidities into the overall prediction algorithm. Adding the COTE score to the BODE index greatly improved the ability to estimate prognosis (Fig 3 in the original article). The authors apparently did not try adding COTE to the GOLD categories, so the predictive value of GOLD + COTE is not known. The addition of comorbidities is a critical piece in understanding the progression of COPD through patients' disease, as is illustrated here. The approach to COPD patients has tended to be disease-specific and not whole-person oriented. That has often led to inadequate management of comorbidities such as coronary artery disease, heart failure, and depression, possibly contributing to earlier deaths. We need more prospective evaluation of the most beneficial whole-person management approaches to the COPD patient.

J. R. Maurer, MD

References

1. Celli BR, Cote C, Marin JM, et al. The body mass index, airflow obstruction, dyspnea, exercise performance (BODE) index in chronic obstructive pulmonary disease. *N Engl J Med.* 2004;350:1005-1012.
2. GOLD. Documents and resources. http://www.goldcopd.org/Guidelines/guidelines-resources.html. Accessed December 29, 2014.
3. Divo M, Cote C, de Torres JP, et al; BODE Collaborative Group. Comorbidities and risk of mortality in patients with chronic obstructive pulmonary disease. *Am J Respir Crit Care Med.* 2012;186:155-161.

Performance of the BODE index in patients with α_1-antitrypsin deficiency-related COPD

Thabut G, Mornex J-F, Pison C, et al (APHP, Paris, France; Hospices Civils de Lyon, France; Clinique Universitaire de Pneumologie CHU Grenoble, France; et al)

Eur Respir J 44:78-86, 2014

The BODE (body mass index, airflow obstruction, dyspnoea and exercise capacity) index is used to decide on referral and transplantation of patients with chronic obstructive pulmonary disease (COPD). The BODE index has not been validated in patients with α_1-antitrypsin deficiency, who account for 15% of COPD patients undergoing lung transplantation. We sought to validate the BODE index in α_1-antitrypsin deficiency-related COPD.

We assessed the prognostic value of the BODE index in 191 patients followed from 2006 to 2012 in a French prospective cohort of patients with α_1-antitrypsin deficiency.

20 patients died during follow-up and 22 underwent lung transplantation. Survival (95% CI) was 93.0% (91.7–94.3%) at 3 years and 76.0% (72.9–79.1%) at 5 years. The 3-year survival was 97.4% (96.6–98.2%), 98.0% (96.7–99.3%), 87.7% (84.5–90.9%) and 75.3% (66.0–84.6%) for patients with BODE index 0–2, 3–4, 5–6 and 7–10, respectively. Survival discrimination of the BODE index was better than with both forced

expiratory volume in 1 s and Global Initiative for Chronic Obstructive Lung Disease classification. Regarding calibration, expected survival by BODE index was noticeably lower than observed survival.

The BODE index showed very good survival discrimination in patients with α_1-antitrypsin deficiency-related COPD. Larger studies are needed to support its use to drive patient referral for lung transplantation.

▶ The BODE index (using measures of body mass index, obstruction, dyspnea, and exercise capacity) was the first multidimensional and now well-validated model designed to predict the progression and approximate survival of patients with chronic obstructive pulmonary disorder (COPD).[1] The value of the index is that it takes into account not only the patient's lung function but also elements of the multisystem nature of the disease, such as exercise capacity and nutritional status. BODE was, however, developed and validated primarily in patients who had smoking-related disease. That cohort of COPD patients is generally at least a decade older than patients with alpha-1 antitrypsin deficiency disease, and they have many of the comorbidities related to smoking such as coronary artery disease. However, because the BODE index has been the most useful and best validated prognosticator for COPD patients, it is often used for alpha-1 antitrypsin-deficient patients to determine when to refer them to transplant centers. Despite the use of BODE in this population, some have suspected that it is not as accurate a prognostic tool as in tobacco-related disease. This study, which is ongoing, uses a national cohort of alpha-1 antitrypsin-deficient emphysema patients and is longitudinally following the cohort with BODE measurements. Although BODE was much better at predicting survival that lung function alone, it was not as sensitive in this population as in the original test populations; the BODE index underestimated survival and will probably require changes to be of optimal use in alpha-1 antitrypsin-deficient patients.

Another study, published this year, authored by Ringbaek et al followed a national cohort of all patients with COPD started on long-term oxygen therapy between January 1994 and December 2010.[2] Alpha-1 antitrypsin-deficient patients in this cohort were on average 17 years younger than other COPD patients and had significantly fewer medical comorbidities. Even adjusting for the comorbidities, however, as well as age and gender, alpha-1 antitrypsin-deficient patients had a significantly lower risk of death. Both types of COPD are systemic diseases in different ways; however, the ubiquitous effects of tobacco clearly result in the greatest whole-body morbidity.

J. R. Maurer, MD

References

1. Celli BR, Cote CG, Marin JM, et al. The body-mass index, airflow obstruction, dyspnea, and exercise capacity index in chronic obstructive pulmonary disease. *N Engl J Med.* 2004;350:1005-1012.
2. Ringbaek TJ, Seersholm N, Perch M, Iversen M, Lange P. Prognosis of patients with alpha1-antitrypsine deficiency on long-term oxygen therapy. *Respir Med.* 2014;108:1189-1194.

The COPD assessment test: a systematic review

Gupta N, Pinto LM, Morogan A, et al (McGill Univ, Montréal, Quebec, Canada)

Eur Respir J 44:873-884, 2014

The COPD assessment test (CAT) is a self-administered questionnaire that measures health-related quality of life. We aimed to systematically evaluate the literature for reliability, validity, responsiveness and minimum clinically important difference (MCID) of the CAT.

Multiple databases were searched for studies analysing the psychometric properties of the CAT in adults with chronic obstructive pulmonary disease. Two reviewers independently screened, selected and extracted data, and assessed methodological quality of relevant studies using the COSMIN checklist.

From 792 records identified, 36 studies were included. The number of participants ranged from 45 to 6469, mean age from 56 to 73 years, and mean forced expiratory volume in 1 s from 39% to 98% predicted. Internal consistency (reliability) was 0.85–0.98, and test–retest reliability was 0.80–0.96. Convergent and longitudinal validity using Pearson's correlation coefficient were: SGRQ-C 0.69–0.82 and 0.63, CCQ 0.68–0.78 and 0.60, and mMRC 0.29–0.61 and 0.20, respectively. Scores differed with GOLD stages, exacerbation and mMRC grades. Mean scores decreased with pulmonary rehabilitation (2.2–3 units) and increased at exacerbation onset (4.7 units). Only one study with adequate methodology reported an MCID of 2 units and 3.3–3.8 units using the anchor-based approach and distribution-based approach, respectively. Most studies had fair methodological quality.

We conclude that the studies support the reliability and validity of the CAT and that the tool is responsive to interventions, although the MCID remains debatable.

▶ In the past decade or so, a major shift in the management of chronic obstructive pulmonary disease (COPD) patients has paralleled an overall shift in medical practice. That change has often been characterized as a shift toward more patient-centric or personalized care. In the case of COPD patients, it has meant a lesser focus on the spirometric measurements and a greater focus on the impact of the disease on the patient, together with his or her lifestyle and family. In fact, in 2011, the Global Obstructive Lung Disease guidelines changed the treatment model from a focus strictly on forced expiratory volume in 1 second (FEV1) to a combination model that included FEV1 but added symptoms, risk of exacerbations, and comorbidities.[1] Measurements of this more "whole patient" impact of disease has necessarily required measurements of health care-related quality of life. Existing tools, such as the St George Respiratory Questionnaire or the Chronic Respiratory Questionnaire, either did not measure all the important disease impacts or were difficult and time-consuming to use. The COPD Assessment Test (CAT) was designed with input from COPD patients, is self-administered and quick (only 8 items), yet it provides a fairly quantitative assessment of health-related quality of life (HRQoL).[2,3] It has recently been the chosen tool in a number of COPD studies to assess HRQoL. The purpose of this systematic review of 36 studies was to "systematically search the literature to evaluate and summarize the psychometric properties of the CAT (reliability, validity, responsiveness, and minimum clinically important difference (MCID)) as a HRQoL instrument used in patients with COPD." In at least 3 and as many as 10 studies, each of these psychometric properties was able to be evaluated. The authors concluded that certain properties, such as responsiveness and validity, need to be further studied in specific populations (such as females, younger patients, and those with mild disease) because those populations were poorly represented in the studies included in the review. However, overall the validity and reliability of the CAT, as well as the responsiveness to interventions, are supported by these studies. A conclusion about the MCID could not be supported because testing of MCID was not robust enough to draw a conclusion. Overall, the CAT appears to be a good measure of HRQoL that is simple and easy to use and meets most psychometric parameters, but it needs additional study because evaluation of MCID is a important outcome in therapeutic trials.

J. R. Maurer, MD

References

1. Documents & Resources. Global Initiative for Chronic Obstructive Lung Disease. www.goldcopd.org/Guidelines/guidelines-resources.html. Accessed December 29, 2014.
2. Jones PW, Harding G, Berry P, Wiklund I, Chen WH, Kline Leidy N. Development and first validation of the COPD assessment test. *Eur Respir J*. 2009;34:648-654.
3. Jones P, Harding G, Wiklund I, Berry P, Leidy N. Improving the process and outcome of care in COPD: development of a standardised assessment tool. *Prim Care Respir J*. 2009;18:208-215.

Physical Activity as a Predictor of Thirty-Day Hospital Readmission after a Discharge for a Clinical Exacerbation of Chronic Obstructive Pulmonary Disease

Chawla H, Bulathsinghala C, Tejada JP, et al (Univ of Connecticut, Farmington)

Ann Am Thorac Soc 11:1203-1209, 2014

Rationale.—Because physical inactivity in chronic obstructive pulmonary disease (COPD) predicts health care use and mortality, we prospectively evaluated the relationship of this variable to the frequency of 30-day readmissions after a hospitalization for an exacerbation.

Methods.—Consented patients discharged after an exacerbation of COPD were asked to wear a GT3X+ accelerometer (ActiGraph, Pensacola, FL) continuously on the wrist for 30 days after hospital discharge. Vector magnitude units (VMU), the sum of movements in three planes over each minute of use, were recorded. Higher physical activity for each minute was defined by a VMU threshold of at least 3,000 counts. Those patients with fewer than 60 minutes/day over the first week were considered inactive.

Measurements and Main Results.—Fifty-four study patients were discharged from the hospital and 38 underwent activity testing. In the latter subgroup, all-cause hospital readmissions within 30 days occurred in 12 patients (32%). Minutes of higher physical activity per day over the first week after discharge were considerably lower in those eventually readmitted than in those who remained as outpatients: 42 ± 14 (SE) versus 114 ± 19 minutes, respectively ($P = 0.02$). In addition, physical activity decreased over time in those who were eventually readmitted, but increased in those who were not readmitted. Those with lower physical activity over Week 1 after discharge were more likely to have 30-day all-cause readmissions than those with higher activity: odds ratio, 6.7, $P = 0.02$. In multivariate testing, both physical inactivity and a history of two or more hospitalizations for exacerbations in the preceding year predicted 30-day readmission.

Conclusions.—These findings underscore the importance of physical activity as a predictor of this type of health care use outcome.

▶ The finding that higher levels of physical activity is an independent predictor of better survivals has recently been reported for a number of chronic illnesses ranging from cancer to cardiac disease to diabetes.[1-3] Exercise capacity measured by a 6-minute walk in 1 of the 4 components of the BODE (body mass index, airway obstruction, dyspnea, and exercise capacity) is one of the best prognostic tools for expected survival in chronic obstructive pulmonary disease (COPD).[4] Furthermore, several studies have consistently identified low levels of physical activity with exacerbations and mortality.[5] This study by Chawla et al identified lower levels of physical activity, probably not surprisingly, as predictive of that group of recently discharged COPD patients who would require readmission. In addition to low levels of activity, decreasing levels of activity postdischarge also predicted both pulmonary and all-cause admissions. This is an important finding because it can identify those patients likely to fall within Medicare's Hospital Readmission Reduction Program, which penalizes hospitals for excessive readmissions within 30 days of discharge. Early identification of at-risk patients should allow increased interventions aimed at increasing levels of activity and keeping them out of hospital—a win-win both for the patient and for the hospitals! However, to achieve this goal, it is important to understand the determinants of physical activity in COPD patients. Although that may seem like a simple task, there is an incomplete understanding of the determinants of physical activity in these patients. A recent systematic review aimed to identify and summarize studies assessing associations between physical activity and its determinants and/or outcomes in COPD patients. Almost all of the 86 studies included in the review were based on low- or very low-quality evidence and often were cross-sectional.[5] Although moderate-level evidence was found relating the impact of low physical activity on mortality and exacerbations, only poor-quality evidence was identified regarding determinants of low physical activity, including the impact of attempted treatments. To design successful interventions to improve physical activity in these patients, much more research is required into the underlying determinants, likely multifactorial, of this problem.

J. R. Maurer, MD

References

1. Nocon M, Hiemann T, Müller-Riemenschneider F, Thalau F, Roll S, Willich SN. Association of physical activity with all-cause and cardiovascular mortality: a systematic review and meta-analysis. *Eur J Cardiovasc Prev Rehabil.* 2008;15: 239-246.
2. Cassileth BR, Yarett I, Lemanne D. Fitness: can exercise lengthen survival in patients with cancer? *The ASCO Post.* 2013;6, http://www.ascopost.com. Accessed December 29, 2014.
3. Sigal RJ, Kenny GP, Wasserman DH, Castaneda-Sceppa C. Physical activity/exercise and type 2 diabetes. *Diabetes Care.* 2004;27:2518-2534.
4. Celli BR, Cote CG, Marin JM, et al. The body-mass index, airflow obstruction, dyspnea, exercise capacity index in chronic obstructive pulmonary disease. *N Engl J Med.* 2004;350:1005-1012.
5. Gimeno-Santos E, Frei A, Steurer-Stey C, on behalf of PROactive consortium. Determinants and outcomes of physical activity in patients with COPD: a systematic review. *Thorax.* 2014;69:731-739.

Coronary artery calcification is increased in patients with COPD and associated with increased morbidity and mortality

Williams MC, for the Evaluation of COPD Longitudinally to Identify Predictive Surrogate Endpoints (ECLIPSE) investigators (Univ of Edinburgh/British Heart Foundation Centre for Cardiovascular Science, UK; et al)
Thorax 69:718-723, 2014

Background.—Coronary artery calcification is pathognomonic of coronary artery disease (CAD). Whether CAD in patients with COPD is linked to lung function, functional capacity and/or clinically relevant outcomes is unknown. The objective was to assess the association between CAD and disease severity, functional capacity and outcomes in patients with COPD.

Methods.—Coronary artery calcium score (CACS; Agatston score) was measured using chest CT in patients with COPD, smokers with normal spirometry and nonsmokers from the Evaluation of COPD Longitudinally to Identify Predictive Surrogate Endpoints (ECLIPSE) study.

Results.—CACS was measured in 942 subjects: 672 with COPD (mean age ± SD, 63 ± 7 years; FEV1 49 ± 16% predicted), 199 smokers with normal spirometry (54 ± 9 years; FEV_1 110 ± 12% predicted) and 71 nonsmokers (55 ± 9 years; FEV_1 114 ± 14% predicted). CACS was higher in patients with COPD than smokers or non-smokers (median (IQR), 128 (492) vs 0 (75) vs 0 (3) Agatston units (AU), $p < 0.001$). In patients with COPD, CACS correlated with age, pack-years, 6 min walking distance, modified Medical Research Council Dyspnoea score and circulating levels of interleukin (IL)-6, IL-8, Clara Cell protein 16, surfactant protein D and peripheral blood neutrophil count, but not with emphysema, exacerbation frequency, % predicted FEV1 or decline in FEV1. CACS was higher in patients with COPD who died than in those who survived until 3-year follow-up (CACS 406 vs 103 AU, $p < 0.001$), and was associated with mortality in a Cox proportional hazards model ($p = 0.036$).

Conclusions.—Patients with COPD have more CAD than controls and this is associated with increased dyspnoea, reduced exercise capacity and increased mortality. These data indicate that the presence of CAD in patients with COPD is associated with poor clinical outcomes (Fig 1).

► Cardiac disease is widely recognized as one of the most common medical comorbidities in patients with chronic obstructive pulmonary disease (COPD). Indeed, the primary differential diagnosis in patients presenting with a respiratory

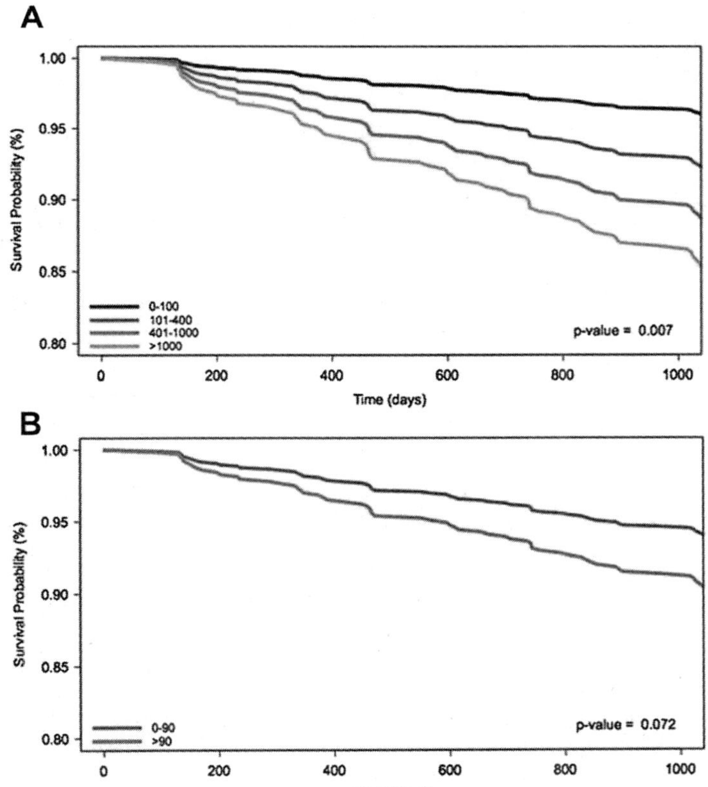

FIGURE 1.—Cox proportional hazards model for patients with COPD and (A) coronary artery calcium score (CACS) (Agatston score)adjusted for age, gender, pack-years, severity of COPD and self-reported cardiovascular disease and (B) CACSP adjusted for pack-years. (Reproduced from Thorax. Williams MC, for the Evaluation of COPD Longitudinally to Identify Predictive Surrogate Endpoints (ECLIPSE) investigators. Coronary artery calcification is increased in patients with COPD and associated with increased morbidity and mortality. *Thorax*. 2014;69:718-723, with permission from the BMJ Publishing Group Ltd.)

decompensation in their health status is often COPD exacerbation versus heart failure. The coexistence of cardiac disease and COPD is not surprising because both have tobacco as a common causative agent. Nevertheless, the relationship between cardiac disease and COPD is complex and poorly studied or understood. For example, COPD remains an independent predictor of coronary artery disease once adjustments are made for smoking and other cardiovascular risk factors.[1] Smoking and coronary disease are associated with low-grade inflammation, oxidative stress, and the downstream effects of circulating inflammatory markers. One way to assess and better define coronary artery disease in COPD patients is to look at coronary artery calcium scores (CACS) on computed tomography (CT) scans. CACS are pathognomonic of coronary artery disease and can help determine the prevalence of coronary artery disease among patients. CACS, although associated with increased mortality in smokers,[2] have not been clearly associated with inflammatory markers.[3] However, CACS is useful in stratifying risk for coronary disease, and this has not been done systematically in COPD patients. The authors sought to determine whether there was a relationship between CACS in these patients and long-term outcomes such as mortality, exacerbations, and FEV_1 (forced expiratory volume in 1 second) decline. They used CT data gathered during the Evaluation of COPD Longitudinally to Identify Predictive Surrogate Endpoints (ECLIPSE) study to do this.[4] Not surprisingly, the incidence of coronary artery calcium was higher in COPD patients than in controls, and higher CACS (Fig 1), an indicator of comorbid coronary artery disease, had worse outcomes. Whether these poorer outcomes are related to COPD, cardiac events, or both is unknown; however, COPD patients are reported to have high cardiovascular disease morbidity and mortality.[5] Further, coronary artery disease is likely undertreated in many COPD patients. CACS may be a good screening test to alert physicians treating COPD to the presence of comorbid coronary artery disease.

J. R. Maurer, MD

References

1. Boschetto P, Beghé B, Fabbri LM, et al. The link between COPD and coronary artery disease—implication for clinical practice. *Respirology.* 2012;17:422-431.
2. Jacobs PC, Prokop M, van der Graaf Y, et al. Comparing coronary artery calcium and thoracic aorta calcium for prediction of all-cause mortality and cardiovascular events on low-dose non-gated computed tomography in a high-risk population of heavy smokers. *Atherosclerosis.* 2010;209:455-462.
3. Jenny NS, Brown ER, Detrano R, et al. Associations of inflammatory markers with coronary artery calcification: results from the Multi-Ethnic Study of Atherosclerosis. *Atherosclerosis.* 2010;209:226-229.
4. Vestbo J, Anderson W, Coxson HO, et al; ECLIPSE investigators. Evaluation of COPD Longitudinally to Identify Predictive Surrogate End-points (ECLIPSE). *Eur Respir J.* 2008;31:869-873.
5. Curkendall SM, Lanes S, de Luise C, et al. Chronic obstructive pulmonary disease severity and cardiovascular outcomes. *Eur J Epidemiol.* 2006;21:803-813.

Efficacy and Safety of a Fixed-Dose Combination of Indacaterol and Glycopyrronium for the Treatment of COPD: A Systematic Review

Rodrigo GJ, Plaza V (Hospital Central de las Fuerzas Armadas, Montevideo, Uruguay; Universitat Autonoma de Barcelona, Spain)

Chest 146:309-317, 2014

Background.—COPD guidelines recommend the combined use of inhaled, long-acting β_2-agonists and long-acting muscarinic antagonists if symptoms are not improved by a single agent. This systematic review assessed the efficacy and safety of the fixed-dose combination of the long-acting β_2-agonist indacaterol and long-acting muscarinic antagonist glycopyrronium (QVA149) compared with its monocomponents (glycopyrronium and indacaterol) and tiotropium for the treatment of moderate to severe COPD.

Methods.—This was a systematic review of randomized, placebo-controlled or crossover trials (3-64 weeks). Primary outcomes were trough FEV_1, severe adverse events, and serious cardiovascular events.

Results.—Five trials (4,842 patients) were included. Compared with tiotropium, QVA149 showed a significant increase in trough FEV_1 (70 mL; $P < .0001$) and a decreased use of rescue medication (−0.63 puffs/d; $P < .0001$). Patients receiving QVA149 had a 19% greater likelihood of experiencing a minimal clinical important difference (MCID) in the number needed to treat for benefit (NNTB) (NNTB = 11) and a 16% greater likelihood of achieving an MCID in the St. George's Respiratory Questionnaire (SGRQ) (NNTB = 11). Similarly, QVA149 vs glycopyrronium showed a significant increase in trough FEV_1 (70 mL; $P < .0001$), a significant reduction in rescue medication use (−0.59; $P < .0001$), and a significant increase in the rate of patients achieving an MCID in the SGRQ (NNTB = 12). QVA149 showed similar levels of safety and tolerability to both comparators. It was not possible to perform a pooled analysis of data comparing QVA149 vs indacaterol.

Conclusions.—Once-daily, inhaled QVA149 showed superior efficacy compared with glycopyrronium and the current standard of care, tiotropium, in patients with moderate to severe COPD.

▶ Bronchodilators, especially long-acting bronchodilators, are the mainstay of pharmacotherapy for chronic obstructive pulmonary disease (COPD). The Global Obstructive Lung Disease (GOLD) Guidelines currently recommend both inhaled long-acting anticholinergic and long-acting beta-2 agonist for virtually all but the mildest COPD patients with minimal symptoms.[1] Currently available long-acting drugs are typically given twice a day. They are administered separately and provide longer symptom improvement than do short-acting drugs and also improve adherence.

The rationale for using both beta-2 agonists and anticholinergic drugs is that they have different mechanisms of action. Several studies have shown the effect to be additive, but in some systematic reviews, the value of both is not as clear.[2,3] In 2013, a new class of bronchodilator drug was approved for use in

Europe and Japan. QVA 149 is both the first combination inhaler of a long-acting beta-2 agonist and a long-acting anticholinergic drug and, additionally, is once-a-day dosing. The current systematic review is intended to summarize studies comparing the QVA 149 combination of indacaterol/glycopyrronium to each of the monocomponents and also to tiotropium, the current long-acting anticholinergic standard of care. It was not possible to do a comparison to indacaterol because there was only 1 available study; QVA 149 compared favorably to both of the anticholinergics as monotherapy. To date, the adverse event profile is similar to that of placebo, and the clinical results of the combination appear at least equal to that of tiotropium or a combination of salmeterol/fluticasone.[4] Novartis, the drug manufacturer, is expected to file for approval in the United States in late 2014 or early 2015. This QVA 149 combination, if it lives up in general use to its preapproval success, could be a significant addition to the COPD pharmacy. It may have particular appeal for those patients who have significant adverse effects or otherwise cannot tolerate inhaled steroids or who have difficulty complying with medication use because it is both once-a-day dosing and requires only 1 inhaler.

J. R. Maurer, MD

References

1. Documents & Resources. Global Initiative for Chronic Obstructive Lung Disease. www.goldcopd.org/Guidelines/guidelines-resources.html. Accessed December 29, 2014.
2. Mahler DA, D'Urzo A, Bateman ED, et al; INTRUST-1 and INTRUST-2 study investigators. Concurrent use of indacaterol plus tiotropium in patients with COPD provides superior bronchodilation compared with tiotropium alone: a randomised, double-blind comparison. *Thorax*. 2012;67:781-788.
3. Kew KM, Dias S, Cates CJ. Long-acting inhaled therapy (beta-agonists, anticholinergics and steroids) for COPD: a network meta-analysis. *Cochrane Database Syst Rev.* 2014;(3):CD010844.
4. Vogelmeier CF, Bateman ED, Pallante J, et al. Efficacy and safety of once-daily QVA149 compared with twice-daily salmeterol-fluticasone in patients with chronic obstructive pulmonary disease (ILLUMINATE): a randomised, double blind, parallel group study. *Lancet Respir Med.* 2013;1:51-60.

Combination Long-Acting β-Agonists and Inhaled Corticosteroids Compared With Long-Acting β-Agonists Alone in Older Adults With Chronic Obstructive Pulmonary Disease

Gershon AS, Campitelli MA, Croxford R, et al (Sunnybrook Health Sciences Centre, Toronto, Ontario, Canada; Inst for Clinical Evaluative Sciences, Toronto, Ontario, Canada; et al)
JAMA 312:1114-1121, 2014

Importance.—Chronic obstructive pulmonary disease (COPD), a manageable respiratory condition, is the third leading cause of death worldwide. Knowing which prescription medications are the most effective in improving health outcomes for people with COPD is essential to maximizing health outcomes.

Objective.—To estimate the long-term benefits of combination long-acting β-agonists (LABAs) and inhaled corticosteroids compared with LABAs alone in a real-world setting.

Design, Setting, and Patients.—Population-based, longitudinal cohort study conducted in Ontario, Canada, from 2003 to 2011. All individuals aged 66 years or older who met a validated case definition of COPD on the basis of health administrative data were included. After propensity score matching, there were 8712 new users of LABA-inhaled corticosteroid combination therapy and 3160 new users of LABAs alone who were followed up for median times of 2.7 years and 2.5 years, respectively.

Exposures.—Newly prescribed combination LABAs and inhaled corticosteroids or LABAs alone.

Main Outcomes and Measures.—Composite outcome of death and COPD hospitalization.

Results.—The main outcome was observed among 5594 new users of LABAs and inhaled corticosteroids (3174 deaths [36.4%]; 2420 COPD hospitalizations [27.8%]) and 2129 new users of LABAs alone (1179 deaths [37.3%]; 950 COPD hospitalizations [30.1%]). New use of LABAs and inhaled corticosteroids was associated with a modestly reduced risk of death or COPD hospitalization compared with new use of LABAs alone (difference in composite outcome at 5 years, −3.7%; 95% CI, −5.7% to −1.7%; hazard ratio [HR], 0.92; 95% CI, 0.88-0.96). The greatest difference was among COPD patients with a codiagnosis of asthma (difference in composite at 5 years, −6.5%; 95% CI, −10.3% to −2.7%; HR, 0.84; 95% CI, 0.77-0.91) and those who were not receiving inhaled long-acting anticholinergic medication (difference in composite at 5 years, −8.4%; 95% CI, −11.9% to −4.9%; HR, 0.79; 95% CI, 0.73-0.86).

Conclusions and Relevance.—Among older adults with COPD, particularly those with asthma and those not receiving a long-acting anticholinergic medication, newly prescribed LABA and inhaled corticosteroid combination therapy, compared with newly prescribed LABAs alone, was associated with a significantly lower risk of the composite outcome of death or COPD hospitalization.

▶ The authors of this study used provincial and national administrative databases to better understand the behavior of physicians in managing elderly patients with chronic obstructive pulmonary disease (COPD). They identified physician-diagnosed COPD in patients aged 66 or older in these databases and obtained pharmacy data on new prescriptions for long-acting beta agonists (LABAs) or LABAs plus inhaled corticosteroids (ICS). A recent systematic review of randomized controlled trials showed that patients treated with LABAs and ICS compared with those treated with LABAs only had fewer disease exacerbations but not fewer hospitalizations or lower mortality.[1] The population in some of the trials reviewed were younger as well and not comparable to the current authors' population, so whether these results can be generalized to the elderly is unclear. In addition, ICS drugs have been shown in multiple studies to increase the rate of pneumonia in users, a particular concern in the elderly who have high rates of community-acquired pneumonia, so the potential impact of this complication is much greater in older populations. In addition, in studying their population, the authors sought to represent the "real world," so they did not exclude patients with other diagnoses such as asthma (who would typically not be included in a COPD study). Asthma and COPD often overlap, especially in the elderly.

The primary outcome was a composite of all-cause mortality and COPD hospitalization. Over the 8-year period of the study of interest in the province, more than 38 000 patients with physician-diagnosed COPD received either a new LABA or LABA-ICS prescription; of those more than 34 000 received LABA-ICS prescriptions, about 10 times the number of new LABA prescriptions. Before propensity matching of the 2 groups, new users of LABAs were older, more likely to use other COPD medications, and more likely to have had a COPD hospitalization within 6 months before the date they entered the study. Before matching new LABA-ICS, users had a lower risk of death or COPD hospitalization compared with new LABA users. Thus, to place things on an equal field, propensity matching was done before the study initiation according to age, sex, codiagnosis of asthma, and COPD duration. Up to 3 LABA + ICS matches were allowed for each LABA-alone match. There are many potential pitfalls in using administrative data such as these. Perhaps in the case of a COPD, an unsubstantiated diagnosis may be put in the chart and carried for years when in fact the patient has a different diagnosis; however, that type of error should have occurred in both groups. As with most administrative studies, we would have more confidence in the findings if a subsequent prospective study confirmed the results. However, in the absence of that, LABA + ICS should not be withheld from patients because of age when the diagnosis and clinical setting are appropriate for their use.

J. R. Maurer, MD

Reference

1. Nannini LJ, Lasserson TJ, Poole P. Combined corticosteroid and long-acting beta(2)-agonist in one inhaler versus long-acting beta(2)-agonists for chronic obstructive pulmonary disease. *Cochrane Database Syst Rev.* 2012;(9):CD006829.

Withdrawal of Inhaled Glucocorticoids and Exacerbations of COPD

Magnussen H, for the WISDOM Investigators (German Ctr for Lung Res, Grosshansdorf, Germany; et al)
N Engl J Med 371:1285-1294, 2014

Background.—Treatment with inhaled glucocorticoids in combination with long-acting bronchodilators is recommended in patients with frequent exacerbations of severe chronic obstructive pulmonary disease (COPD). However, the benefit of inhaled glucocorticoids in addition to two long-acting bronchodilators has not been fully explored.

Methods.—In this 12-month, double-blind, parallel-group study, 2485 patients with a history of exacerbation of COPD received triple therapy consisting of tiotropium (at a dose of 18 μg once daily), salmeterol (50 μg twice daily), and the inhaled glucocorticoid fluticasone propionate (500 μg twice daily) during a 6-week run-in period. Patients were then randomly assigned to continued triple therapy or withdrawal of fluticasone in three steps over a 12-week period. The primary end point was the time to the first moderate or severe COPD exacerbation. Spirometric findings, health status, and dyspnea were also monitored.

Results.—As compared with continued glucocorticoid use, glucocorticoid withdrawal met the prespecified noninferiority criterion of 1.20 for the upper limit of the 95% confidence interval (CI) with respect to the first moderate or severe COPD exacerbation (hazard ratio, 1.06; 95% CI, 0.94 to 1.19). At week 18, when glucocorticoid withdrawal was complete, the adjusted mean reduction from baseline in the trough forced expiratory volume in 1 second was 38 ml greater in the glucocorticoid-withdrawal group than in the glucocorticoid-continuation group ($P<0.001$); a similar between-group difference (43 ml) was seen at week 52 ($P=0.001$). No change in dyspnea and minor changes in health status occurred in the glucocorticoid-withdrawal group.

Conclusions.—In patients with severe COPD receiving tiotropium plus salmeterol, the risk of moderate or severe exacerbations was similar among those who discontinued inhaled glucocorticoids and those who continued glucocorticoid therapy. However, there was a greater decrease in lung function during the final step of glucocorticoid withdrawal. (Funded by Boehringer Ingelheim Pharma; WISDOM ClinicalTrials.gov number, NCT00975195.)

▶ Recurrent exacerbations in patients with chronic obstructive pulmonary disease (COPD) decrease health-related quality of life and often result in a decline in lung function. Inhaled corticosteroids decrease the rate of exacerbations and are often used in patients with recurrent exacerbations. Because many of these patients also have severe or very severe airway obstruction, they are usually receiving multiple types of bronchodilator therapy as well, particularly long-acting beta-agonists (LABAs) and long-acting muscarinic antagonists (LAMAs). LAMAs have recently been shown to decrease the number of exacerbations as well. Inhaled corticosteroids are important drugs in the management of these very ill patients but have some annoying and serious side effects and some potential risks, including serious pneumonia.[1] Interestingly, as drugs for COPD come available, the approach is generally to add them to existing regimens, particularly in the more seriously ill patients. Magnusson et al reasoned that, because both inhaled corticosteroids and muscarinic antagonists have been shown to reduce exacerbations, maybe it is possible to use only bronchodilator therapy (LABAs + LAMAs) and get a therapeutic result equivalent to the use of all 3 drugs. They designed a robust, double-blinded prospective randomized trial to test this. In 1 arm, the standard doses of all 3 drugs were given, whereas in the other arm, standard doses of all 3 drugs were given initially. Then the dose of inhaled corticosteroids was gradually reduced to zero over a 12-week period. Patients were followed for 1 year, and the primary end point was first moderate or exacerbation. Serious adverse events, including pneumonia, cardiac events, stroke, and death, were similar in the 2 groups; however, the steroid withdrawal group had a significant decrease in lung function compared with the nonwithdrawal group (Fig 2 in the original article) and a worsening of health status that was assessed by the St George Respiratory Questionnaire and the modified Medical Research Council dyspnea scale. The changes were considered generally below the level of clinical significance. So what does all this mean? It seems that it is possible to remove inhaled steroids in patients with severe and very severe disease on double long-acting bronchodilator therapy without an increase in exacerbations. However, this is done at a cost of reduced lung function and worsened quality, which may not be clinically significant across a large study population but will be in some individual patients. Care providers can be fairly confident that in patients who have steroid-related complications or intolerance, who cannot afford steroids, or who want to reduce their medications, this change can be made without serious adverse events. However, decisions should be made in partnership with the patient and his or her preferences.

J. R. Maurer, MD

Reference

1. Suissa S, Patenaude V, Lapi F, Ernst P. Inhaled corticosteroids in COPD and the risk of serious pneumonia. *Thorax*. 2013;68:1029-1036.

Predictors of Chronic Obstructive Pulmonary Disease Exacerbation Reduction in Response to Daily Azithromycin Therapy

Han MK, Tayob N, Murray S, et al (Univ of Michigan Health System, Ann Arbor; et al)

Am J Respir Crit Care Med 189:1503-1508, 2014

Rationale.—Daily azithromycin decreases acute exacerbations of chronic obstructive pulmonary disease (AECOPD), but long-term side effects are unknown.

Objectives.—To identify the types of exacerbations most likely to be reduced and clinical subgroups most likely to benefit from azithromycin, 250 mg daily, added to usual care.

Methods.—Enrollment criteria included irreversible airflow limitation and AECOPD requiring corticosteroids, emergency department visit, or hospitalization in the prior year or use of supplemental oxygen. Recurrent events and cumulative incidence analyses compared treatment received for AECOPD by randomization group, stratified by subgroups of interest. Cox proportional hazards models estimated treatment effects in subgroups adjusted for age, sex, smoking status, FEV_1% predicted, concomitant COPD medications, and oxygen use.

Measurements and Main Results.—Azithromycin was most effective in reducing AECOPD requiring both antibiotic and steroid treatment (n = 1,113; cumulative incidence analysis, $P = 0.0002$; recurrent events analysis, $P = 0.002$). No difference in treatment response by sex ($P = 0.75$), presence of chronic bronchitis ($P = 0.19$), concomitant inhaled therapy ($P = 0.29$), or supplemental oxygen use ($P = 0.23$) was observed. Older age and milder Global Initiative for Chronic Obstructive Lung Disease stage were associated with better treatment response ($P = 0.02$ and 0.04, respectively). A significant interaction between treatment and current smoking was seen ($P = 0.03$) and azithromycin did not reduce exacerbations in current smokers (hazard ratio, 0.99; 95% confidence interval, 0.71–1.38; $P = 0.95$).

Conclusions.—Azithromycin is most effective in preventing AECOPD requiring both antibiotic and steroid treatment. Adjusting for confounders, we saw no difference in efficacy by sex, history of chronic bronchitis, oxygen use, or concomitant COPD therapy. Greater efficacy was seen in older patients and milder Global Initiative for Chronic Obstructive Lung Disease stages. We found little evidence of treatment effect among current smokers. Clinical trial registered with www.clinicaltrials.gov (NCT0011986 and NCT00325897).

▶ The COPD Clinical Research Network reported in 2011 that azithromycin used daily for a year significantly reduced the number of acute exacerbations of chronic obstructive pulmonary disease (COPD) in at-risk patients.[1] However, that report also included a significant downside. There was a significant risk of hearing loss and also colonization of the nasopharynx with azithromycin-resistant organisms. Thus, because azithromycin is not an entirely benign approach to reduction of exacerbations and adds significant cost to maintenance therapy, the investigators reanalyzed the data to determine whether there were specific patient demographics/characteristics or specific types of exacerbations that benefited more from azithromycin use. Identifying such subgroups might allow a more targeted approach to azithromycin prophylaxis. This reanalysis yielded the following information: (1) azithromycin appeared most effective in preventing the most severe exacerbations, (2) it seemed more useful in older patients and milder disease, and (3) it did not appear to have a significant impact in smokers. The only real guidance this reanalysis gives in deciding which patients might not benefit from azithromycin and should therefore probably be offered the drug with caution given its significant side effects—that is, current smokers. A retrospective secondary analysis is always fraught with potential bias, and therefore the relative benefits of azithromycin in different patients needs to be studied prospectively. Currently, the ongoing prospective studies are addressing intermittent dosing as a means of reducing side effects and may be able to identify as well the most appropriate groups for treatment. However, the study we need should predefine subgroups of patients, possibly using those identified in this analysis, and prospectively study them to determine the positive impact vs the potential harm of azithromycin.

J. R. Maurer, MD

Reference

1. Albert RK, Connett J, Bailey WC, et al; COPD Clinical Research Network. Azithromycin for prevention of exacerbations of COPD. *N Engl J Med.* 2011;365: 689-698.

Benefits of High-Dose N-Acetylcysteine to Exacerbation-Prone Patients With COPD

Tse HN, Raiteri L, Wong KY, et al (Kwong Wah Hosp, Hong Kong, SAR; Innovation & Med Sciences, Vicenza, Italy; Wong Tai Sin Hosp, Hong Kong)
Chest 146:611-623, 2014

Background.—Although high-dose N-acetylcysteine (NAC) has been suggested to reduce COPD exacerbations, it is unclear which category of patients with COPD would benefit most from NAC treatment. The objective of this study was to compare the effect of high-dose NAC (600 mg bid) between high-risk and low-risk Chinese patients with COPD.

Methods.—Patients with spirometry-confirmed stable COPD were randomized to treatment with either NAC 600 mg bid or placebo in addition to their usual treatments. Patients were followed up every 16 weeks for a total of 1 year. Further analysis was performed according to each patient's exacerbation risk at baseline as defined by the current GOLD (Global Initiative for Chronic Obstructive Lung Disease) strategy to analyze the effect of high-dose NAC in high-risk and low-risk patients.

Results.—Of the 120 patients with COPD randomized (men, 93.2%; mean age, 70.8 ± 0.74 years; prebronchodilator FEV_1, 53.9 ± 2.0%; baseline characteristics comparable between treatment groups), 108 (NAC, 52; placebo, 56) completed the 1-year study. For high-risk patients (n = 89), high-dose NAC compared with placebo significantly reduced exacerbation frequency (0.85 vs 1.59 [*P* = .019] and 1.08 vs 2.22 [*P* = .04] at 8 and 12 months, respectively), prolonged time to first exacerbation (*P* = .02), and increased the probability of being exacerbation free at 1 year (51.3% vs 24.4%, *P* = .013). This beneficial effect of high-dose NAC vs placebo was not significant in low-risk patients.

Conclusions.—High-dose NAC (600 mg bid) for 1 year reduces exacerbations and prolongs time to first exacerbation in high-risk but not in low-risk Chinese patients with COPD.

Trial Registry.—ClinicalTrials.gov; No.: NCT01136239; URL: www.clinicaltrials.gov.

► N-Acetylcysteine (NAC) is an old drug that has had many lives. It has long been used as a mucolytic with varied results in pulmonary patients, particularly those with high sputum production. It has been an important hepatocyte protector in acute acetaminophen and other hepatic poisoning, has been used to protect kidney function when iodine-contrast is used for imaging, and was briefly the drug of choice in the treatment of idiopathic pulmonary fibrosis. In countries outside the United States, NAC is used much more commonly for chronic obstructive pulmonary disease (COPD), and a number of studies have suggested it may be effective in reducing the number of acute exacerbations. Several Cochrane Reviews have been done on this topic, but the latest one in 2012 concluded that newer evidence may suggest less impact on exacerbation frequency than previously thought.[1] NAC has anti-inflammatory and antioxidant properties and theoretically may be of benefit both as a mucolytic and anti-inflammatory. The authors suggest that one reason for previous studies showing mixed results in decreasing numbers of exacerbations is that too low a dose of NAC was used.[2] The current report is actually a post-hoc analysis of a study completed and reported by the authors in 2013.[3] In that study, they showed some reduction in exacerbation rate. This study reanalyzes that data and states the reduction in exacerbation rate according to severity of disease. The results show that the bulk of impact of high dose NAC was in the more severe patients. NAC is a low side effect, inexpensive drug. It would be useful to have such a drug in the armamentarium of drugs for COPD if, in fact, it works. More study with high dosing in ethnically diverse populations is warranted.

J. R. Maurer, MD

References

1. Poole P, Black PN, Cates CJ. Mucolytic agents for chronic bronchitis or chronic obstructive pulmonary disease. *Cochrane Database Syst Rev.* 2012;(8):CD00128.
2. Decramer M, Rutten-van Molken M, Dekhuijzen PN, et al. Effects of N-acetylcysteine on outcomes in chronic obstructive pulmonary disease (Bronchitis Randomized on NAC Cost-Utility Study, BRONCUS): a randomized placebo-controlled trial. *Lancet.* 2005;365:1552-1560.
3. Tse HN, Raiteri L, Wong KY, et al. High dose N-acetylcysteine in stable COPD: the 1-year, double-blind, randomized, placebo-controlled HIACE study. *Chest.* 2013;144:106-118.

Breathlessness, Functional Status, Distress, and Palliative Care Needs Over Time in Patients With Advanced Chronic Obstructive Pulmonary Disease or Lung Cancer: A Cohort Study

Weingaertner V, on behalf of the PAALiativ Project (Univ Hosp of Cologne, Germany)

J Pain Symptom Manage 48:569-581, 2014

Context.—Breathlessness is a distressing symptom in advanced disease. Understanding its patterns, burden, and palliative care (PC) needs over time is important to improve patients' quality of life.

Objectives.—To describe and compare the courses of refractory breathlessness, functional status, distress, and PC needs in patients with advanced chronic obstructive pulmonary disease (COPD) or lung cancer (LC) over time.

Methods.—This was a cohort study of patients with COPD (Stage III/IV) or LC. Data were assessed monthly with up to 12 telephone interviews, using the modified Borg Scale, Karnofsky Performance Status Scale,

Distress Thermometer, and Palliative care Outcome Scale as outcomes measures. Descriptive analysis compared all outcomes between COPD and LC at baseline and over time (forward from study entry and backward from death).

Results.—A total of 82 patients (50 COPD and 32 LC), mean (SD) age of 67.2 (7.8), and 36% female were included (8 COPD and 23 LC deceased). The patients with COPD perceived higher levels of breathlessness and distress at lower functional status steadily over time. The LC patients' breathlessness, distress, and PC needs increased, whereas functional status decreased toward death. The PC needs were similar between disease groups. Breathlessness was negatively correlated with functional status (COPD = mean $r = -0.20$, $P = 0.012$; LC = mean $r = -0.277$, $P = 0.029$) and positively correlated with PC needs in COPD patients (mean $r = 0.343$, $P < 0.001$). Death was significantly predicted by diagnosis (LC: hazard ratio =7.84, $P < 0.001$) and functional status (10% decline: hazard ratio =1.52, $P = 0.001$).

Conclusion.—The PC needs of patients with advanced COPD are comparable with LC patients, and breathlessness severity and distress are even higher. The care for COPD patients requires further improvement to address symptom burden and PC needs.

▶ In 2008, the American Thoracic Society clinical policy statement recognizing the need for more formalized palliative care for end-stage lung disease and critical care patients more or less gave permission for a different, but proactive, approach to the management of progressive, advanced disease. The problem was that, because palliative care was so rarely offered to end-stage lung disease patients, other than cancer patients, there were no guidelines or care pathways available for management. We are beginning to see a series of studies that assess the disease burden of end-stage pulmonary patients, the level of need, and in what areas and formulation of appropriate palliative care plans. Weingaertner and her colleagues prospectively followed 2 cohorts of patients, 1 with chronic obstructive pulmonary disorder (COPD) and the other with lung cancer. Needs were similar except that the level of dyspnea in COPD patients was more severe, created more distress and more functional impairment, and was present throughout the palliative care period. In lung cancer patients, the dyspnea was initially less and increased as the patient approached death. Unfortunately, adequate tools or approaches for managing this dyspnea are not available in many palliative care regimens, which tend to be focused on pain control. Schroedl et al conducted interviews with patients admitted to hospital with acute exacerbations of COPD to help determine their unmet healthcare needs, including preparation for end of life. The major findings were 1) only half understood the severity of their disease, 2) breathlessness was universal and severe, 3) they were unable to participate in desired activities, 4) most had depression and/or anxiety, 5) most were socially limited and felt confined to their homes, and 6) half expressed a fear of the future.[1] This study concluded that the many unmet needs might best be handled by integrating specialist palliative care into the COPD care model. The attention being paid to this long-neglected area is overdue, but necessary and welcome. Chronic lung disease is, after all, the fourth most common cause of death in our country.

J. R. Maurer, MD

Reference

1. Schroedl CJ, Yountz SE, Szmuilowicz E, Hutchison PJ, Rosenberg SR, Kalhan R. A qualitative study of unmet healthcare needs in chronic obstructive pulmonary disease: a potential role for specialist palliative care? *Ann Am Thorac Soc.* 2014;11:1433-1438.

3 Lung Cancer

Introduction

Lung cancer is the leading cause of cancer death around the world. In 2014, 72 330 women and 86 930 men died from lung cancer in the United States.[1] While death rates in men have been falling over the past 15 years and in women appear finally to be stabilizing, more people in the United States die from lung cancer annually than from breast, colorectal, and prostate cancers combined. Lung cancer overall 5-year survival at present is 18%, which, while creeping in the right direction, continues to be dismal in comparison to these other common solid tumors.[1]

The observed improvements in death rates from lung cancer are largely attributed to reductions in tobacco use. While other lung cancer risks are well described, more than 90% of lung cancer is felt to be attributable to smoking.[1-4] Unfortunately, with approximately 19% of the adult population in the United States still habitually smoking, lung cancer as well as all the other smoking-related diseases, notably cardiovascular disease, cerebrovascular disease, and chronic obstructive pulmonary disease, will continue to be prevalent and deadly for the foreseeable future. Smoking invokes an enormous morbidity; based on National Health Interview Survey (NHIS) and National Health and Nutrition Examination Survey (NHANES) data, Rostron and colleagues estimate that 14 million persons in the United States had at least 1 serious smoking-induced illness in 2009.[4] Jha and Peto outline 3 simple and vital messages to give to smokers: 1) The risk is big, and there is a lot to lose. 2) The loss is worse for those who die in middle age (so quit early!). 3) Quitting will help you live longer.[5]

Reductions in death rates for breast, colorectal, and prostate cancers are largely attributed to early detection and advances in treatment. Though controversy continues to be generated about screening and early detection for these cancers, screening is nonetheless widely accepted and practiced in the broad medical community.[6] In 2014, the discussion has shifted away from *whether* we should be doing lung cancer screening with low-dose CT scanning (LDCT) to *how to implement* cost-effective screening in our communities.[7,8] The United States Preventive Services Task Force (USPSTF), American Cancer Society (ACS), American College of Chest Physicians (ACCP), American Thoracic Society (ATS), American Association for Thoracic Surgery (AATS), National Comprehensive Cancer Network (NCCN), and American Society for Clinical Oncology (ASCO) all have issued guidelines or statements endorsing lung cancer screening with LDCT.[6,8-11] There is agreement among all of these societies and institutions that screening should be offered to patients who meet the criteria of the NLST: ages 55-74, with a 30 pack-year smoking history, either currently smoking or having quit within the prior 15 years.[12] However, there continues to be debate about screening in patients who do not meet these criteria, particularly in patients whose risk can be estimated to be equivalent or higher to the study population of NLST, as there is no evidence base demonstrating that screening in these individuals will result in a reduction in lung cancer mortality.[10,11,13-16] Several useful reviews are available this year to guide physicians through the process of developing and implementing comprehensive programs for lung cancer screening, with an emphasis on "program," as screening for lung cancer involves much more than a simple LDCT.[8,15,16] The current statement on lung cancer screening from the Centers for Medicare and Medicaid Services (CMS) recommends establishing metrics of performance. A policy statement from ACCP and ATS recommends the first of such metrics, including 1) screening should be targeted to a population matching that of the National Lung Screening Trial (NLST) and 2) reading of LDCT must be done using a structured, algorithmic approach.[8] Given the potential risks to individual patients of false positive results and the consequences thereof, and the potential enormous cost of screening to the nation, evaluation of quality metrics of lung cancer screening as it is generalized to the broad community will be necessary and important.

As lung cancer screening is incorporated into practice, the perennial challenge of the evaluation of pulmonary nodules will be amplified because of the sheer numbers of nodules that will inevitably be found. This area of pulmonary medicine has become even more complex for several reasons. 1) Most of the nodules identified by screening are NOT cancers, and so we need evaluative tools, both invasive and noninvasive, to minimize unnecessary potentially harmful and costly evaluation.[17,18] 2) We have a growing appreciation that nodule density may reflect biologic behavior, but we don't have any reliable means for measuring either density or behavior. 3) There is not uniform agreement on what nodule size should be used to define "abnormal," and moreover there is not uniform agreement on even how to measure nodule size.[19,20] 4) New tools, including nodule volume measurement, are becoming available, but we do not as yet know how to incorporate this information into clinical management.[21] The management of small, early stage cancers is also receiving needed attention, as lung-sparing surgical approaches may be a reasonable alternative in some patients.[22,23]

Screening may eventually shift the distribution of lung cancer stage toward early disease, but the burden of disease now and for the near future will remain at advanced stages. The encouraging news is that we continue to see steady advances in treatment options for patients with Stage III and IV lung NSCLC. It is increasingly recognized that many, and in fact the majority, of adenocarcinomas of the lung have oncogenic driver mutations that may be potentially targetable.[24] Molecular testing should be part of standard evaluation in patients with advanced lung adenocarcinoma, as identification of mutations in the epidermal growth factor receptor (*EGFR*) gene and rearrangements in the anaplastic lymphoma kinase (*ALK*) gene may substantively change the first-line approach from standard chemotherapy to targeted therapies.[25-27]

Lung cancer as a field is experiencing exciting times. Screening is on the brink of dissemination to the community, new diagnostic tools are being incorporated into practice, and scientific discoveries are being translated to treatment. Though the burden of disease is enormous and mortality still much too high, applications of new knowledge are finally beginning to result in measurable improvements in outcomes. There is still a long road ahead, but compared to a decade ago, the future appears much more hopeful.

Lynn T. Tanoue, MD

References

1. Siegel R, Ma J, Zou Z, Jemal A. Cancer statistics, 2014. *CA Cancer J Clin.* 2014; 64:9-29.
2. Denholm R, Schuz J, Straif K, et al. Is previous respiratory disease a risk factor for lung cancer? *Am J Respir Crit Care Med.* 2014;190:549-559.
3. McCunney RJ, Li J. Radiation risks in lung cancer screening programs: a comparison with nuclear industry workers and atomic bomb survivors. *Chest.* 2014;145: 618-624.
4. Rostron BL, Chang CM, Pechacek TF. Estimation of cigarette smoking-attributable morbidity in the United States. *JAMA Intern Med.* 2014;174:1922-1928.
5. Jha P, Peto R. Global effects of smoking, of quitting, and of taxing tobacco. *N Engl J Med.* 2014;370:60-68.
6. Smith RA, Manassaram-Baptiste D, Brooks D, et al. Cancer screening in the United States, 2014: a review of current American Cancer Society guidelines and current issues in cancer screening. *CA Cancer J Clin.* 2014;64:30-51.
7. Black WC, Gareen IF, Soneji SS, et al. Cost-effectiveness of CT screening in the National Lung Screening Trial. *N Engl J Med.* 2014;371:1793-1802.
8. Mazzone P, Powell CA, Arenberg D, et al. Components necessary for high quality lung cancer screening: American College of Chest Physicians and American Thoracic Society Policy Statement. *Chest.* 2015;147:295-303.
9. Moyer VA. Screening for lung cancer: U.S. Preventive Services Task Force Recommendation Statement. *Ann Intern Med.* 2014;160:330-338.
10. NCCN Clinical Practice Guidelines in Oncology: Non-small Cell Lung Cancer. http://nccn.org. Accessed October 14, 2009.
11. Jaklitsch MT, Jacobson FL, Austin JH, et al. The American Association for Thoracic Surgery guidelines for lung cancer screening using low-dose computed tomography scans for lung cancer survivors and other high-risk groups. *J Thorac Cardiovasc Surg.* 2012;144:33-38.
12. Aberle DR, Adams AM, Berg CD, et al. Reduced lung-cancer mortality with low-dose computed tomographic screening. *N Engl J Med.* 2011;365:395-409.
13. Ollier M, Chamoux A, Naughton G, Pereira B, Dutheil F. Chest CT scan screening for lung cancer in asbestos occupational exposure: a systematic review and meta-analysis. *Chest.* 2014;145:1339-1346.
14. Tammemagi MC, Katki HA, Hocking WG, et al. Selection criteria for lung-cancer screening. *N Engl J Med.* 2013;368:728-736.
15. Tanoue LT, Tanner NT, Gould MK, Silvestri GA. Lung cancer screening. *Am J Respir Crit Care Med.* 2015;191:19-33.

16. Gould MK. Clinical practice. Lung-cancer screening with low-dose computed tomography. *N Engl J Med.* 2014;371:1813-1820.
17. Kinsey CM, Arenberg DA. Endobronchial ultrasound-guided transbronchial needle aspiration for non-small cell lung cancer staging. *Am J Respir Crit Care Med.* 2014;189:640-649.
18. Deppen SA, Blume JD, Kensinger CD, et al. Accuracy of FDG-PET to diagnose lung cancer in areas with infectious lung disease: a meta-analysis. *JAMA.* 2014;312:1227-1236.
19. Yip R, Henschke CI, Yankelevitz DF, Smith JP. CT screening for lung cancer: alternative definitions of positive test result based on the national lung screening trial and international early lung cancer action program databases. *Radiology.* 2014;273:591-596.
20. Henschke CI, Yip R, Yankelevitz DF, Smith JP, International Early Lung Cancer Action Program I. Definition of a positive test result in computed tomography screening for lung cancer: a cohort study. *Ann Intern Med.* 2013;158:246-252.
21. Mehta HJ, Ravenel JG, Shaftman SR, et al. The utility of nodule volume in the context of malignancy prediction for small pulmonary nodules. *Chest.* 2014; 145:464-472.
22. Altorki NK, Yip R, Hanaoka T, et al. Sublobar resection is equivalent to lobectomy for clinical stage 1A lung cancer in solid nodules. *J Thorac Cardiovasc Surg.* 2014;147:754-762.
23. Tsutani Y, Miyata Y, Nakayama H, et al. Appropriate sublobar resection choice for ground glass opacity-dominant clinical stage IA lung adenocarcinoma: wedge resection or segmentectomy. *Chest.* 2014;145:66-71.
24. Kris MG, Johnson BE, Berry LD, et al. Using multiplexed assays of oncogenic drivers in lung cancers to select targeted drugs. *JAMA.* 2014;311:1998-2006.
25. Leighl NB, Rekhtman N, Biermann WA, et al. Molecular testing for selection of patients with lung cancer for epidermal growth factor receptor and anaplastic lymphoma kinase tyrosine kinase inhibitors: American Society of Clinical Oncology endorsement of the College of American Pathologists/International Association for the study of lung cancer/association for molecular pathology guideline. *J Clin Oncol.* 2014;32:3673-3679.
26. Lindeman NI, Cagle PT, Beasley MB, et al. Molecular testing guideline for selection of lung cancer patients for EGFR and ALK tyrosine kinase inhibitors: guideline from the College of American Pathologists, International Association for the Study of Lung Cancer, and Association for Molecular Pathology. *J Mol Diagn.* 2013;15:415-453.
27. Solomon BJ, Mok T, Kim DW, et al. First-line crizotinib versus chemotherapy in ALK-positive lung cancer. *N Engl J Med.* 2014;371:2167-2177.

Epidemiology of Lung Cancer

Cancer Statistics, 2014

Siegel R, Ma J, Zou Z, et al (American Cancer Society, Atlanta, GA; Information Management Services, Inc, Silver Spring, MD; et al)

CA Cancer J Clin 64:9-29, 2014

Each year, the American Cancer Society estimates the numbers of new cancer cases and deaths that will occur in the United States in the current year and compiles the most recent data on cancer incidence, mortality, and survival. Incidence data were collected by the National Cancer Institute, the Centers for Disease Control and Prevention, and the North American Association of Central Cancer Registries and mortality data were

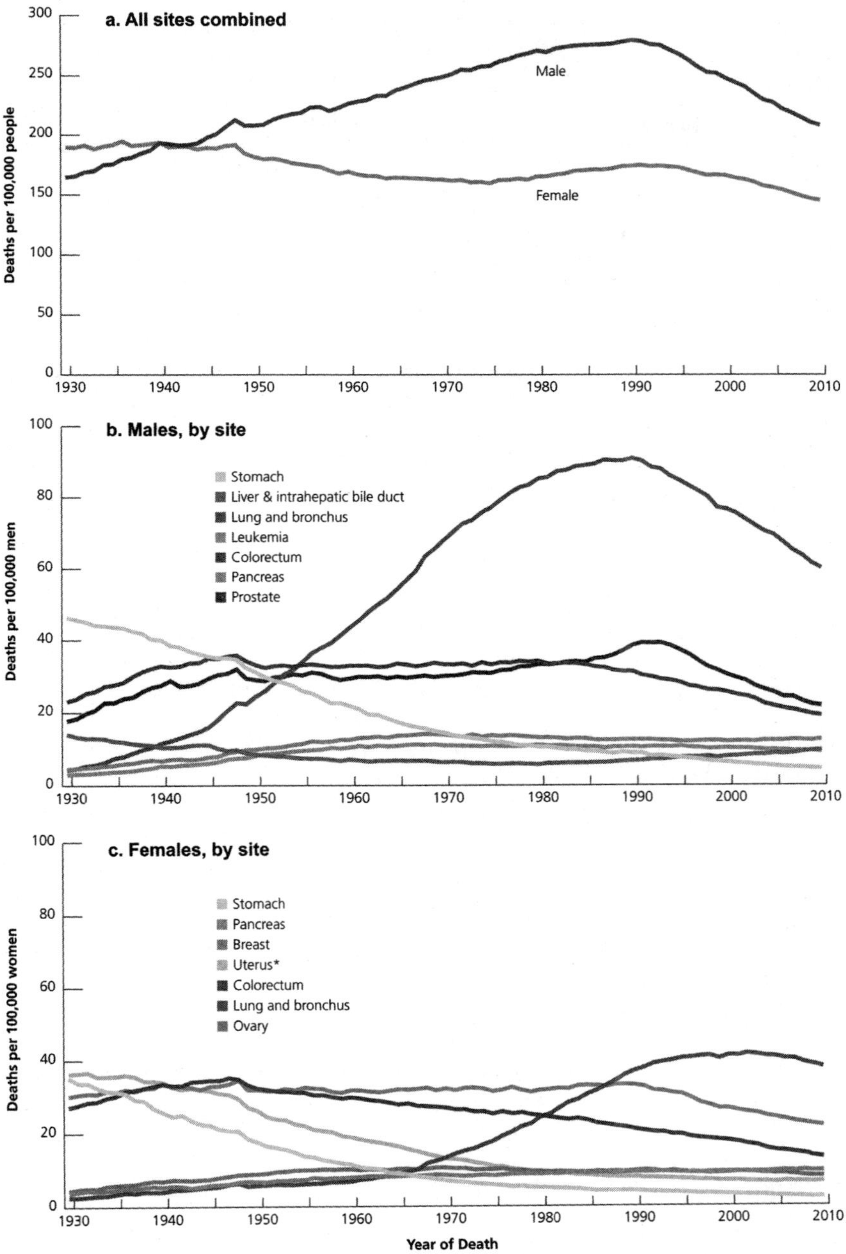

FIGURE 6.—Trends in Death Rates Overall and for Selected Sites by Sex, United States, 1930 to 2010. Rates are age adjusted to the 2000 US standard population. Due to changes in International Classification of Diseases (ICD) coding, numerator information has changed over time. Rates for cancers of the lung and bronchus, colorectum, liver, uterus, and ovary are affected by these changes. *Uterus includes uterine cervix and uterine corpus. (Reprinted from Siegel R, Ma J, Zou Z, et al. Cancer statistics, 2014. *CA Cancer J Clin*. 2014;64:9-29, with permission from CA: A Cancer Journal for Clinicians and John Wiley and Sons, www.interscience.wiley.com.)

collected by the National Center for Health Statistics. A total of 1,665,540 new cancer cases and 585,720 cancer deaths are projected to occur in the United States in 2014. During the most recent 5 years for which there are data (2006-2010), delay-adjusted cancer incidence rates declined slightly in men (by 0.6% per year) and were stable in women, while cancer death rates decreased by 1.8% per year in men and by 1.4% per year in women. The combined cancer death rate (deaths per 100,000 population) has been continuously declining for 2 decades, from a peak of 215.1 in 1991 to 171.8 in 2010. This 20% decline translates to the avoidance of approximately 1,340,400 cancer deaths (952,700 among men and 387,700 among women) during this time period. The magnitude of the decline in cancer death rates from 1991 to 2010 varies substantially by age, race, and sex, ranging from no decline among white women aged 80 years and older to a 55% decline among black men aged 40 years to 49 years. Notably, black men experienced the largest drop within every 10-year age group. Further progress can be accelerated by applying existing cancer control knowledge across all segments of the population (Fig 6).

▶ As has unfortunately been the case for several decades, lung cancer was the leading cause of cancer death in both men and women in the United States in 2014. Although more new cases of breast cancers in women and more new cases of prostate cancer in men were diagnosed, more people of both sexes died from lung cancer this year than from breast, prostate, and colorectal cancers combined. In 2014, lung cancer claimed an estimated 159 260 American lives—86 930 men and 72 330 women. Fig 6 demonstrates trends in death rates overall and for selected sites for men and women in the United States from 1930 to 2010. The total number of overall deaths has been decreasing steadily over the past 20 years (Fig 6, top panel), a substantial portion of which is the result of the steady decrease in lung cancer deaths in men (Fig 6, middle panel). In women, the lung cancer death rate does seem finally to be decreasing slightly (Fig 6, bottom panel). Notably, death rates for the 4 leading causes of cancer death—lung, breast, prostate, and colorectal—are now all declining. Although the reductions in lung cancer death rates among both men and women are largely due to reduction in tobacco use, reductions in death rates for breast, prostate, and colorectal cancers are generally attributed to early detection and treatment advances.[1-4] It will be interesting over the coming years to observe the impact of lung cancer screening on lung cancer incidence and death rates as screening is introduced into medical practice.[5]

L. T. Tanoue, MD

References

1. Jemal A, Thun MJ, Ries LA, et al. Annual report to the nation on the status of cancer, 1975–2005, featuring trends in lung cancer, tobacco use, and tobacco control. *J Natl Cancer Inst.* 2008;100:1672-1694.
2. Berry DA, Cronin KA, Plevritis SK, et al. Effect of screening and adjuvant therapy on mortality from breast cancer. *N Engl J Med.* 2005;353:1784-1792.
3. Etzioni R, Tsodikov A, Mariotto A, et al. Quantifying the role of PSA screening in the US prostate cancer mortality decline. *Cancer Causes Control.* 2008;19:175-181.

4. Edwards BK, Ward E, Kohler BA, et al. Annual report to the nation on the status of cancer, 1975–2006, featuring colorectal cancer trends and impact of interventions (risk factors, screening, and treatment) to reduce future rates. *Cancer.* 2010; 116:544-573.
5. Moyer VA. Screening for Lung Cancer: U.S. Preventive Services Task Force Recommendation Statement. *Ann Intern Med.* 2014;160:330-338.

Is Previous Respiratory Disease a Risk Factor for Lung Cancer?

Denholm R, Schüz J, Straif K, et al (International Agency for Res on Cancer, Lyon, France; et al)

Am J Respir Crit Care Med 190:549-559, 2014

Rationale.—Previous respiratory diseases have been associated with increased risk of lung cancer. Respiratory conditions often co-occur and few studies have investigated multiple conditions simultaneously.

Objectives.—Investigate lung cancer risk associated with chronic bronchitis, emphysema, tuberculosis, pneumonia, and asthma.

Methods.—The SYNERGY project pooled information on previous respiratory diseases from 12,739 case subjects and 14,945 control subjects from 7 case–control studies conducted in Europe and Canada. Multivariate logistic regression models were used to investigate the relationship between individual diseases adjusting for co-occurring conditions, and patterns of respiratory disease diagnoses and lung cancer. Analyses were stratified by sex, and adjusted for age, center, ever-employed in a high-risk occupation, education, smoking status, cigarette pack-years, and time since quitting smoking.

Measurements and Main Results.—Chronic bronchitis and emphysema were positively associated with lung cancer, after accounting for other respiratory diseases and smoking (e.g., in men: odds ratio [OR], 1.33; 95% confidence interval [CI], 1.20–1.48 and OR, 1.50; 95% CI, 1.21–1.87, respectively). A positive relationship was observed between lung cancer and pneumonia diagnosed 2 years or less before lung cancer (OR, 3.31; 95% CI, 2.33–4.70 for men), but not longer. Co-occurrence of chronic bronchitis and emphysema and/or pneumonia had a stronger positive association with lung cancer than chronic bronchitis "only." Asthma had an inverse association with lung cancer, the association being stronger with an asthma diagnosis 5 years or more before lung cancer compared with shorter.

Conclusions.—Findings from this large international case–control consortium indicate that after accounting for co-occurring respiratory diseases, chronic bronchitis and emphysema continue to have a positive association with lung cancer.

▶ This is a report from the SYNERGY project, which is a consortium of international lung cancer case-control studies that collected information on occupational and smoking histories. Thirteen of the participating SYNERGY centers also collected information on self-reported previous respiratory disease, including chronic bronchitis, emphysema, tuberculosis, pneumonia, and asthma. The study population included 12 739 case subjects and 14 945 controls. Of the respiratory diseases studied, emphysema had the strongest association with lung cancer. Pneumonia had a positive association, with the relationship being stronger if pneumonia were diagnosed less than 2 years before the lung cancer diagnosis. No association was observed between tuberculosis and lung cancer. For men, chronic bronchitis, emphysema, and pneumonia were associated with an increased risk of lung cancer, compared with persons with no previous respiratory diagnoses. For women, emphysema and pneumonia were associated with increased lung cancer risk.

One of the main points of this report is the observation that co-occurrence of chronic bronchitis, emphysema, and/or pneumonia was common. The presence of more than 1 of these diseases resulted in a stronger association with lung cancer than each individually. Co-occurrence of more than one respiratory disease was observed in 50% to 83% of cases and 40% to 83% of controls. Although previous respiratory disease is not at present a criterion for lung cancer screening, the identification of groups at higher risk may influence surveillance in the future.

L. T. Tanoue, MD

Radiation Risks in Lung Cancer Screening Programs: A Comparison With Nuclear Industry Workers and Atomic Bomb Survivors

McCunney RJ, Li J (Massachusetts Inst of Technology, Cambridge)
Chest 145:618-624, 2014

The National Lung Cancer Screening Trial (NLST) demonstrated that screening with low-dose CT (LDCT) scan reduced lung cancer and overall mortality by 20% and 7%, respectively. The LDCT scanning involves an approximate 2-mSv dose, whereas full-chest CT scanning, the major diagnostic study used to follow up nodules, may involve a dose of 8 mSv. Radiation associated with CT scanning and other diagnostic studies to follow up nodules may present an independent risk of lung cancer. On the basis of the NLST, we estimated the incidence and prevalence of nodules detected in screening programs. We followed the Fleischner guidelines for follow-up of nodules to assess cumulative radiation exposure over 20- and 30-year periods. We then evaluated nuclear worker cohort studies and atomic bomb survivor studies to assess the risk of lung cancer from radiation associated with long-term lung cancer screening programs. The findings indicate that a 55-year-old lung screening participant may experience a cumulative radiation exposure of up to 280 mSv over a 20-year period and 420 mSv over 30 years. These exposures exceed those of nuclear workers and atomic bomb survivors. This assessment suggests that long-term (20-30 years) LDCT screening programs are associated with nontrivial cumulative radiation doses. Current lung cancer screening protocols, if conducted over 20- to 30-year periods, can independently increase the risk of lung cancer beyond cigarette smoking as a result of cumulative radiation exposure. Radiation exposures from LDCT screening

and follow-up diagnostic procedures exceed lifetime radiation exposures among nuclear power workers and atomic bomb survivors.

▶ Exposure to diagnostic radiation is one of the potential harms of lung cancer screening with low-dose computed tomography (LDCT) scanning. The consensus opinion of the National Academy of Science Committee to Assess the Biological Effects of Ionizing Radiation (BEIR VII) is that radiation exposure is cumulative over a lifetime and that the relation between radiation exposure and resulting health effects is linear with no threshold.[1] The expected effective radiation dose of a single LDCT is in the range of 1.5 to 2.0 mSv, compared with an average of 8 mSv for a single regular dose chest computed tomography (CT) scan.[2] In the National Lung Screening Trial (NLST), participants received an average radiation exposure of 8 mSv over 3 years of screening.[3]

Although the benefit from reduction in lung cancer mortality should outweigh potential harm from radiation in patients meeting NLST criteria, the balance of benefit and harm might be adversely affected in younger patients who could potentially receive more cumulative radiation over many years of screening. McCunney and Li estimated the potential worst-case scenarios for cumulative radiation exposure of a 55-year-old lung cancer screening participant, who was screened over the course of 20 to 30 years and who had a new small (false-positive) nodule detected every 2 to 4 years that required radiographic monitoring. This scenario is not hard to imagine, given the high rate of new nodule identification in the screening population. They assumed that full-dose CT scans would be required for follow-up monitoring of such nodules. Table 2 in the original article demonstrates the estimated radiation exposure from screening and follow-up CT scans over the projected duration of screening. Total radiation exposure ranged from 160 to 420 mSv. This exceeds the radiation exposure experienced by atomic bomb survivors, as well as occupational standards for nuclear industry workers.

We know the potential exists for carcinogenic effects of diagnostic radiation. Bach and colleagues estimate that approximately 1 radiation-associated cancer death will result per 2500 persons screened.[3] The concerning cumulative radiation exposure projected by McCunney and Li does not take into consideration current practice that LDCT can reasonably be used in place of full-dose CT for follow-up of screening-detected lung nodules or that technology to substantively decrease the amount of radiation incurred for imaging studies is already available. Further, in this study, a nodule size of > 4 mm was deemed abnormal; that threshold is being reconsidered by the screening community.[4-7] With these changes, adherence to standardized algorithmic nodule evaluation, and careful consideration of how nodule size and density influence intensity of follow-up, the number of follow-up imaging studies should be minimized. Nonetheless, the concerns raised by this analysis are real, thought provoking, and highlight the importance of performing both screening and nodule evaluation rigorously and efficiently.

L. T. Tanoue, MD

References

1. National Research Council, ed. Health Risks from Exposure to Low Levels of Ionizing Radiation, BEIR VII. Washington, DC: National Academy Press; 2005.
2. Smith-Bindman R, Lipson J, Marcus R, et al. Radiation dose associated with common computed tomography examinations and the associated lifetime attributable risk of cancer. *Arch Intern Med.* 2009;169:2078-2086.
3. Bach PB, Mirkin JN, Oliver TK, et al. Benefits and harms of CT screening for lung cancer: a systematic review. *JAMA.* 2012;307:2418-2429.
4. Mazzone P, Powell CA, Arenberg D, et al. Components necessary for high quality lung cancer screening: American College of Chest Physicians and American Thoracic Society Policy Statement. *Chest.* 2015;147:295-303.
5. Henschke CI, Yip R, Yankelevitz DF, Smith JP, International Early Lung Cancer Action Program Investigators. Definition of a positive test result in computed tomography screening for lung cancer: a cohort study. *Ann Intern Med.* 2013; 158:246-252.
6. Lung-RADS Version 1.0 Assessment Categories Release date: April 28, 2014. American College of Radiology. 2014. http://www.acr.org/~/media/ACR/Documents/PDF/QualitySafety/Resources/LungRADS/AssessmentCategories.pdf. Accessed March 9, 2015.
7. Naidich DP, Bankier AA, MacMahon H, et al. Recommendations for the management of subsolid pulmonary nodules detected at CT: a statement from the Fleischner Society. *Radiology.* 2013;266:304-317.

Tobacco-related Issues

Global Effects of Smoking, of Quitting, and of Taxing Tobacco

Jha P, Peto R (Univ of Toronto, Ontario, Canada; Univ of Oxford, UK)
N Engl J Med 370:60-68, 2014

Background.—If current global smoking patterns continue, about 50% of all the young men and 10% of all the young women now living will become smokers and few will stop. As a result the annual number of deaths attributable to tobacco will increase from about 5 million in 2010 to over 10 million in a few decades. Tobacco will be associated with about 1 billion deaths in this century, mostly in low- and middle-income countries and half before these individuals reach age 70 years. The 2013 World Health Assembly issued a call to governments to reduce the prevalence of smoking by a third by 2015 and thereby avoid over 200 million deaths from tobacco. Such a reduction could be achieved if the inflation-adjusted price of cigarettes doubled, since price is a key factor in the initiation and cessation of smoking behavior. Without large price increases, it is unlikely that the desired reduction in smoking will be achieved.

Smoking Effects and Cessation.—Mortality among middle-aged cigarette smokers is two to three times that of similar persons who never smoked. Life span is reduced by an average of 10 years. Many of those who die are still in middle age and lose many years of life. The good news is that stopping smoking is an effective intervention. Persons who begin smoking in early adulthood but stop by age 30, 40, or even 50 years gain about 10, 9, and 6 years of life, respectively, compared to those who continue to smoke. Persons who stop smoking before age 40 years avoid more than 90% of the excess risk for death during the next few decades compared to those who continue to smoke.

Pricing Effects.—Tobacco-control programs that use price and non-price interventions can increase smoking cessation rates and discourage the initiation of smoking. The two pricing approaches are specific excise taxes on tobacco and ad valorem (added value) taxes. Of these, the specific excise taxes exert a substantial, rapid effect on cigarette consumption. Higher taxes are especially effective for poorer or less educated individuals and may prevent young persons from taking up the habit.

Smuggling can be a concern with higher tobacco taxes. Using specific excise taxes on tobacco, employing stronger tax administration strategies, and instituting efforts to control smuggling can limit the problem. Even with some smuggling, large tax increases tend to substantially reduce consumption while raising revenue, which can then be used in health-promotion activities.

Other effective interventions include bans on advertising, the use of plain packaging for tobacco products, and the removal of all brand images. Pictorial warnings can be placed on the packages to convey the danger of smoking even to illiterate persons, who account for half of the deaths from tobacco in India. Bans on advertising should be comprehensive and include all direct and indirect promotions. This has the added advantage of severing the media from any dependence on the tobacco industry. Among populations with many long-term smokers, low-cost epidemiologic studies showing linkages between tobacco use and premature death may inform political movements against tobacco use as well as provide information for individuals who smoke.

Conclusions.—Many countries use non-price interventions, but few use large increases in specific excise taxes on tobacco to reduce smoking. However, studies show that a key component of effective and realistic strategies to significantly reduce smoking is a large increase in the price of cigarettes.

▶ Global mortality and morbidity related to cigarette smoking are staggering. In 2010, there were an estimated 5 million tobacco-attributable deaths in the world. On average, 50% of men and 10% of women begin smoking at young ages, and relatively few quit. The health burden of these individuals will increase as they age, with resultant morbidity and premature death. The World Health Organization (WHO) estimates that if current smoking prevalence continues, 1 billion persons during this century will die of tobacco-related diseases.[1,2]

In this review, Jha and Peto identify 3 key messages for smokers in the 21st century:

1. The risk is big, and there is a lot to lose. In middle age, mortality among smokers is 2 to 3 times what would be expected, leading to an average reduction in life span of about 10 years, as demonstrated in Fig 1 in the original article.
2. The loss is worse for those who die of tobacco-related disease in middle age. Those smokers who die in middle age have a loss of life expectancy of about 20 years of life compared with never smokers.

3. Quitting works. People who stop smoking at ages 30, 40, or 50 gain, on average, 10, 9, and 6 years of life expectancy, respectively, compared with people who continue smoking.[3]

The World Health Assembly of WHO estimates that a reduction in smoking prevalence by one-third by 2025 will save 200 million tobacco-related deaths over the rest of the century. The challenge is, how do we achieve that goal? Jha and Peto offer the following observations and recommendations on interventions that have reliably resulted in decreasing tobacco consumption:

1. Large increases in specific tobacco taxes are rapid and effective curbs.[4-6]
2. Taxes must consistently result in high cost to the consumer to achieve the desired effect.
3. Comprehensive curtailing advertising and plain packaging of cigarettes.
4. Bans on smoking in public places.
5. Raising political awareness.
6. Providing information, including data about premature death, to individual smokers.
7. Physician support, telephone- or Internet-based counseling.
8. Pharmacologic treatments.

As individual physicians and healthcare providers, we may not feel empowered to enact most of these interventions. Nonetheless, the combined voice is powerful, and we should lend ours to achieve these goals.

L. T. Tanoue, MD

References

1. Jha P. Avoidable global cancer deaths and total deaths from smoking. *Nat Rev Cancer.* 2009;9:655-664.
2. WHO Report on the Global Tobacco Epidemic, 2013. *Enforcing Bans on Tobacco Advertising, Promotion and Sponsorship*. Geneva, Switzerland: World Health Organization; 2013.
3. Pirie K, Peto R, Reeves GK, Green J, Beral V; Million Women Study Collaborators. The 21st century hazards of smoking and benefits of stopping: a prospective study of one million women in the UK. *Lancet.* 2013;381:133-141.
4. Effectiveness of Tax and Price Policies for Tobacco Control. *IARC Handbook of Cancer Prevention, Volume 14*. Lyon, France: International Agency for Research on Cancer; 2011.
5. Levy DT, Hyland A, Higbee C, Remer L, Compton C. The role of public policies in reducing smoking prevalence in California: results from the California tobacco policy simulation model. *Health Policy.* 2007;82:167-185.
6. Pizacani B, Mosbaek C, Hedberg K, et al. Decline in cigarette consumption following implementation of a comprehensive tobacco prevention and education program - Oregon, 1996–1998 (Reprinted from MMWR, vol 48, pg 140–143, 1999). *JAMA.* 1999;281:1483-1484.

Estimation of Cigarette Smoking-Attributable Morbidity in the United States

Rostron BL, Chang CM, Pechacek TF, et al (US Food and Drug Administration, Silver Spring, MD; Ctrs for Disease Control and Prevention, Atlanta, GA)
JAMA Intern Med 174:1922-1928, 2014

Importance.—Cigarette smoking has been found to harm nearly every bodily organ and is a leading cause of preventable disease, but current estimates of smoking-attributable morbidity by condition for the United States are generally unavailable.

Objective.—To estimate the burden of major medical conditions attributable to cigarette smoking in the United States.

Design, Setting, and Participants.—The disease burden of smoking was estimated using population-attributable risk calculations, taking into account the uncertainty of estimates. Population estimates came from 2009 US Census Bureau data and smoking prevalence, disease prevalence, and disease relative risk estimates came from National Health Interview Survey data for surveyed adults from 2006 through 2012. National Health and Nutrition Examination Survey spirometry data obtained from medical examination of surveyed adults from 2007 through 2010 was used to adjust for underreporting of chronic obstructive pulmonary disease.

Exposures.—Smoking status was assessed from self-reported National Health Interview Survey data.

Main Outcomes and Measures.—The number of adults 35 years and older who had had a major smoking-attributable disease by sex and condition and the total number of these conditions were estimated for the United States in 2009.

Results.—Using National Health Interview Survey data, we estimated that 6.9 million (95% CI, 6.5-7.4 million) US adults had had a combined 10.9 million (95% CI, 10.3-11.5 million) self-reported smoking-attributable medical conditions. Using chronic obstructive pulmonary disease prevalence estimates obtained from National Health and Nutrition Examination Survey self-reported and spirometry data, we estimated that US adults had had a combined 14.0 million (95% CI, 12.9-15.1 million) smoking-attributable conditions in 2009.

Conclusions and Relevance.—We estimate that US adults have had approximately 14 million major medical conditions that were attributable to smoking. This figure is generally conservative owing to the existence of other diseases and medical events that were not included in these estimates. Cigarette smoking remains a leading cause of preventable disease in the United States, underscoring the need for continuing and vigorous smoking-prevention efforts.

▶ Smoking is the most common cause of preventable death in the United States and around the world. The Centers for Disease Control and Prevention (CDC) in 2000 had estimated that 8.6 million individuals in the United States had 12.7 million smoking-attributable conditions.[1] This new study demonstrates that this was an underestimate. Using data from the National Health Interview Survey (NHIS) from 2006 to 2012 and informed by recent National Health and Nutrition Examination Survey (NHANES) data analyzing the degree of underreporting of chronic obstructive pulmonary disease (COPD), Rostron and colleagues estimate that 14 million persons in the United States had at least 1 serious smoking-induced illness in 2009. The enormous increase in the appreciated magnitude of cigarette-attributable morbidity largely relates to a more accurate assessment of the prevalence of COPD, which is underestimated by self-report as in NHIS, and more accurately estimated by self-report supplemented by spirometry data, as was achieved in NHANES.

Table 4 in the original article outlines the estimated number of lifetime cases of smoking-attributable morbidity by sex and condition in 2009. Of note, women accounted for 57% of cases of COPD, although their smoking prevalence was 4% to 5% less than that of men.[2] This raises again the question of whether women are more susceptible to respiratory complications of smoking, specifically COPD, which inevitably leads to the question of whether women are also more susceptible to the development of lung cancer related to smoking.

The bottom line is that 40 million American still smoke. Tobacco control, at a health policy level, in our legislatures and communities, and in our offices, must continue to be a public health priority.

L. T. Tanoue, MD

References

1. Centers for Disease Control and Prevention (CDC). Cigarette smoking-attributable morbidity—United States, 2000. *MMWR Morb Mortal Wkly Rep.* 2003;52:842-844.
2. Schroeder SA. Even more illness caused by smoking than previously estimated. *JAMA Intern Med.* 2014;174:1928-1929.

Electronic Cigarettes: A Position Statement of the Forum of International Respiratory Societies

Schraufnagel DE, on behalf of the Forum of International Respiratory Societies (Univ of Illinois at Chicago; et al)
Am J Respir Crit Care Med 190:611-618, 2014

Background.—Awareness and usage of electronic cigarettes has exponentially increased during the last few years, especially among young people and women in some countries. The rapid acceptance of electronic cigarettes may be attributed in part to the perception created by marketing and the popular press that they are safer than combustible cigarettes.

Goals.—To alert and advise policy makers about electronic cigarettes and their potential hazards.

Methods.—Using The Union's position paper on electronic cigarettes as the starting template, the document was written using an iterative process. Portions of the manuscript have been taken directly from the position papers of participating societies.

Results.—Because electronic cigarettes generate less tar and carcinogens than combustible cigarettes, use of electronic cigarettes may reduce disease caused by those components. However, the health risks of electronic cigarettes have not been adequately studied. Studies looking at whether electronic cigarettes can aid smoking cessation have had inconsistent results. Moreover, the availability of electronic cigarettes may have an overall adverse health impact by increasing initiation and reducing cessation of combustible nicotine delivery products.

Conclusions.—The health and safety claims regarding electronic nicotine delivery devices should be subject to evidentiary review. The potential benefits of electronic cigarettes to an individual smoker should be weighed against potential harm to the population of increased social acceptability of smoking and use of nicotine, the latter of which has addictive power and untoward effects. As a precaution, electronic nicotine delivery devices should be restricted or banned until more information about their safety is available. If they are allowed, they should be closely regulated as medicines or tobacco products.

▶ Electronic cigarettes have been rapidly introduced into the culture of our communities. Patients frequently ask me if it is "OK" to smoke electronic cigarettes to help them quit smoking. Recently, a patient wanted to know why he could not "vape" his electronic cigarette in our hospital healing garden. This statement by Schraufnagel and colleagues represents the stance on electronic cigarettes of the Forum of International Respiratory Societies (FIRS), whose member societies include the Asociación Latinoamericana del Tórax (ALAT), the American College of Chest Physicians (ACCP), the American Thoracic Society (ATS), the Asian Pacific Society of Respirology (APSR), the European Respiratory Society (ERS), the International Union Against Tuberculosis and Lung Disease (The Union), and the Pan African Thoracic Society (PATS). The FIRS statement summarizes all the relevant concerns about electronic cigarettes as follows:

- "The health risks of electronic cigarettes have not been adequately studied.
- The addictive power of nicotine and its untoward effects should not be underestimated.
- The potential benefits of electronic nicotine delivery devices, including harm reduction and as an aid to smoking cessation, have not been well studied.
- Potential benefits to an individual smoker should be weighed against harm to the population of increased social acceptability of smoking and use of nicotine.
- Health and safety claims regarding electronic nicotine delivery devices should be subject to evidentiary review.
- Adverse health effects for nonsmokers exposed to the emissions of electronic cigarettes cannot be excluded.
- Electronic nicotine delivery devices should be restricted or banned, at least until more information about their safety is available.
- If electronic nicotine delivery devices are permitted, they should be regulated as medicines and subject to the same evidentiary review as other medicines.

- If electronic nicotine delivery devices are not regulated as medicines, they should be regulated as tobacco products.
- Research, supported by sources other than the tobacco or electronic cigarette industry, should be performed to determine the impact of electronic nicotine delivery devices on health in a wide variety of settings.
- The patterns of use and the consequences at the population level of electronic nicotine delivery devices should be monitored.
- All information derived from this research should be conveyed to the public in a clear manner."

L. T. Tanoue, MD

Hidden Formaldehyde in E-Cigarette Aerosols

Jensen RP, Luo W, Pankow JF, et al (Portland State Univ, OR)
N Engl J Med 372:392-394, 2015

Background.—The usual liquids in e-cigarettes are solutions of propylene glycol, glycerol, or both; nicotine; and flavorings. Nuclear magnetic resonance (NMR) spectroscopy shows that formaldehyde-containing hemiacetals can be formed during "vaping" and may pose a health risk for e-cigarette users.

Methods.—A commercial sample of e-liquid was vaporized using a tank system e-cigarette that featured a variable-voltage battery. The aerosolized liquid was then collected and analyzed for the presence of formaldehyde-releasing agents. The results were extrapolated to indicate what exposure to formaldehyde a daily user of e-cigarettes might experience.

Results.—The simulated vaping consumed 5 to 11 mg of e-liquid with each puff, with 2 to 6 mg of liquid collected in the NMR spectroscopy tube. The limit for detecting formaldehyde was about 0.1 μg per 10 puffs. At 3.3 V, no measurable amount of formaldehyde was formed. At 5.0 V, the mean amount of formaldehyde was 380 μg per 10 puffs. The high-voltage results were extrapolated for an e-cigarette user vaping at a rate of 3 ml/day. This amounted to the user inhaling 14.4 mg/day of formaldehyde, which is conservative, since not all the liquid was collected during testing and no gas-phase formaldehyde was included. Conventional cigarettes expose users to a daily dose of 150 μg per cigarette, or 3 mg per pack of 20 cigarettes. Among persons weighing 70 kg, the incremental lifetime cancer risk associated with long-term cigarette smoking at 1 pack a day is estimated to be 9×10^{-4}. If inhaling formaldehyde-releasing agents is assumed to carry the same risk per unit of formaldehyde as the risk associated with inhaling gaseous formaldehyde, long-term vaping carries an incremental lifetime cancer risk of 4.2×10^{-3}, which is 5 to 15 times as high as the risk with long-term smoking, depending on what calculation basis is used. Formaldehyde-releasing agents may also be deposited in the respiratory tract more readily than gaseous formaldehyde and increase the user's cancer risk.

Conclusions.—Formaldehyde-releasing agents are used as industrial biocides. More than 2% of the total solvent molecules in vaped e-cigarettes have been shown to convert to these agents, so there are higher concentrations of formaldehyde-releasing agents than of nicotine in vaped e-cigarettes. How these agents act when they enter the respiratory tract is as yet unknown, but formaldehyde is a known carcinogen.

▶ Electronic cigarettes (e-cigarettes) are inhalational nicotine delivery devices. E-liquids typically are solutions of nicotine and propylene glycol and/or glycerol, flavored with various chemicals to make "vaping" more pleasurable. Their exact chemical contents are unknown because e-cigarettes are not regulated by the Food and Drug Administration. "Higher quality" e-cigarettes use variable voltage batteries to deliver different intensities of vapor, flavor, throat sensation, and nicotine.

Formaldehyde is a degradation product of propylene glycol. The reaction of formaldehyde with propylene glycol and glycerol during vaporization produces hemiacetals, which are formaldehyde-releasing agents. Using nuclear magnetic resonance spectroscopy, Jensen and colleagues analyzed a commercial e-liquid vaporized with the use of a variable voltage battery e-cigarette. They demonstrated that significant concentrations of formaldehyde-releasing agents are generated by e-cigarette vaping at high voltage, which may result in substantially more exposure of the airways to formaldehyde than conventional cigarettes (Fig 1 in the original article).

This report is part of a growing body of literature raising serious concerns about potential health hazards of e-cigarettes.[1,2] Formaldehyde is an International Agency for Research on Cancer group 1 carcinogen. E-cigarettes, like conventional cigarettes, should be strictly regulated.

L. T. Tanoue, MD

References

1. Schraufnagel DE, Blasi F, Drummond MB, et al. Electronic cigarettes. A position statement of the forum of international respiratory societies. *Am J Respir Crit Care Med.* 2014;190:611-618.
2. Vardavas CI, Anagnostopoulos N, Kougias M, Evangelopoulou V, Connolly GN, Behrakis PK. Short-term pulmonary effects of using an electronic cigarette: impact on respiratory flow resistance, impedance, and exhaled nitric oxide. *Chest.* 2012; 141:1400-1406.

Lung Cancer Screening

Components Necessary for High Quality Lung Cancer Screening: American College of Chest Physicians and American Thoracic Society Policy Statement

Mazzone P, Powell CA, Arenberg D, et al (Cleveland Clinic, OH; Icahn School of Medicine at Mount Sinai, NY; Univ of Michigan, Ann Arbor; et al)
Chest 147:295-303, 2015

Lung cancer screening with a low dose chest CT scan can result in more benefit than harm when performed in settings committed to developing and maintaining high quality programs. This project aimed to identify the components of screening that should be a part of all lung cancer screening programs. To do so, committees with expertise in lung cancer screening were assembled by the Thoracic Oncology Network of the ACCP and the Thoracic Oncology Assembly of the ATS. Lung cancer program components were derived from evidence-based reviews of lung cancer screening, and supplemented by expert opinion. This statement was developed and modified based on iterative feedback of the committees. Nine essential components of a lung cancer screening program were identified. Within these components twenty one Policy Statements were developed and translated into criteria that could be used to assess the qualification of a program as a screening facility. Two additional Policy Statements related to the need for multi-society governance of lung cancer screening were developed. High quality lung cancer screening programs can be developed within the presented framework of nine essential program components outlined by our committees. This document has been formally endorsed by several professional organizations (ACCP, ATS, American Association of Thoracic Surgery, American Cancer Society, American Society of Preventive Oncology).

▶ Much of the controversy and concern relating to lung cancer screening with low-dose computed tomography (CT) scanning revolves around the balance between the benefit and potential harms of screening. The benefit is straightforward: Lung cancer screening performed properly in the appropriate population results in a reduction in mortality from lung cancer.[1,2] The potential harms are less straightforward, although well appreciated, the most prominent of which are a high rate of abnormal results of which the large majority are false-positive findings, the potential for complications of invasive and noninvasive testing related to those findings, the appreciation of the enormous potential cost of screening, and concern about cost-effectiveness.

This policy statement was generated by a committee of experts in lung cancer screening representing the American College of Chest Physicians (ACCP) and American Thoracic Society (ATS). The committee identified nine essential components of a high-quality lung cancer screening program:

1. Who is offered lung cancer screening?
2. How often, and for how long, to screen?
3. How the CT is performed?
4. Lung nodule identification
5. Structured reporting
6. Lung nodule management algorithms
7. Smoking cessation
8. Patient and provider education
9. Data collection

Using the evidence base for each component, the committee developed policy statements outlining assessment criteria for measuring program quality. (See the table in article by Tanoue et al, reproduced here.) These policy statements may potentially inform the performance metrics by which the quality of a lung cancer screening program is measured. The committee already suggested 2 such metrics: 1) for component 1 (Who is offered lung cancer screening?), at least 90% of all screened subjects must match the program's stated policy, the evidence base for which indicates that screening should be limited to persons identified at high enough risk of developing lung cancer that potential benefit outweighs potential harm. These individuals would at a minimum meet the criteria of the National Lung Screening Trial cohort or the screening population recommended by the US Preventive Task Force.[1,3] For component 5 (Structured reporting), the selected structured CT scan reporting system identified by the screening program should be used for at least 90% of CT screen reports.

The components and policy statements are likely to serve as the platform informing the development of other metrics that will be used to measure quality and performance of screening programs. The policy statement has been endorsed by ACCP, ATS, the American Association of Thoracic Surgery, the American Cancer Society, and the American Society of Preventive Oncology.

L. T. Tanoue, MD

References

1. Aberle DR, Adams AM, Berg CD, et al. Reduced lung-cancer mortality with low-dose computed tomographic screening. *N Engl J Med.* 2011;365:395-409.
2. de Koning HJ, Meza R, Plevritis SK, et al. Benefits and harms of computed tomography lung cancer screening strategies: a comparative modeling study for the U.S. Preventive SERVICES Task Force. *Ann Intern Med.* 2014;160:311-320.
3. Moyer VA. Screening for lung cancer: U.S. Preventive Services Task Force recommendation statement. *Ann Intern Med.* 2014;160:330-338.

Cost-Effectiveness of CT Screening in the National Lung Screening Trial

Black WC, for the National Lung Screening Trial Research Team (Dartmouth–Hitchcock Med Ctr, Lebanon, NH; et al)

N Engl J Med 371:1793-1802, 2014

Background.—The National Lung Screening Trial (NLST) showed that screening with low-dose computed tomography (CT) as compared with chest radiography reduced lung-cancer mortality. We examined the cost-effectiveness of screening with low-dose CT in the NLST.

Methods.—We estimated mean life-years, quality-adjusted life-years (QALYs), costs per person, and incremental cost-effectiveness ratios (ICERs) for three alternative strategies: screening with low-dose CT, screening with radiography, and no screening. Estimations of life-years were based on the number of observed deaths that occurred during the trial and the projected survival of persons who were alive at the end of the trial. Quality adjustments were derived from a subgroup of participants who were selected to complete quality-of-life surveys. Costs were based on utilization rates and Medicare reimbursements. We also performed analyses of subgroups defined according to age, sex, smoking history, and risk of lung cancer and performed sensitivity analyses based on several assumptions.

Results.—As compared with no screening, screening with low-dose CT cost an additional $1,631 per person (95% confidence interval [CI], 1,557 to 1,709) and provided an additional 0.0316 life-years per person (95% CI, 0.0154 to 0.0478) and 0.0201 QALYs per person (95% CI, 0.0088 to 0.0314). The corresponding ICERs were $52,000 per life-year gained (95% CI, 34,000 to 106,000) and $81,000 per QALY gained (95% CI, 52,000 to 186,000). However, the ICERs varied widely in subgroup and sensitivity analyses.

Conclusions.—We estimated that screening for lung cancer with low-dose CT would cost $81,000 per QALY gained, but we also determined that modest changes in our assumptions would greatly alter this figure. The determination of whether screening outside the trial will be cost-effective will depend on how screening is implemented. (Funded by the National Cancer Institute; NLST ClinicalTrials.gov number, NCT00047385.)

▶ The National Lung Screening Trial (NLST) is the largest randomized study evaluating lung cancer screening with low-dose computed tomography (CT) scanning (LDCT).[1] The study population included more than 50 000 persons aged 55 to 74 years, with a history of at least 30 pack-years of smoking and who were either currently smoking or had quit within 15 years of study enrollment. NLST achieved a 20% reduction in lung cancer mortality in the group screened with annual LDCT compared with the group screened with chest radiography. The results of NLST comprise the largest portion of the evidence base on which current screening recommendations are based.

This study by Black and colleagues is the long-awaited cost-effectiveness analysis of NLST. Cost-effectiveness is one of the controversial aspects of implementing lung cancer screening. Early estimates of cost-effectiveness varied widely, from as low as $2500 per quality-adjusted life-year (QALY) to as high as $2 million per QALY.[2,3] The cost-effectiveness of LDCT screening for lung cancer in NLST was estimated as $81 000/QALY. Screening was more cost-effective in women ($46 000/QALY) than men ($147 000 per QALY), in current smokers ($43 000 per QALY) than former smokers ($615 000 per QALY), and in those at the highest 2 quintiles of risk of developing lung cancer than in the 3 lowest quintiles of risk. Other factors influencing cost-effectiveness included the cost of the LDCT scan, the number of follow-up scans performed for positive findings, and mortality related to surgeries performed for nodules. Concern has been raised that the tight monitoring of these factors in NLST may not generalize to the broader community, in which case screening may be less cost-effective. Given the potential enormous cost of screening to the nation, cost-effectiveness of lung cancer screening will continue to be closely scrutinized.

L. T. Tanoue, MD

References

1. Aberle DR, Berg CD, Black WC, et al. The National Lung Screening Trial: overview and study design. *Radiology.* 2011;258:243-253.
2. Mahadevia PJ, Fleisher LA, Frick KD, Eng J, Goodman SN, Powe NR. Lung cancer screening with helical computed tomography in older adult smokers: a decision and cost-effectiveness analysis. *JAMA.* 2003;289:313-322.
3. Wisnivesky JP, Mushlin AI, Sicherman N, Henschke C. The cost-effectiveness of low-dose CT screening for lung cancer: preliminary results of baseline screening. *Chest.* 2003;124:614-621.

CT Screening for Lung Cancer: Alternative Definitions of Positive Test Result Based on the National Lung Screening Trial and International Early Lung Cancer Action Program Databases

Yip R, Henschke CI, Yankelevitz DF, et al (Icahn School of Medicine at Mount Sinai, Levy Place, NY; et al)

Radiology 273:591-596, 2014

Purpose.—To determine the usefulness of alternative nodule size thresholds in a population undergoing computed tomographic (CT) screening for lung cancer and to compare the reported International Early Lung Cancer Action Program (I-ELCAP) results with the National Lung Screening Trial (NLST) results.

Materials and Methods.—The institutional review board approved this retrospective analysis. Informed consent was obtained according to HIPAA compliance. Findings in the CT cohort in the NLST of 25 813 participants who underwent baseline CT in 2002–2004 were reviewed. The frequency of solid and part-solid pulmonary nodules and the lung cancer diagnoses using an alternative nodule threshold of 5.0, 6.0, 7.0, 8.0, and 9.0 mm were determined. Proportional reduction in the frequency of positive results and their 95% confidence intervals using each of the alternative thresholds were calculated.

Results.—The frequency of positive results in the baseline round in the CT arm of the NLST using the definition of a positive result of any parenchymal, solid or part-solid, noncalcified nodule of 5.0 mm or larger was 15.8% (4080 of 25 813). Using alternative thresholds of 6.0, 7.0, 8.0, and 9.0 mm, the frequencies of positive results were 10.5% (2700 of 25 813, 7.2% (1847 of 25 813), 5.3% (1362 of 25 813), and 4.1% (1007 of 25 813), respectively, and the corresponding proportional reduction in additional CT scans would have been 33.8% (1380 of 1480), 54.7% (2233 of 4080), 66.6% (2718 of 4080), and 73.8% (3013 of 4080), respectively. Concomitantly, the proportion of lung cancer diagnoses determined within the first 12 months would be delayed up to 9 months for 0.9% (two of 232), 2.6% (six of 232), 6.0% (14 of 232), and 9.9% (23 of 232) of the patients, respectively.

Conclusion.—The NLST results are similar to those previously reported for the I-ELCAP and suggest that, even for high-risk participants in the

NLST, higher thresholds of nodule size should be considered and prospectively evaluated.

▶ The high prevalence of pulmonary nodules on low-dose computed tomography (LDCT) scans done for lung cancer screening has prompted a critical discussion of what nodule size threshold should be used to define "abnormal." Including a nodule of any size as a positive finding, or even using a very small size threshold, identifies an inordinate number of abnormalities and increases the false-positive rate. Using a larger threshold size incurs the risk of delaying or even missing early-stage cancer diagnoses. In the early LDCT screening studies, when *any* nodule was considered a positive finding, the rates of abnormal results were extremely high.[1,2] In the National Lung Screening Trial (NLST), 4 mm was chosen as the cutoff; nodules > 5 mm were deemed abnormal.[3] Using this definition, 39.1% of the population screened in NLST had at least 1 positive finding identified over the 3 years of screening. The American College of Radiology recently proposed that nodules of different densities should have different size thresholds defining positive findings on the baseline screen: > 6 mm for solid nodules, > 6 mm for part-solid nodules, and > 20 mm for pure ground-glass nodules.[4] This discussion is further muddied by the fact that different groups have used different means of measuring nodule size. The International Early Lung Cancer Action Project (I-ELCAP) defines nodule size as the average of the maximum length and width on a single transaxial image, using computer-aided detection, whereas NLST used a 1-dimensional linear measurement of nodule diameter.[3,5]

This study investigates the impact of alternative definitions of "positive result" on the outcomes of NLST. Yip and colleagues compared the frequency of positive results and delays in cancer diagnosis that would have resulted in NLST if the threshold of abnormality were set at > 6, 7, 8, or 9 mm compared with the original definition of > 5 mm. Table 1 in the original article demonstrates the distributions of NLST participants and cancers diagnosed stratified by the diameter of the largest noncalcified nodule (NCN) on the baseline screening LDCT. Of the 234 total cancers diagnosed on baseline scans, 23 (10%) occurred in nodules of 5 to 9 mm diameter. As can be seen in Table 2 of the original article, which demonstrates number of positive results and lung cancer diagnoses in the first year of scanning according to the different threshold definitions, the frequency of positive results decreased progressively from 15.8% in the 5-mm threshold group to 4.1% in the 9-mm threshold group, which resulted in the percentage of lung cancer diagnoses among the total abnormal findings increasing from 5.7% to 19.6%. In other words, raising the threshold size definition of "abnormal" resulted in a significant decrease in the number of false-positive results. On the flip side, increasing the threshold size to 6, 7, 8, and 9 mm would have resulted in a decrease in the total number of participants diagnosed with lung cancer to 230, 226, 218, and 209, respectively. Theoretically, those cancers that would not have been identified on the baseline scan because of the increase in threshold size would eventually be diagnosed because of growth over the ensuing years of screening. Furthermore, because they were all small (< 9 mm diameter), it seems unlikely that a delay in diagnosis would likely result in worse long-term outcomes. The important caveat is that this would be reliably true only if all patients returned for follow-up screening.

Determining what nodule size should define a positive finding on LDCT screening merits continued focused discussion, given the important implications this has on rates of false-positive findings and new lung cancer diagnoses. Nodule volume measurements are increasingly a part of this debate.[6,7] Standardization of the threshold size for a positive finding will help ensure that a conscious, cost-effective balance is achieved between maximizing early detection to decrease lung cancer deaths and minimizing potential harm and cost associated with false-positive results.

L. T. Tanoue, MD

References

1. Henschke CI, McCauley DI, Yankelevitz DF, et al. Early Lung Cancer Action Project: overall design and findings from baseline screening. *Lancet*. 1999;354:99-105.
2. Swensen SJ, Jett JR, Hartman TE, et al. CT screening for lung cancer: five-year prospective experience. *Radiology*. 2005;235:259-265.
3. Aberle DR, Adams AM, Berg CD, et al. Reduced lung-cancer mortality with low-dose computed tomographic screening. *N Engl J Med*. 2011;365:395-409.
4. Lung-RADS Version 1.0 Assessment Categories Release date: April 28, 2014. American College of Radiology; 2014. http://www.acr.org/~/media/ACR/Documents/PDF/QualitySafety/Resources/LungRADS/AssessmentCategories.pdf. Accessed March 9, 2015.
5. Henschke CI, Yip R, Yankelevitz DF, Smith JP, International Early Lung Cancer Action Program Investigators. Definition of a positive test result in computed tomography screening for lung cancer: a cohort study. *Ann Intern Med*. 2013;158:246-252.
6. Veronesi G, Maisonneuve P, Bellomi M, et al. Estimating overdiagnosis in low-dose computed tomorgraphy screening for lung cancer: a cohort study. *Ann Intern Med*. 2012;157:776-784.
7. Mehta HJ, Ravenel JG, Shaftman SR, et al. The utility of nodule volume in the context of malignancy prediction for small pulmonary nodules. *Chest*. 2014;145:464-472.

Lung Cancer Screening

Tanoue LT, Tanner NT, Gould MK, et al (Yale School of Medicine, New Haven, CT; Med Univ of South Carolina, Charleston; Kaiser Permanente Res, Palo Alto, CA)

Am J Respir Crit Care Med 191:19-33, 2015

The United States Preventive Services Task Force recommends lung cancer screening with low-dose computed tomography (LDCT) in adults of age 55 to 80 years who have a 30 pack-year smoking history and are currently smoking or have quit within the past 15 years. This recommendation is largely based on the findings of the National Lung Screening Trial. Both policy-level and clinical decision-making about LDCT screening must consider both the potential benefits of screening (reduced mortality from lung cancer) and possible harms. Effective screening requires an appreciation that screening should be limited to individuals at high risk of death from lung cancer, and that the risk of harm related to false positive findings, overdiagnosis, and unnecessary invasive testing is real. A comprehensive understanding of these aspects of screening will inform appropriate implementation, with the objective that an evidence-based and systematic approach to screening will help to reduce the enormous mortality burden of lung cancer.

► The National Lung Screening Trial (NLST) demonstrated that annual screening for lung cancer with low-dose chest computed tomography scanning prevents a significant number of lung cancer deaths compared with screening with chest radiograph.[1] The Prostate, Lung, Colorectal, and Ovarian Screening Study (PLCO) demonstrated that annual screening for lung cancer with chest radiograph was no more effective than no screening.[2] The results of both of these studies were published in 2011. Since then, a wealth of information relating to lung cancer screening has been generated considering the balance between benefit and potential harm, which population is at high enough risk of lung cancer to warrant screening, cost-effectiveness, and how screening should be implemented in the general population. Many of these topics are still hotly debated, but the recent United States Preventive Services Task Force recommendation supporting screening and the anticipated approval for lung cancer screening by the Centers for Medicare Services indicate that lung cancer screening in the broad community is going to be a reality.[3] This concise clinical review provides a comprehensive discussion of the topics noted here, all of which are relevant and important in making decisions about screening for individual patients. The review includes a synopsis of the American College of Chest Physicians and the American Thoracic Society policy statement on screening, which outlines the components necessary for high-quality lung cancer screening and provides a roadmap for the standards and performance metrics that are likely to be mandated for screening programs (Table 3 in the original article).[4]

L. T. Tanoue, MD

References

1. Aberle DR, Adams AM, Berg CD, et al. Reduced lung-cancer mortality with low-dose computed tomographic screening. *N Engl J Med.* 2011;365:395-409.
2. Oken MM, Hocking WG, Kvale PA, et al; PLCO Project Team. Screening by chest radiograph and lung cancer mortality: the Prostate, Lung, Colorectal, and Ovarian (PLCO) randomized trial. *JAMA.* 2011;306:1865-1873.
3. Moyer VA. Screening for Lung Cancer: U.S. Preventive Services Task Force recommendation statement. *Ann Intern Med.* 2014;160:330-338.
4. Mazzone P, Powell CA, Arenberg D, et al. Components necessary for high quality lung cancer screening: American College of Chest Physicians and American Thoracic Society Policy Statement. *Chest.* 2015;147:295-303.

Cancer Screening in the United States, 2014: A Review of Current American Cancer Society Guidelines and Current Issues in Cancer Screening

Smith RA, Manassaram-Baptiste D, Brooks D, et al (American Cancer Society, Atlanta, GA)

CA Cancer J Clin 64:30-51, 2014

Each year the American Cancer Society publishes a summary of its guidelines for early cancer detection, a report on data and trends in cancer screening rates, and select issues related to cancer screening. In this issue of the journal, we summarize current American Cancer Society cancer screening guidelines. In addition, the latest data on the use of cancer screening from the National Health Interview Survey is described, as are several issues related to screening coverage under the Patient Protection and Affordable Care Act, including the expansion of the Medicaid program (Table 5).

▶ The American Cancer Society (ACS) publishes yearly updated guidelines on cancer screening. This year's update includes a recommendation for lung cancer screening with low-dose chest computed tomography. The recommendation specifically states that healthcare providers with access to high-quality lung cancer screening centers should initiate a discussion about lung cancer screening with their patients aged 55 to 74 years who have at least a 30 pack-year history of smoking and are currently smoking or have quit within the past 15 years. These patient criteria match the entry criteria of the National Lung Screening Trial (NLST).[1] The guidelines point out that patients undergoing lung cancer screening should be in relatively good health and that, when possible, screening should

TABLE 5.—Key Discussion Points for the Process of Shared Decision-Making Related to Screening for Early Lung Cancer Detection With LDCT

- Benefit: Screening with LDCT has been shown to substantially reduce the risk of dying from lung cancer.
- Limitations: LDCT will not detect all lung cancers or all lung cancers early, and not all patients who have a lung cancer detected by LDCT will avoid death from lung cancer.
- Harms: There is a significant chance of a false-positive result, which will require additional periodic testing and, in some instances, an invasive procedure to determine whether an abnormality is lung cancer or some nonlung-related incidental finding. Fewer than one in 1000 patients with a false-positive result experience a major complication resulting from a diagnostic workup. Death within 60 d of a diagnostic evaluation has been documented, but is rare and most often occurs in patients with lung cancer.

Helping individuals clarify their personal values can facilitate effective decision-making:

- Individuals who value the opportunity to reduce their risk of dying from lung cancer and who are willing to accept the risks and costs associated with undergoing LDCT and the relatively high likelihood of the need for further tests, even tests that have the rare but real risk of complications and death, may opt to be screened with LDCT every year.
- Individuals who place a greater value on avoiding testing that carries a high risk of false-positive results and a small risk of complications, and who understand and accept that they are at a much higher risk of death from lung cancer than from screening complications, may opt not to be screened with LDCT.

LDCT indicates low-dose helical computed tomography.

be performed in an organized screening program by a multidisciplinary team skilled in the evaluation of abnormal lung lesions, which are prevalent on screening examinations.

Table 5 outlines the discussion points the ACS recommends for the purpose of shared decision making with patients relating to lung cancer screening. The ACS recommends that clinicians not discuss lung cancer screening with patients who do not meet the criteria outlined here. That statement is tempered by the suggestion that, for patients whose lung cancer risk is felt to approximate or exceed the risk of the NLST study population but who do not meet NLST criteria, clinicians should use their best judgment in deciding whether to initiate a screening discussion.

L. T. Tanoue, MD

Reference

1. Aberle DR, Adams AM, Berg CD, et al. Reduced lung-cancer mortality with low-dose computed tomographic screening. *N Engl J Med.* 2011;365:395-409.

Chest CT Scan Screening for Lung Cancer in Asbestos Occupational Exposure: A Systematic Review and Meta-analysis

Ollier M, Chamoux A, Naughton G, et al (Univ Hosp CHU G. Montpied, Clermont-Ferrand, France; Australian Catholic Univ, Fitzroy, Victoria, Australia)
Chest 145:1339-1346, 2014

Objective.—Lung cancer is the most frequent malignant asbestos-related pathology and remains the most fatal cancer of industrialized countries. In heavy smokers, early detection of lung cancer with chest CT scan leads to a 20% mortality reduction. However, the use of CT scan screening for early detection of lung cancer in asbestos-exposed workers requires further investigation. This study aimed to determine whether CT scan screening in asbestos-exposed workers is effective in detecting asymptomatic lung cancer using a systematic review and meta-analysis.

Methods.—We reviewed all cohort studies involving chest CT scan screening in former asbestos-exposed workers. The search strategy used the following keywords: "asbestos," "lung cancer," "screening," and "occupation*" or "work." Databases were PubMed, Cochrane Library, Science Direct, and Embase.

Results.—Seven studies matched our inclusion criteria. Baseline screening detected 49 asymptomatic lung cancers among 5,074 asbestos-exposed workers. Of the 49 reported lung cancers, at least 18 were in the earliest stage (stage I), accessible to complete removal surgery. The prevalence of all lung cancers detected by CT scan screening in asbestos-exposed workers was 1.1% (95% CI, 0.6%-1.8%).

Conclusions.—CT scan screening in asbestos-exposed workers is effective in detecting asymptomatic lung cancer. Detection of lung cancer in asbestos-exposed workers using CT scanning is at least equal to the prevalence in heavy smokers (1%; 95% CI, 0.09%-1.1%) and also shared a similar proportion of stage I diagnoses. Screening asbestos-exposed workers could reduce mortality in proportions previously observed among heavy smokers and, thus, should not be neglected, particularly for individuals combining both exposures.

▶ At present, there is no guideline recommendation to screen individuals with occupational asbestos exposure for lung cancer. There is broad acceptance that parenchymal lung disease associated with asbestos (asbestosis) is a risk factor for lung cancer and acknowledgment that the combination of asbestos exposure and cigarette smoking increases lung cancer risk. Whether asbestos exposure without accompanying parenchymal lung disease and in the absence of smoking increases lung cancer risk is controversial, and methods to reliably estimate the intensity of asbestos exposure are lacking.[1,2] Although asbestos is now banned from use in the United States, the long delay between exposure and disease makes previous occupational exposure, even several decades ago, a continuing concern. In this meta-analysis of 7 studies, including 5074 asbestos-exposed workers who underwent chest computed tomography (CT) screening for lung cancer, the prevalence of lung cancer at the baseline screen was 1.1% (range 0.4%—4.28%). This is in the range of the prevalence of lung cancer at the baseline screening CT in the National Lung Screening Trial (NLST).[3]

The current US Preventive Services Task Force recommendation for lung cancer screening does not consider factors other than age and smoking history. Other lung cancer risks, such as occupational exposure or family history of lung cancer, are not included in the decision of who should be screened. The reason for this is that those risks were not considered in the National Lung Screening Trial, and so the evidence base supporting screening for such individuals is lacking. The discomfort with not screening such patients is evident in the screening recommendations of the National Comprehensive Cancer Network (NCCN), which recommends screening be extended to persons > 50 years of age with > 20 pack-years smoking and 1 additional risk factor (radon exposure, occupational exposure, personal history of cancer, family history of lung cancer, chronic obstructive pulmonary disease [COPD], pulmonary fibrosis), and the American Association of Thoracic Surgery (AATS), which recommends screening be extended to persons aged 50 to 79 with > 20 pack-years of smoking and another risk for lung cancer (COPD, environmental or occupational exposure, prior cancer or radiation therapy, or family history of lung cancer).[4,5] These recommendations of NCCN and AATS have no evidence base to prove that screening in these groups decreases lung cancer mortality. Although extending eligibility for screening to populations beyond NLST might prevent a greater number of lung cancer deaths, it is likely to be less efficient. The legitimate concern is that the inherent potential harms of screening as well as the resultant decrease in cost-efficiency may outweigh any benefit of decreased lung cancer deaths in populations at lower risk.

What is the right answer, then, for patients whom we perceive are at increased risk for lung cancer based on factors beyond age and smoking? What do we do with patients whose lung cancer risk based on available risk assessment tools is in the range of that of the NLST population, but who do not meet NLST criteria? What about screening in persons with occupational asbestos exposure? The answers to these difficult questions are not known because there have been no large randomized studies evaluating the effect of screening on lung cancer mortality in non-NLST populations. Simply proving that lung cancer risk exists in those populations is not sufficient to assume that screening will be effective. Ideally, large randomized controlled trials should be performed to address the efficacy of screening in populations whose risk can be estimated as high enough to warrant screening but for whom no data as to mortality outcomes related to screening are currently available.

L. T. Tanoue, MD

References

1. Balmes JR. Asbestos and lung cancer: what we know. *Am J Respir Crit Care Med.* 2013;188:8-9.
2. Markowitz SB, Levin SM, Miller A, Morabia A. Asbestos, asbestosis, smoking, and lung cancer. New findings from the North American insulator cohort. *Am J Respir Crit Care Med.* 2013;188:90-96.
3. Aberle DR, Adams AM, Berg CD, et al. Reduced lung-cancer mortality with low-dose computed tomographic screening. *N Engl J Med.* 2011;365:395-409.
4. NCCN Clinical Practice Guidelines in Oncology (NCCN Guidelines). Lung Cancer Screening. 2014. www.nccn.org/professionals/physician_gls/pdf/lung_screening.pdf. Accessed January 30, 2015.
5. Jaklitsch MT, Jacobson FL, Austin JH, et al. The American Association for Thoracic Surgery guidelines for lung cancer screening using low-dose computed tomography scans for lung cancer survivors and other high-risk groups. *J Thorac Cardiovasc Surg.* 2012;144:33-38.

Diagnostic Evaluation

The Utility of Nodule Volume in the Context of Malignancy Prediction for Small Pulmonary Nodules

Mehta HJ, Ravenel JG, Shaftman SR, et al (Univ of Florida College of Medicine, Gainesville, FL; Med Univ of South Carolina, Charleston; et al)
Chest 145:464-472, 2014

Background.—An estimated 150,000 pulmonary nodules are identified each year, and the number is likely to increase given the results of the National Lung Screening Trial. Decision tools are needed to help with the management of such pulmonary nodules. We examined whether adding any of three novel functions of nodule volume improves the accuracy of an existing malignancy prediction model of CT scan-detected nodules.

Methods.—Swensen's 1997 prediction model was used to estimate the probability of malignancy in CT scan-detected nodules identified from a sample of 221 patients at the Medical University of South Carolina between 2006 and 2010. Three multivariate logistic models that included a novel function of nodule volume were used to investigate the added predictive value. Several measures were used to evaluate model classification performance.

Results.—With use of a 0.5 cutoff associated with predicted probability, the Swensen model correctly classified 67% of nodules. The three novel models suggested that the addition of nodule volume enhances the ability to correctly predict malignancy; 83%, 88%, and 88% of subjects were correctly classified as having malignant or benign nodules, with significant net improved reclassification for each ($P < .0001$). All three models also performed well based on Nagelkerke R^2, discrimination slope, area under the receiver operating characteristic curve, and Hosmer-Lemeshow calibration test.

Conclusions.—The findings demonstrate that the addition of nodule volume to existing malignancy prediction models increases the proportion of nodules correctly classified. This enhanced tool will help clinicians to risk stratify pulmonary nodules more effectively.

▶ Evaluation of the solitary pulmonary nodule is bread-and-butter pulmonary medicine. Pulmonary nodules are incredibly common; a widely quoted annual incidence of 150 000 pulmonary nodules per year is likely a gross underestimate because this figure was based on community studies done in the pre-computed tomography (CT) era.[1] Lung cancer screening undoubtedly will cause the number of pulmonary nodules identified to dramatically increase because nodules are so prevalent among screened populations. In the National Lung Screening Trial, 39.1% of all participants had at least 1 nodule discovered over 3 years of screening.[2] The fact that 96% of these nodules were not cancer highlights the need for better tools to help identify the small minority of nodules that actually are malignant.

This study by Mehta and colleagues builds on a validated prediction model developed by Swensen and colleagues for estimating the probability of malignancy for a solitary pulmonary nodule.[3] The variables in the Swensen model include patient age, smoking history, history of cancer, nodule diameter, nodule edge characteristic (spiculation), and location in the lung (upper or lower lobe). Mehta and colleagues added automated nodule volume, nodule volume to diameter ratio, or sphericity index as an additional variable. These new models were applied to 221 subjects with 233 nodules newly identified nodules with diameter < 15 mm, who were followed for a minimum of 2 years. Malignancy was established by surgical resection or needle biopsy; benignity was inferred by CT scan stability for at least 2 years. Each of the enhanced new models outperformed the original Swensen model in predicting malignancy, correctly classifying more subjects as having malignant lesions than the Swensen model.

It is worth noting that nodule volume adds more information than simple linear diameter. Diameter does not take into consideration all 3 dimensions of a nodule and may be less reliable in nodules that are irregularly shaped or spiculated. Nodule volume calculation is increasingly available with newer-generation CT software, although it is not yet part of routine radiographic description of pulmonary nodules and may not be as reliable in part-solid or ground glass nodules. This approach by Mehta and colleagues is of particular interest because it was developed in patients with small nodules, the patient group that is most likely to increase as lung cancer screening becomes more widely practiced. More reliable predictive tools may both help avoid unnecessary invasive interventions in patients with small benign pulmonary nodules and facilitate prompt management in patients who actually do have cancer.

L. T. Tanoue, MD

References

1. Holin SM, Dwork RE, Glaser S, Rikli AE, Stocklen JB. Solitary pulmonary nodules found in a community-wide chest roentgenographic survey; a five-year follow-up study. *Am Rev Tuberc.* 1959;79:427-439.
2. Aberle DR, Adams AM, Berg CD, et al. Reduced lung-cancer mortality with low-dose computed tomographic screening. *N Engl J Med.* 2011;365:395-409.
3. Swensen SJ, Silverstein MD, Ilstrup DM, Schleck CD, Edell ES. The probability of malignancy in solitary pulmonary nodules. Application to small radiologically indeterminate nodules. *Arch Intern Med.* 1997;157:849-855.

How many names for a rose: Inconsistent classification of multiple foci of lung cancer due to ambiguous rules

Fonseca A, Detterbeck FC (Yale School of Medicine, New Haven, CT)
Lung Cancer 85:7-11, 2014

Objectives.—Stage classification is important because it allows consistent definition of patient groups, and thus provides a foundation for comparison of outcomes. For patients with multiple pulmonary foci of lung cancer, however, the classification rules are ambiguous and confusing.

Materials and Methods.—We surveyed experts and clinicians who regularly evaluate patients with lung cancer to see how similar or different their interpretation of the official stage classification was for such patients.

Results.—We found a great deal of inconsistency in how four clinical scenarios were classified. No method of classification was chosen by a majority when there were more than two choices allowed by the classification rules. In a scenario with pulmonary foci of cancer of different histologic types, 86% classified this as separate primary cancers and 14% as multifocal lung cancer.

Conclusion.—The marked variability in classification must be taken into account when interpreting reported outcomes of patients with multiple pulmonary foci of lung cancer.

▶ One of the most challenging aspects of lung cancer staging is the evaluation and designation of pulmonary nodules separate from the primary tumor, which fall under the umbrella of "additional pulmonary nodules." The first step in this evaluation is determined by the clinical assessment of the relationship of the additional nodule(s) to the primary tumor. If the assessment is that the separate nodule is related to the primary tumor, then the nodule is defined in the context of its anatomic relationship to the dominant lesion, as T3 (satellite nodule, same lobe as primary tumor), T4 (ipsilateral nodule, lobe other than that of the primary tumor), or M1a (contralateral nodule).[1] If the separate nodule is suspected or proved to be malignant but is not felt to be related to the primary tumor, then the clinical and staging assessment becomes less clear. The variable nomenclature for this situation includes synchronous lung cancers, second primary lung cancers, multiple foci of lung cancer, and so on. Although definitions for synchronous primary lung cancers have been proposed by Martini and Melamed[2] and Detterbeck et al[3] and may be used reasonably consistently, definitions for other subgroups of additional pulmonary nodules are lacking. Inconsistencies in staging may follow, which can have significant clinical implications because staging is often used, correctly or not, as a basic roadmap for treatment. This article discusses the complexities of the classification of additional pulmonary nodules and addresses some of the nuances that may complicate staging for these patients. It is an interesting discussion of an area of uncertainty that still exists despite the extensive database of patients that informed the 2010 international lung cancer staging reclassification[4] and points out the importance of informed tumor board discussion in situations that do not fit standard staging definitions.

L. T. Tanoue, MD

References

1. Detterbeck FC, Boffa DJ, Tanoue LT. The new lung cancer staging system. *Chest.* 2009;136:260-271.
2. Martini N, Melamed MR. Multiple primary lung cancers. *J Thorac Cardiovasc Surg.* 1975;70:606-612.
3. Detterbeck FC, Postmus PE, Tanoue LT. The stage classification of lung cancer: Diagnosis and Management of Lung Cancer, 3rd ed: American College of Chest Physicians evidence-based clinical practice guidelines. *Chest.* 2013;143:e191S-e210S.
4. Goldstraw P, Crowley J, Chansky K, et al. The IASLC Lung Cancer Staging Project: proposals for the revision of the TNM stage groupings in the forthcoming (seventh) edition of the TNM Classification of malignant tumours. *J Thorac Oncol.* 2007;2:706-714.

Endobronchial Ultrasound–guided Transbronchial Needle Aspiration for Non–Small Cell Lung Cancer Staging

Kinsey CM, Arenberg DA (Univ of Vermont College of Medicine, Burlington; Univ of Michigan Health System, Ann Arbor)
Am J Respir Crit Care Med 189:640-649, 2014

Real-time endobronchial ultrasound-guided transbronchial needle aspiration (EBUS-TBNA) is an established technique for invasive mediastinal staging of non-small cell lung cancer (NSCLC). Needle-based techniques are now recommended as a first-line diagnostic modality for mediastinal staging. Accurate performance of systematic staging with EBUS-TBNA requires a detailed knowledge of mediastinal anatomy. This examination begins at the N3 lymph nodes, progressing through the N2 and N1 lymph node stations, unless a higher station lymph node is positive for malignant cells by rapid on-site cytologic examination. Objective methods of identifying EBUS-TBNA targets include sampling any lymph node station with a visible lymph node or with a lymph node greater than 5 mm in short axis. Three passes per station or the use of rapid on-site cytologic examination with identification of diagnostic material (tumor or lymphocytes) up to five passes are well-established techniques. Obtaining sufficient tissue for molecular profiling may require performing more than three passes. The operating characteristics of EBUS-TBNA are similar to mediastinoscopy. However, mediastinoscopy should be considered in the setting of a negative EBUS-TBNA and a high posterior probability of N2 or N3 involvement.

▶ Accurate staging of lung cancer is essential to achieving best patient care. Endobronchial ultrasound-guided (EBUS) needle aspiration (NA) is increasingly used to stage lung cancer. An extensive systematic literature review of studies to inform the most recent American College of Chest Physicians lung cancer guidelines evaluated the performance characteristics of EBUS for mediastinal staging, predominantly in patients with discrete mediastinal lymph node enlargement.[1] The overall median sensitivity of EBUS was 89%. The evidence base supported 2 important recommendations in which endoscopic techniques were felt to be superior to mediastinoscopy or surgical staging: 1) patients with high suspicion of N2,3 involvement, either by discrete mediastinal lymph node enlargement or positron emission tomography (PET) uptake, and 2) patients with an intermediate suspicion of N2,3 involvement based on a radiographically normal mediastinum (by computed tomography and/or PET) and a central tumor or N1 lymph node enlargement.

This review by Kinsey and Arenberg rigorously describes the approach to mediastinal staging with EBUS-NA. The review thoroughly describes the advantages and limitations of EBUS mediastinal staging, including recommendations for number of lymph node passes to achieve accuracy for histologic diagnosis as well as molecular analysis, the role of rapid on-site cytologic examination, and the appropriate sequence for nodal sampling. Careful planning can facilitate the efficient establishment of diagnosis and staging in a single procedure. The authors also point out that, in cases in which EBUS-NA is negative but the clinical suspicion of malignant mediastinal nodal involvement is high, further staging with a surgical technique should be pursued.

L. T. Tanoue, MD

Reference

1. Silvestri GA, Gonzalez AV, Jantz MA, et al. Methods for staging non-small cell lung cancer: diagnosis and management of lung cancer, 3rd ed: American College of Chest Physicians evidence-based clinical practice guidelines. *Chest*. 2013;143: e211S-e250S.

Cost effectiveness of endosonography versus surgical staging in potentially resectable lung cancer: a health economics analysis of the ASTER trial from a European perspective

Rintoul RC, Glover MJ, Jackson C, et al (Papworth Hosp, Cambridge, UK; Brunel Univ, Middlesex, UK; Inst of Public Health, Cambridge, UK; et al)
Thorax 69:679-681, 2014

In the ASTER study, mediastinal staging was more accurate for patients randomised to combined endobronchial and endoscopic ultrasound, followed by surgical staging if endoscopy was negative, versus surgical staging alone. Here, we report survival, quality of life and cost effectiveness up to 6 months, for the UK, The Netherlands and Belgium, separately. Survival in the two arms of the study was similar. In all three countries, the endosonography strategy had slightly higher quality-adjusted life years over 6 months, and was cheaper. Therefore, based on clinical accuracy and cost effectiveness, we conclude that mediastinal staging should commence with endosonography.

▶ The ASTER study was a prospective, randomized, controlled trial performed in Belgium, the Netherlands, and the United Kingdom. Patients with suspected non-small cell lung cancer (NSCLC) requiring mediastinal staging based on findings on computed tomography (CT) and positron emission tomography/CT were randomized to surgical staging alone or to combined endoscopic and endobronchial ultrasound followed by surgical staging if endosonography was negative. In the endosonography arm, sensitivity was 94%, compared with 79% in the surgical staging arm. Twenty percent of patients required surgical staging after initial endosonography.

There was little difference between patients from the 3 countries in quality-of-life measurements at 2 and 6 months after randomization. When combined with survival at 6 months, there was an overall mean increase in quality-adjusted survival related to endosonographic staging, resulting in an overall increase in quality adjusted life years. Staging procedures and thoracotomy were the main drivers of cost. Although there were variations in median length of stay after thoracotomy, in the proportion of patients who had additional treatment after surgery, and in the frequency of admission to hospital during the follow-up period, the endosonographic approach was associated with lower cost in all 3 countries. The conclusion was that endosonography is more cost-effective than surgery as the initial approach to staging of the mediastinum.

L. T. Tanoue, MD

Accuracy of FDG-PET to Diagnose Lung Cancer in Areas With Infectious Lung Disease: A Meta-analysis

Deppen SA, Blume JD, Kensinger CD, et al (Veterans Affairs Hosp, Nashville, TN; Vanderbilt Univ Med Ctr, Nashville, TN; et al)
JAMA 312:1227-1236, 2014

Importance.—Positron emission tomography (PET) combined with fludeoxyglucose F 18 (FDG) is recommended for the noninvasive diagnosis of pulmonary nodules suspicious for lung cancer. In populations with endemic infectious lung disease, FDG-PET may not accurately identify malignant lesions.

Objectives.—To estimate the diagnostic accuracy of FDG-PET for pulmonary nodules suspicious for lung cancer in regions where infectious lung disease is endemic and compare the test accuracy in regions where infectious lung disease is rare.

Data Sources and Study Selection.—Databases of MEDLINE, EMBASE, and the Web of Science were searched from October 1, 2000, through April 28, 2014. Articles reporting information sufficient to calculate sensitivity and specificity of FDG-PET to diagnose lung cancer were included. Only studies that enrolled more than 10 participants with benign and malignant lesions were included. Database searches yielded 1923 articles, of which 257 were assessed for eligibility. Seventy studies were included in the analysis. Studies reported on a total of 8511 nodules; 5105 (60%) were malignant.

Data Extraction and Synthesis.—Abstracts meeting eligibility criteria were collected by a research librarian and reviewed by 2 independent reviewers. Hierarchical summary receiver operating characteristic curves were constructed. A random-effects logistic regression model was used to summarize and assess the effect of endemic infectious lung disease on test performance.

Main Outcome and Measures.—The sensitivity and specificity for FDG-PET test performance.

Results.—Heterogeneity for sensitivity ($I^2 = 87\%$) and specificity ($I^2 = 82\%$) was observed across studies. The pooled (unadjusted) sensitivity was 89% (95% CI, 86%-91%) and specificity was 75% (95% CI, 71%-79%). There was a 16 percentage point–lower average adjusted specificity in regions with endemic infectious lung disease (61% [95% CI, 49%-72%]) compared with nonendemic regions (77% [95% CI, 73%-80%]). Lower specificity was observed when the analysis was limited to rigorously conducted and well-controlled studies. In general, sensitivity did not change appreciably by endemic infection status, even after adjusting for relevant factors.

Conclusions and Relevance.—The accuracy of FDG-PET for diagnosing lung nodules was extremely heterogeneous. Use of FDG-PET combined with computed tomography was less specific in diagnosing malignancy in populations with endemic infectious lung disease compared with nonendemic regions. These data do not support the use of FDG-PET to diagnose lung cancer in endemic regions unless an institution achieves test performance accuracy similar to that found in nonendemic regions.

▶ Positron emission tomography (PET) is increasingly being incorporated into the evaluation of lung nodules. Newer generation PET-computed tomography (CT) scanners allow the functional information of PET to be hybridized with the more precise anatomic information of CT scanning. It is well appreciated that PET imaging cannot distinguish among neoplasia, inflammation, and infection. For the purposes of nodule evaluation, this may be particularly problematic in areas of endemic infectious disease. Internationally, tuberculosis is a common cause of pulmonary nodules. In the United States, fungal diseases are more common causes of pulmonary nodules, with endemic histoplasmosis, coccidioidomycosis, and blastomycosis being present in different parts of the country.

The American College of Chest Physicians lung cancer guidelines on the evaluation of solitary pulmonary nodules recommends that functional imaging, preferably PET, be performed to characterize solid indeterminate nodules measuring >8 mm in diameter with low to moderate pretest probability of malignancy.[1] Patients whose nodules demonstrate moderate or intense uptake would go on to nonsurgical biopsy or surgical resection. This meta-analysis by Deppen and colleagues included 70 studies evaluating PET in the evaluation of pulmonary nodules. Ten of these studies, including 1431 individuals, reported on endemic infectious lung disease. Average specificity for lung cancer in these patients was 61%, compared with 77% in patients with pulmonary nodules in nonendemic regions.

This study points out that, in regions with high prevalence of endemic infectious disease, the specificity of PET to identify malignant pulmonary nodules is decreased. Relying on PET but failing to recognize this decrease in sensitivity could lead to unnecessary invasive interventions for lung nodules of infectious etiology. The use of PET scanning in the evaluation of solitary pulmonary nodules in areas of endemic infectious disease should be tempered by this consideration.

L. T. Tanoue, MD

Reference

1. Gould MK, Donington J, Lynch WR, et al. Evaluation of individuals with pulmonary nodules: when is it lung cancer? Diagnosis and Management of Lung Cancer, 3rd ed: American College of Chest Physicians evidence-based clinical practice guidelines. *Chest*. 2013;143:e93S-e120S.

Assessing the Usefulness of ^{18}F-fluorodeoxyglucose PET-CT Scan After Stereotactic Body Radiotherapy for Early-Stage Non-small Cell Lung Cancer

Pastis NJ Jr, Greer TJ, Tanner NT, et al (Med Univ of South Carolina, Charleston)
Chest 146:406-411, 2014

Background.—Although stereotactic body radiation therapy (SBRT) is an established treatment option for early-stage lung cancer, there are no guidelines for reassessing patients for local treatment failure or intrathoracic recurrence after treatment. This study reports the sensitivity, specificity, and positive and negative predictive values for ^{18}F-fluorodeoxyglucose (FDG) PET-CT scanning when used to evaluate patients after SBRT.

Methods.—Charts were reviewed of all patients who received SBRT and a subsequent FDG PET-CT scan at a university hospital over a 5-year period. Pretreatment and 3-month posttreatment tumor characteristics on PET-CT scan and outcome data (adverse events from SBRT, need for repeat biopsy, rate of local treatment failure and recurrent disease, and all-cause mortality) were recorded.

Results.—Eighty-eight patients were included in the study. Fourteen percent of patients (12 of 88) had positive 3-month PET scans. Of the positive results, 67% (eight of 12) were true positives. Eighty-six percent (76 of 88 patients) had negative 3-month FDG PET-CT scans, with 89% (68 of 76) true negatives. FDG PET-CT scan performed 3 months after SBRT for nonsmall cell lung cancer (NSCLC) had a sensitivity of 50% (95% CI, 0.26-0.75), a specificity of 94% (95% CI, 0.89-1.0), a positive predictive value of 67% (95% CI, 0.4-0.93), and a negative predictive value of 89% (95% CI, 0.83- 0.96).

Conclusions.—FDG PET-CT scan 3 months after treatment of NSCLC with SBRT was a specific but insensitive test for the detection of recurrence or treatment failure. Serial CT scans should be used for early surveillance following SBRT, whereas FDG PET-CT scans should be reserved to define suspected metastatic disease or to evaluate new abnormalities on CT scan, or for possible reassessment later in the follow-up period after radiation-related inflammation subsides.

▶ Surveillance patterns after treatment for lung cancer vary widely, reflecting the absence of rigorous long-term studies to inform best practices and likely also reflecting the appreciation that relapse is common. The patients in this study by Pastis and colleagues were enrolled in a Radiation Therapy Oncology Group (RTOG) trial evaluating stereotactic body radiotherapy (SBRT) for medically inoperable early-stage non-small cell lung cancer (NSCLC); 95% of the patients had Stage I disease. The RTOG study protocol required positron emission tomography/computed tomography (PET-CT) imaging 3 months posttreatment. Of the 88 patients included in the study, 12 had abnormal 3-month PET-CT scans, of which 8 were true positives. Of the 76 patients with negative PET-CT scans, 68 were true negatives. The sensitivity and specificity of PET-CT performed 3 months after SBRT were 50% and 94%, respectively.

This study points out the fallibility of PET-CT imaging in this setting, particularly in the lack of reliability in identifying cancer recurrence. The poor sensitivity is somewhat surprising. If anything, PET-CT might have been anticipated to be less specific because many patients develop inflammation related to radiation pneumonitis in the area of SBRT, which might have been anticipated to cause increased ^{18}F-fluorodeoxyglucose uptake and false-positive findings. Based on these results, PET-CT imaging should not be used routinely for follow-up of early-stage NSCLC treated with SBRT, at least not at the 3-month posttreatment time point. Surveillance of patients who have undergone curative-intent SBRT for early-stage NSCLC should probably be managed in the same manner as patients who have undergone curative intent surgical resection, that is, with chest CT scan every 6 months for the first 2 years and yearly thereafter.[1] PET-CT in these patients may be better utilized as an adjunct to CT in the evaluation of new abnormalities in the primary tumor bed or in identifying metastatic disease.

L. T. Tanoue, MD

Reference

1. Colt HG, Murgu SD, Korst RJ, Slatore CG, Unger M, Quadrelli S. Follow-up and surveillance of the patient with lung cancer after curative-intent therapy: diagnosis and management of lung cancer, 3rd ed: American College of Chest Physicians evidence-based clinical practice guidelines. *Chest.* 2013;143:e437S-e454S.

Lung Cancer Treatment

Appropriate Sublobar Resection Choice for Ground Glass Opacity-Dominant Clinical Stage IA Lung Adenocarcinoma: Wedge Resection or Segmentectomy

Tsutani Y, Miyata Y, Nakayama H, et al (Hiroshima Univ, Japan; Kanagawa Cancer Ctr, Yokohama, Japan; et al)
Chest 145:66-71, 2014

Background.—The purpose of this multicenter study was to characterize ground glass opacity (GGO)-dominant clinical stage IA lung adenocarcinomas and evaluate prognosis of these tumors after sublobar resection, such as segmentectomy and wedge resection.

Methods.—We evaluated 610 consecutive patients with clinical stage IA lung adenocarcinoma who underwent complete resection after preoperative high-resolution CT scanning and ^{18}F-fluorodeoxyglucose PET/CT scanning and revealed 239 (39.2%) that had a >50% GGO component.

Results.—GGO-dominant tumors rarely exhibited pathologic invasiveness, including lymphatic, vascular, or pleural invasion and lymph node metastasis. There was no significant difference in 3-year recurrence-free survival (RFS) among patients who underwent lobectomy (96.4%), segmentectomy (96.1%), and wedge resection (98.7%) of GGO-dominant tumors (P =.44). Furthermore, for GGO-dominant T1b tumors, 3-year RFS was similar in patients who underwent lobectomy (93.7%), segmentectomy (92.9%), and wedge resection (100%, P =.66). Two of 84 patients (2.4%) with GGO-dominant T1b tumors had lymph node metastasis. Multivariate Cox analysis showed that tumor size, maximum standardized uptake value on ^{18}F-fluorodeoxyglucose PET/CT scan, and surgical procedure did not affect RFS in GGO-dominant tumors.

Conclusions.—GGO-dominant clinical stage IA lung adenocarcinomas are a uniform group of tumors that exhibit low-grade malignancy and have an extremely favorable prognosis. Patients with GGO-dominant

clinical stage IA adenocarcinomas can be successfully treated with wedge resection of a T1a tumor and segmentectomy of a T1b tumor.

▶ Recommendations for management of small pulmonary nodules are increasingly taking nodule density into consideration. Radiographic distinctions between solid, part-solid (subsolid), and pure ground-glass (GGO) densities have informed a growing clinical sense that nodule density may reflect tumor biological behavior and prognosis. With an appreciation that overdiagnosis in lung cancer does exist, the behavior of most pure ground-glass nodules, although still potentially some form of adenocarcinoma, is typically indolent.[1,2] The biological behavior of part-solid nodules is less clear, and the uncertainty of prognosis for this group is reflected in the recommendations of the American College of Radiology and American College of Chest Physicians for closer monitoring and lower threshold for intervention than for pure ground-glass lesions.[3-6]

This study by Tsutani and colleagues addresses the impact of different surgical approaches on outcomes in patients with surgically resected clinical Stage IA tumors with GGO predominance, defined as nodules with a consolidation/tumor ratio (ie, solid component diameter/total diameter) of < 50% on thin-section CT scanning. Among 610 consecutive patients with clinical Stage IA lung adenocarcinomas treated at 4 centers in Japan, 239 met this definition. For these patients, there was no difference between lobectomy, segmentectomy, or wedge resection in 3-year recurrence-free survival or overall survival. GGO-dominant tumors rarely had pathologically invasive tumors or lymph node metastases (Table 4 in the original article).

The authors conclude that sublobar resection should be performed for patients with GGO-dominant clinical Stage IA tumors. Although there was no difference in outcomes between segmentectomy and wedge resection, they specifically recommend segmentectomy over wedge because of advantages of segmentectomy in securing sufficient surgical margins and achieving adequate assessment of hilar lymph nodes. The authors acknowledge that a major limitation of this study is its retrospective design because the choice of resection type was at the discretion of the individual surgeon. They point out that 2 clinical trials comparing surgical results between lobectomy and sublobar resection for clinical Stage 1A non-small cell lung cancer (NSCLC) are being conducted by the Cancer and Leukemia Group B and the Japan Clinical Oncology Group/West Japan Oncology Group, the results of which should more clearly inform the proper surgical approach to patients with small, early-stage NSCLC, including distinctions made on the basis of radiographic tumor density.

L. T. Tanoue, MD

References

1. Patz EF Jr, Pinsky P, Gatsonis C, et al; NLST Overdiagnosis Manuscript Writing Team. Overdiagnosis in low-dose computed tomography screening for lung cancer. *JAMA Intern Med.* 2014;174:269-274.
2. Bach PB, Jett JR, Pastorino U, Tockman MS, Swensen SJ, Begg CB. Computed tomography screening and lung cancer outcomes. *JAMA.* 2007;297:953-961.

3. Lung-RADS Version 1.0 Assessment Categories Release date: April 28, 2014. American College of Radiology; 2014. http://www.acr.org/~/media/ACR/Documents/PDF/QualitySafety/Resources/LungRADS/AssessmentCategories.pdf. Accessed March 9, 2015.
4. Naidich DP, Bankier AA, MacMahon H, et al. Recommendations for the management of subsolid pulmonary nodules detected at CT: a statement from the Fleischner Society. *Radiology.* 2013;266:304-317.
5. Detterbeck FC, Mazzone PJ, Naidich DP, Bach PB. Screening for lung cancer: diagnosis and management of lung cancer, 3rd ed: American College of Chest Physicians evidence-based clinical practice guidelines. *Chest.* 2013;143:e78S-e92S.
6. Gould MK, Donington J, Lynch WR, et al. Evaluation of individuals with pulmonary nodules: when is it lung cancer? Diagnosis and management of lung cancer, 3rd ed: American College of Chest Physicians evidence-based clinical practice guidelines. *Chest.* 2013;143:e93S-e120S.

Sublobar resection is equivalent to lobectomy for clinical stage 1A lung cancer in solid nodules

Altorki NK, for the I-ELCAP Investigators (NY Presbyterian Hosp/Weill Cornell Med College; et al)
J Thorac Cardiovasc Surg 147:754-764, 2014

Objectives.—A single randomized trial established lobectomy as the standard of care for the surgical treatment of early-stage non—small cell lung cancer. Recent advances in imaging/staging modalities and detection of smaller tumors have once again rekindled interest in sublobar resection for early-stage disease. The objective of this study was to compare lung cancer survival in patients with non—small cell lung cancer with a diameter of 30 mm or less with clinical stage 1 disease who underwent lobectomy or sublobar resection.

Methods.—We identified 347 patients diagnosed with lung cancer who underwent lobectomy (n = 294) or sublobar resection (n = 53) for non—small cell lung cancer manifesting as a solid nodule in the International Early Lung Cancer Action Program from 1993 to 2011. Differences in the distribution of the presurgical covariates between sublobar resection and lobectomy were assessed using unadjusted *P* values determined by logistic regression analysis. Propensity scoring was performed using the same covariates. Differences in the distribution of the same covariates between sublobar resection and lobectomy were assessed using adjusted *P* values determined by logistic regression analysis with adjustment for the propensity scores. Lung cancer—specific survival was determined by the Kaplan—Meier method. Cox survival regression analysis was used to compare sublobar resection with lobectomy, adjusted for the propensity scores, surgical, and pathology findings, when adjusted and stratified by propensity quintiles.

Results.—Among 347 patients, 10-year Kaplan—Meier for 53 patients treated by sublobar resection compared with 294 patients treated by lobectomy was 85% (95% confidence interval, 80-91) versus 86% (confidence interval, 75-96) (*P* =.86). Cox survival analysis showed no significant difference between sublobar resection and lobectomy when adjusted for propensity scores or when using propensity quintiles ($P = .62$ and $P = .79$, respectively). For those with cancers 20 mm or less in diameter, the 10-year rates were 88% (95% confidence interval, 82-93) versus 84% (95% confidence interval, 73-96) ($P = .45$), and Cox survival analysis showed no significant difference between sublobar resection and lobectomy using either approach ($P = .42$ and $P = .52$, respectively).

Conclusions.—Sublobar resection and lobectomy have equivalent survival for patients with clinical stage IA non–small cell lung cancer in the context of computed tomography screening for lung cancer.

▶ The only randomized study to date comparing lobectomy to limited or sublobar resection (segmentectomy or wedge resection) for early stage non-small cell lung cancer (NSCLC) was performed by the Lung Cancer Study Group (LCSG) in the 1980s.[1] That study demonstrated a 3-fold increase in local recurrence rate and a 50% increase in cancer-related deaths in patients undergoing limited resection compared with lobectomy. On the basis of these results, lobectomy has been the surgical approach of choice for early-stage NSCLC. However, the LCSG findings have been questioned as still reliable because the study predated the use of computed tomography (CT) imaging. Lung cancer tumors diagnosed by plain chest radiography were inevitably larger and, given the limitation of staging modalities at that time, undetected metastatic disease may have been present. Twenty to 30 years later, routine access to CT imaging has resulted in the identification of smaller tumors, with an increasing number of such tumors anticipated with lung cancer screening. This has refueled the ongoing debate among thoracic surgeons as to the optimal approach to surgical resection for early stage NSCLC. The field is further muddied by the fact that limited or sublobar resection is an umbrella term, including anatomic segmentectomy and wedge resection. These are generally not regarded as oncologically equivalent operations because segmentectomy is superior to wedge resection in terms of achieving sufficient surgical margins and ability to assess the hilar lymph nodes.

This study by Altorki and colleagues describes a series of 347 patients with early-stage NSCLC identified on low-dose CT screening, treated with either lobectomy or sublobar resection. All of the cancers were small (< 3 cm), solid nodules radiographically. In a nonrandomized fashion, 294 patients underwent lobectomy, and 53 underwent sublobar resection (16 segmentectomy and 37 wedge resection). Eighty-seven percent of the nodules treated with lobectomy and 94% of the nodules treated with sublobar resection were < 20 mm in diameter, so the majority of these cancers were stage IA. There was no difference between lobectomy and sublobar resection in 10-year survival, which was very good in both groups (86% and 85%, respectively). However, within the sublobar resection group, no recurrences occurred in the segmentectomy group, whereas 27% of patients who underwent wedge resection had cancer recurrence.

This study is limited by being retrospective and nonrandomized but does suggest that, for small, solid stage I NSCLC identified by screening, sublobar resection and lobectomy have similar survival outcomes. This finding mirrors the report by Tsutani and colleagues that follows in this section, that sublobar resection and lobectomy have similar outcomes in patients with ground-glass dominant stage 1A NSCLC.[2] As our ability to find and successfully treat early-stage NSCLC has improved, we are increasingly aware that these patients are at risk for second or even third lung cancers. Consideration of lung-sparing surgical approaches is therefore important, particularly as the generalization of screening to the broader community is anticipated to increase the numbers of early-stage cancers identified.

L. T. Tanoue, MD

References

1. Ginsberg RJ, Rubinstein LV. Randomized trial of lobectomy versus limited resection for T1 N0 non-small cell lung cancer. Lung Cancer Study Group. *Ann Thorac Surg*. 1995;60:615-622.
2. Tsutani Y, Miyata Y, Nakayama H, et al. Appropriate sublobar resection choice for ground glass opacity-dominant clinical stage IA lung adenocarcinoma: wedge resection or segmentectomy. *Chest*. 2014;145:66-71.

Molecular Approach to Lung Cancer

Molecular Testing for Selection of Patients With Lung Cancer for Epidermal Growth Factor Receptor and Anaplastic Lymphoma Kinase Tyrosine Kinase Inhibitors: American Society of Clinical Oncology Endorsement of the College of American Pathologists/International Society for the Study of Lung Cancer/Association of Molecular Pathologists Guideline

Leighl NB, Rekhtman N, Biermann WA, et al (Princess Margaret Cancer Centre, Toronto, Ontario, Canada; Memorial Sloan Kettering Cancer Ctr, NY; Einstein Med Ctr Montgomery, East Norriton, PA; et al)
J Clin Oncol 32:3673-3679, 2014

Purpose.—The College of American Pathologists (CAP), the International Society for the Study of Lung Cancer (IASLC), and the Association of Molecular Pathologists (AMP) guideline on molecular testing for the selection of patients with lung cancer for epidermal growth factor receptor (EGFR) and anaplastic lymphoma kinase (ALK) tyrosine kinase inhibitors was considered for endorsement.

Methods.—American Society of Clinical Oncology (ASCO) staff reviewed the CAP/IASLC/AMP guideline for developmental rigor; an ASCO ad hoc review panel of experts reviewed the guideline content.

Results.—The ASCO panel concurred that the recommendations are clear, thorough, and based on the most relevant scientific evidence in this content area and present options that will be acceptable to patients. The CAP/IASLC/AMP guideline comprises 37 recommendations (evidence grade A or B), expert consensus opinions, or suggestions that address the following five principal questions: (1) When should molecular testing be performed? (2) How should *EGFR* testing be performed? (3) How should *ALK* testing be performed? (4) Should other genes be routinely tested in lung adenocarcinoma? (5) How should molecular testing be implemented and operationalized?

Conclusion.—The ASCO review panel endorses the CAP/IASLC/AMP guideline. This guideline represents an important advance toward standardization of *EGFR* and *ALK* testing practices and is of major clinical relevance in advancing the care of patients with lung cancer. In the Discussion section, the ASCO review panel highlights three evolving areas: advances in ALK testing methodology, considerations for selecting appropriate populations for molecular testing, and emergence of other targetable molecular alterations.

► The American Society of Clinical Oncology (ASCO) recently endorsed the guideline for molecular testing of patients with lung cancer developed jointly by the College of American Pathologists, the International Association for the Study of Lung Cancer, and the Association for Molecular Pathology.[1] This guideline is discussed previously in this section. Of note, ASCO specifically comments on the suggestion in the guideline that "encourages" *EGFR* and *ALK* testing in patients with Stage I, II, and III lung cancers. It is important to recognize that targeted therapies are of proven benefit only in advanced stage (ie, predominantly Stage IV) *EGFR*-mutant or *ALK*-rearranged adenocarcinomas. Although it may be argued that molecular testing done in early-stage resected cancers could facilitate rapid initiation of treatment in the event of recurrence, the reality is that many of these patients may never recur. Furthermore, in many, if not most, cases in which recurrence is suspected, a repeat confirmatory biopsy will be performed, and so other opportunities for molecular testing will likely arise. Lastly, molecular testing is costly, and cost-effectiveness would demand that testing not be performed if the information gained will not affect treatment. In sum, at present molecular testing should be included in the evaluation of patients with advanced non-small cell lung cancer but should not be performed routinely for patients with early-stage lung cancer. This area of interest will continue to evolve as more targeted therapies become available.

L. T. Tanoue, MD

Reference

1. Lindeman NI, Cagle PT, Beasley MB, et al; College of American Pathologists International Association for the Study of Lung Cancer and Association for Molecular Pathology. Molecular testing guideline for selection of lung cancer patients for EGFR and ALK tyrosine kinase inhibitors: guideline from the College of American Pathologists, International Association for the Study of Lung Cancer, and Association for Molecular Pathology. *J Mol Diagn.* 2013;15:415-453.

Phase III Study of Afatinib or Cisplatin Plus Pemetrexed in Patients With Metastatic Lung Adenocarcinoma With *EGFR* Mutations

Sequist LV, Yang JC-H, Yamamoto N, et al (Massachusetts General Hosp and Harvard Med School, Boston, MA; Natl Taiwan Univ Hosp, Taipei; Shizuoka Cancer Ctr, Japan; et al)

J Clin Oncol 31:3327-3334, 2013

Purpose.—The LUX-Lung 3 study investigated the efficacy of chemotherapy compared with afatinib, a selective, orally bioavailable ErbB family blocker that irreversibly blocks signaling from epidermal growth factor receptor (EGFR/ErbB1), human epidermal growth factor receptor 2 (HER2/ErbB2), and ErbB4 and has wide-spectrum preclinical activity against *EGFR* mutations. A phase II study of afatinib in *EGFR* mutation—positive lung adenocarcinoma demonstrated high response rates and progression-free survival (PFS).

Patients and Methods.—In this phase III study, eligible patients with stage IIIB/IV lung adenocarcinoma were screened for *EGFR* mutations. Mutation-positive patients were stratified by mutation type (exon 19 deletion, L858R, or other) and race (Asian or non-Asian) before two-to-one random assignment to 40 mg afatinib per day or up to six cycles of cisplatin plus pemetrexed chemotherapy at standard doses every 21 days. The primary end point was PFS by independent review. Secondary end points included tumor response, overall survival, adverse events, and patient-reported outcomes (PROs).

Results.—A total of 1,269 patients were screened, and 345 were randomly assigned to treatment. Median PFS was 11.1 months for afatinib and 6.9 months for chemotherapy (hazard ratio [HR], 0.58; 95% CI, 0.43 to 0.78; $P = .001$). Median PFS among those with exon 19 deletions and L858R *EGFR* mutations ($n = 308$) was 13.6 months for afatinib and 6.9 months for chemotherapy (HR, 0.47; 95% CI, 0.34 to 0.65; $P = .001$). The most common treatment-related adverse events were diarrhea, rash/acne, and stomatitis for afatinib and nausea, fatigue, and decreased appetite for chemotherapy. PROs favored afatinib, with better control of cough, dyspnea, and pain.

Conclusion.—Afatinib is associated with prolongation of PFS when compared with standard doublet chemotherapy in patients with advanced lung adenocarcinoma and *EGFR* mutations.

▶ Driver mutations in the epidermal growth factor receptor (EGFR) gene are present in approximately 10% to 15% of patients with adenocarcinoma of the lung.[1] Tumors expressing these mutations are dependent on EGFR pathway signaling and are thereby rendered susceptible to inhibition by selective EGFR inhibition. The prototype-targeted therapies that accomplish this are gefitinib and erlotinib, oral small molecule EGFR tyrosine kinase inhibitors (TKIs). EGFR TKIs are now considered first-line treatment for patients with advanced stage adenocarcinoma of the lung with sensitizing EGFR mutations.[2]

EGFR is one of the ErbB family of receptor tyrosine kinases, which includes human epidermal growth factor (EGFR, HER1, ErbB1), HER2 (Neu, ErbB2), HER3 (ErbB3), and HER4 (ErbB4). Afatinib is an oral agent that irreversibly binds HER1 and HER2. This study by Sequist and colleagues summarizes the international LUX-Lung 3 phase III clinical trial, the largest prospective, randomized trial comparing first-line (ie, initial treatment) EGFR-targeted therapy with platinum-based chemotherapy (cisplatin/pemetrexed) in patients with advanced stage EGFR-mutant non-small cell lung cancer (NSCLC).

Fig 2 in the original article summarizes the end points of the study. Panel C demonstrates that 72% of patients were East Asian, 68% were never-smokers, and 65% were women, the typical phenotype of patient with EGFR-mutant tumors. Panel A demonstrates progression-free survival in the entire study population; panel B demonstrates progression-free survival in the 308 patients with the common EGFR mutations that would be anticipated to have response to TKIs (exon 19 deletions and exon 21 L858R point mutation). In both groups, there was a significant benefit in progression-free survival with treatment with afatinib compared to chemotherapy. This study supports the use of EGFR TKIs as initial therapy for patients with advanced EGFR mutation-positive NSCLC.

Patients with EGFR-mutated tumors invariably have disease progression at some point. The inevitability of relapse has highlighted the need for new approaches to targeted therapies. Afatinib is of interest in this regard because irreversible inhibition of the EGFR signaling pathway is one such approach, and furthermore, it appears that afatinib may also have benefit in treatment of EGFR-mutated tumors that are failing treatment with erlotinib due to acquisition of T790M mutation, the most common cause of EGFR TKI resistance. Newer generation therapies building on the biologic vulnerabilities of known molecular targets are increasingly of interest as the population of patients relapsing on treatment with first-generation targeted therapies grows.

L. T. Tanoue, MD

References

1. Cancer Genome Atlas Research Network. Comprehensive molecular profiling of lung adenocarcinoma. *Nature*. 2014;511:543-550.
2. Mok TS, Wu YL, Thongprasert S, et al. Gefitinib or carboplatin-paclitaxel in pulmonary adenocarcinoma. *N Engl J Med*. 2009;361:947-957.

First-Line Crizotinib versus Chemotherapy in *ALK*-Positive Lung Cancer

Solomon BJ, for the PROFILE 1014 Investigators (MacCallum Cancer Centre, Melbourne, Victoria, Australia; et al)
N Engl J Med 371:2167-2177, 2014

Background.—The efficacy of the ALK inhibitor crizotinib as compared with standard chemotherapy as first-line treatment for advanced ALK-positive non–small-cell lung cancer (NSCLC) is unknown.

Methods.—We conducted an open-label, phase 3 trial comparing crizotinib with chemotherapy in 343 patients with advanced *ALK*-positive nonsquamous NSCLC who had received no previous systemic treatment for advanced disease. Patients were randomly assigned to receive oral crizotinib at a dose of 250 mg twice daily or to receive intravenous chemotherapy (pemetrexed, 500 mg per square meter of body-surface area, plus either cisplatin, 75 mg per square meter, or carboplatin, target area under the curve of 5 to 6 mg per milliliter per minute) every 3 weeks for up to six cycles. Crossover to crizotinib treatment after disease progression was permitted for patients receiving chemotherapy. The primary end point was progression-free survival as assessed by independent radiologic review.

Results.—Progression-free survival was significantly longer with crizotinib than with chemotherapy (median, 10.9 months vs. 7.0 months; hazard ratio for progression or death with crizotinib, 0.45; 95% confidence interval [CI], 0.35 to 0.60; $P<0.001$). Objective response rates were 74% and 45%, respectively ($P<0.001$). Median overall survival was not reached in either group (hazard ratio for death with crizotinib, 0.82; 95% CI, 0.54 to 1.26; $P=0.36$); the probability of 1-year survival was 84% with crizotinib and 79% with chemotherapy. The most common adverse events with crizotinib were vision disorders, diarrhea, nausea, and edema, and the most common events with chemotherapy were nausea, fatigue, vomiting, and decreased appetite. As compared with chemotherapy, crizotinib was associated with greater reduction in lung cancer symptoms and greater improvement in quality of life.

Conclusions.—Crizotinib was superior to standard first-line pemetrexed-plus-platinum chemotherapy in patients with previously untreated advanced *ALK*-positive NSCLC. (Funded by Pfizer; PROFILE 1014 ClinicalTrials.gov number, NCT01154140.)

▶ Rearrangements of the anaplastic lymphoma kinase (ALK) gene are the third most common lung cancer oncogenic driver mutations. Compared with the general population with non-small cell lung cancer (NSCLC), patients with ALK-rearranged lung cancers tend to be younger and with minimal or no smoking history, and their tumors typically demonstrate adenocarcinoma histology. Crizotinib is an oral small-molecule tyrosine kinase inhibitor of ALK kinase. In a prior randomized phase 3 study of patients with advanced ALK-positive NSCLC who had failed first-line treatment with platinum-based chemotherapy, crizotinib was demonstrated be superior to standard second-line chemotherapy with pemetrexed or docetaxol.[1]

This study reports results of PROFILE 1014, an ongoing international, multicenter, randomized, open-label, phase 3 clinical trial comparing crizotinib as first-line treatment for advanced ALK-positive NSCLC vs standard platinum-based chemotherapy (cis- or carbo-platin/pemetrexed). This is the first reported randomized trial comparing crizotinib to standard chemotherapy as initial treatment for patients with advanced ALK-positive NSCLC. As can be seen in the figure (panels A and B), median progression-free survival was significantly longer in the crizotinib-treated group (10.9 months vs 7.0 months with chemotherapy). Overall survival was similar in both groups, neither of which had reached median overall survival at the time of the report. Crizotinib was also associated with better quality of life than chemotherapy.

The identification of targetable oncogenic driver mutations is revolutionizing the treatment of advanced lung cancer. For decades, the standard first-line approach to patients with Stage IV NSCLC has been platinum-based chemotherapy. The first dramatic change to this approach was the demonstration that in patients with advanced epidermal growth factor receptor (EGFR)-mutated adenocarcinoma, first-line treatment with EGFR tyrosine kinase inhibitors is superior to standard chemotherapy.[2-4] The findings of Solomon and colleagues similarly suggest that in patients with advanced ALK-rearranged NSCLC, first-line targeted ALK kinase inhibition is superior to standard chemotherapy. Although ALK-rearrangements are present in only 3 to 5% of all patients with NSCLC, for this identifiable minority of patients, targeted therapy may have an enormous benefit on both survival and quality of life.

L. T. Tanoue, MD

References

1. Shaw AT, Kim DW, Nakagawa K, et al. Crizotinib versus chemotherapy in advanced ALK-positive lung cancer. *N Engl J Med*. 2013;368:2385-2394.
2. Mok TS, Wu YL, Thongprasert S, et al. Gefitinib or carboplatin-paclitaxel in pulmonary adenocarcinoma. *N Engl J Med*. 2009;361:947-957.
3. Sequist LV, Yang JC, Yamamoto N, et al. Phase III study of afatinib or cisplatin plus pemetrexed in patients with metastatic lung adenocarcinoma with EGFR mutations. *J Clin Oncol*. 2013;31:3327-3334.
4. Maemondo M, Inoue A, Kobayashi K, et al. Gefitinib or chemotherapy for non-small-cell lung cancer with mutated EGFR. *N Engl J Med*. 2010;362:2380-2388.

Ceritinib in *ALK*-Rearranged Non–Small-Cell Lung Cancer

Shaw AT, Kim D-W, Mehra R, et al (Massachusetts General Hosp, Boston; Seoul Natl Univ Hosp, South Korea; Fox Chase Cancer Ctr, Philadelphia, PA; et al)

N Engl J Med 370:1189-1197, 2014

Background.—Non–small-cell lung cancer (NSCLC) harboring the anaplastic lymphoma kinase gene (*ALK*) rearrangement is sensitive to the ALK inhibitor crizotinib, but resistance invariably develops. Ceritinib (LDK378) is a new ALK inhibitor that has shown greater antitumor potency than crizotinib in preclinical studies.

Methods.—In this phase 1 study, we administered oral ceritinib in doses of 50 to 750 mg once daily to patients with advanced cancers harboring genetic alterations in *ALK*. In an expansion phase of the study, patients received the maximum tolerated dose. Patients were assessed to determine the safety, pharmacokinetic properties, and antitumor activity of ceritinib. Tumor biopsies were performed before ceritinib treatment to identify resistance mutations in *ALK* in a group of patients with NSCLC who had had disease progression during treatment with crizotinib.

Results.—A total of 59 patients were enrolled in the dose-escalation phase. The maximum tolerated dose of ceritinib was 750 mg once daily; dose-limiting toxic events included diarrhea, vomiting, dehydration, elevated aminotransferase levels, and hypophosphatemia. This phase was followed by an expansion phase, in which an additional 71 patients were treated, for a total of 130 patients overall. Among 114 patients with NSCLC who received at least 400 mg of ceritinib per day, the overall response rate was 58% (95% confidence interval [CI], 48 to 67). Among 80 patients who had received crizotinib previously, the response rate was 56% (95% CI, 45 to 67). Responses were observed in patients with various resistance mutations in *ALK* and in patients without detectable mutations. Among patients with NSCLC who received at least 400 mg of ceritinib per day, the median progression-free survival was 7.0 months (95% CI, 5.6 to 9.5).

Conclusions.—Ceritinib was highly active in patients with advanced, *ALK*-rearranged NSCLC, including those who had had disease progression during crizotinib treatment, regardless of the presence of resistance mutations in *ALK*. (Funded by Novartis Pharmaceuticals and others; ClinicalTrials.gov number, NCT01283516.)

▶ Chromosomal rearrangements of the anaplastic lymphoma kinase gene (ALK) gene have been demonstrated in a number of human cancers, including non-small cell lung cancer (NSCLC), anaplastic large cell lymphoma, and breast cancer. ALK rearrangements lead to the expression of ALK fusion genes, with resultant constitutive ALK kinase activation.[1] The most common ALK fusion oncogene in NSCLC is echinoderm microtubule-associated protein-like 4 (EML4)-ALK, which is identified in approximately 3% to 5% of patients with NSCLC; this translates into approximately 8000 patients in the United States annually. The typical clinical phenotype is a younger age at presentation, with little or absent smoking history, and tumors of adenocarcinoma histology.

EML4-ALK is an oncogenic "driver." Tumor cells constitutively express ALK, which regulates cell growth and survival pathway and renders these cells highly sensitive to ALK kinase inhibition. The small molecule ALK tyrosine kinase inhibitor (TKI), crizotinib, is approved for second-line treatment of advanced ALK-rearranged NSCLC and has recently demonstrated efficacy as first-line therapy.[2] However, benefit with crizotinib is predictably limited because most patients will relapse within 12 months due to development of acquired resistance, a situation parallel to the acquired resistance observed in epidermal growth factor receptor (EGFR)-mutated NSCLC treated with EGFR TKIs.[1,3] Addressing this inevitable progression has become one of the major challenges of the new era of molecularly targeted therapies.

Ceritinib is another oral, small-molecule TKI of ALK and is a more potent enzymatic inhibitor of ALK kinase than crizotinib. In preclinical studies, ceritinib demonstrated activity against both crizotinib-sensitive and crizotinib-resistant tumors.[4,5] This study by Shaw and colleagues is a phase I study of ceritinib in patients with locally advanced or metastatic ALK-rearranged cancers. Of the 130 patients in this clinical trial, 122 (94%) had NSCLC, of which 80 (68%)

had disease progression on crizotinib. Treatment of this subgroup with ceritinib resulted in a median progression-free survival of 6.9 months. This suggests that patients with advanced ALK-rearranged NSCLC who initially respond but then have disease progression on crizotinib may still benefit from more potent ALK inhibition by a different kinase inhibitor. These results merit confirmation in larger randomized trials.

From a pulmonary perspective, it is well documented that tyrosine kinase inhibition in the setting of EGFR-mutated adenocarcinoma can be associated with interstitial lung disease. In many cases, the toxicity panel of new oncology drugs will be imperfectly defined until many patients are treated, particularly with the pressure to "fast track" cancer drugs through regulatory channels. In this Phase I study, 4 cases of interstitial lung disease were identified that were felt possibly related to ceritinib. Although all resolved with discontinuation of the drug and "administration of standard treatments," we need to be cognizant of the potential for toxicities that may not be evident until these new therapies are generalized to the broader population.

L. T. Tanoue, MD

References

1. Katayama R, Shaw AT, Khan TM, et al. Mechanisms of acquired crizotinib resistance in ALK-rearranged lung cancers. *Sci Transl Med.* 2012;4:120ra117.
2. Solomon BJ, Mok T, Kim DW, et al. First-line crizotinib versus chemotherapy in ALK-positive lung cancer. *N Engl J Med.* 2014;371:2167-2177.
3. Doebele RC, Pilling AB, Aisner DL, et al. Mechanisms of resistance to crizotinib in patients with ALK gene rearranged non-small cell lung cancer. *Clin Cancer Res.* 2012;18:1472-1482.
4. Marsilje TH, Pei W, Chen B, et al. Synthesis, structure-activity relationships, and in vivo efficacy of the novel potent and selective anaplastic lymphoma kinase (ALK) inhibitor 5-chloro-N2-(2-isopropoxy-5-methyl-4-(piperidin-4-yl)phenyl)-N4-(2-(isopropylsulf onyl)phenyl)pyrimidine-2,4-diamine (LDK378) currently in phase 1 and phase 2 clinical trials. *J Med Chem.* 2013;56:5675-5690.
5. Friboulet L, Li N, Katayama R, et al. The ALK inhibitor ceritinib overcomes crizotinib resistance in non-small cell lung cancer. *Cancer Discov.* 2014;4:662-673.

Molecular Testing Guideline for Selection of Lung Cancer Patients for EGFR and ALK Tyrosine Kinase Inhibitors: Guideline from the College of American Pathologists, International Association for the Study of Lung Cancer, and Association for Molecular Pathology

Lindeman NI, Cagle PT, Beasley MB, et al (Brigham & Women's Hosp, Boston, MA; The Methodist Hosp, Houston, TX; Mount Sinai Med Ctr, NY; et al)
J Mol Diagn 15:415-453, 2013

Objective.—To establish evidence-based recommendations for the molecular analysis of lung cancers that are required to guide *EGFR*- and *ALK*-directed therapies, addressing which patients and samples should be tested, and when and how testing should be performed.

TABLE 3.—Summary of Guideline Recommendations

Section I: When Should Molecular Testing of Lung Cancers Be Performed?

Question 1: Which Patients Should Be Tested for *EGFR* Mutations and *ALK* Rearrangements?

1.1a: Recommendation: *EGFR* molecular testing should be used to select patients for EGFR-targeted TKI therapy, and patients with lung adenocarcinoma should not be excluded from testing on the basis of clinical characteristics.

1.1b: Recommendation: *ALK* molecular testing should be used to select patients for ALK-targeted TKI therapy, and patients with lung adenocarcinoma should not be excluded from testing on the basis of clinical characteristics.

1.2: Recommendation: In the setting of lung cancer resection specimens, *EGFR* and *ALK* testing is recommended for adenocarcinomas and mixed lung cancers with an adenocarcinoma component, regardless of histologic grade. In the setting of fully excised lung cancer specimens, *EGFR* and *ALK* testing is not recommended in lung cancers that lack any adenocarcinoma component, such as pure squamous cell carcinomas, pure small cell carcinomas, or large cell carcinomas lacking any immunohistochemistry (IHC) evidence of adenocarcinoma differentiation.

1.3: Recommendation: In the setting of more limited lung cancer specimens (biopsies, cytology) where an adenocarcinoma component cannot be completely excluded, *EGFR* and *ALK* testing may be performed in cases showing squamous or small cell histology but clinical criteria (eg, young age, lack of smoking history) may be useful in selecting a subset of these samples for testing.

1.4: Recommendation: To determine *EGFR* and *ALK* status for initial treatment selection, primary tumors or metastatic lesions are equally suitable for testing.

1.5: Expert consensus opinion: For patients with multiple, apparently separate, primary lung adenocarcinomas, each tumor may be tested but testing of multiple different areas within a single tumor is not necessary.

Question 2: When Should a Patient Specimen Be Tested for *EGFR* Mutation or *ALK* Rearrangement?

2.1a: Recommendation: *EGFR* mutation testing should be ordered at the time of diagnosis for patients presenting with advanced-stage disease (stage IV according to the 7th edition TNM staging system) who are suitable for therapy or at time of recurrence or progression in patients who originally presented with lower-stage disease but were not previously tested.

2.1b: Suggestion: *ALK* rearrangement testing should be ordered at the time of diagnosis for patients presenting with advanced-stage disease (stage IV according to the 7th edition TNM staging system) who are suitable for therapy or at time of recurrence or progression in patients who originally presented with lower-stage disease but were not previously tested.

2.2a: Expert consensus opinion: *EGFR* testing of tumors at diagnosis from patients presenting with stage I, II, or III disease is encouraged but the decision to do so should be made locally by each laboratory, in collaboration with its oncology team.

2.2b: Expert consensus opinion: *ALK* testing of tumors at diagnosis from patients presenting with stage I, II, or III disease is encouraged, but the decision to do so should be made locally by each laboratory, in collaboration with its oncology team.

2.3: Recommendation: Tissue should be prioritized for *EGFR* and *ALK* testing.

Question 3: How Rapidly Should Test Results Be Available?

3.1: Expert consensus opinion: *EGFR* and *ALK* results should be available within 2 weeks (10 working days) of receiving the specimen in the testing laboratory.

3.2: Expert consensus opinion: Laboratories with average turnaround times beyond 2 weeks need to make available a more rapid test—either in-house or through a reference laboratory—in instances of clinical urgency.

3.3: Expert consensus opinion: Laboratory departments should establish processes to ensure that specimens that have a final histopathologic diagnosis are sent to outside molecular pathology laboratories within 3 working days of receiving requests and to intramural molecular pathology laboratories within 24 hours.

Section II: How Should *EGFR* Testing Be Performed?

Question 4: How Should Specimens Be Processed for *EGFR* Mutation Testing?

4.1: Expert consensus opinion: Pathologists should use formalin-fixed, paraffin-embedded (FFPE) specimens or fresh, frozen, or alcohol-fixed specimens for PCR-based *EGFR* mutation tests. Other tissue treatments (eg, acidic or heavy metal fixatives, or decalcifying solutions) should be avoided in specimens destined for *EGFR* testing.

4.2: Expert consensus opinion: Cytologic samples are also suitable for *EGFR* and *ALK* testing, with cell blocks being preferred over smear preparations.

Question 5: What Are the Specimen Requirements for *EGFR* Testing?

5.1: Expert consensus opinion: Pathologists should determine the adequacy of specimens for *EGFR* testing by assessing cancer cell content and DNA quantity and quality.

5.2: Expert consensus opinion: Each laboratory should establish the minimum proportion and number of cancer cells needed for mutation detection during validation.

5.3: Expert consensus opinion: A pathologist should assess the tumor content of each specimen and either perform, or guide a trained technologist to perform, microdissection for tumor cell enrichment as needed.

Question 6: How Should *EGFR* Testing Be Performed?

6.1: Recommendation: Laboratories may use any validated *EGFR* testing method with sufficient performance characteristics.

6.2: Expert consensus opinion: Laboratories should use *EGFR* test methods that are able to detect mutations in specimens with at least 50% cancer cell content, although laboratories are strongly encouraged to use (or have available at an external reference laboratory) more sensitive tests that are able to detect mutations in specimens with as little as 10% cancer cells.

6.3: Expert consensus opinion: Clinical *EGFR* mutation testing should be able to detect all individual mutations that have been reported with a frequency of at least 1% of *EGFR*-mutated lung adenocarcinomas.

6.4: Recommendation: Immunohistochemistry for total *EGFR* is not recommended for selection of *EGFR* TKI therapy.

6.5: Recommendation: *EGFR* copy number analysis (ie, FISH or CISH) is not recommended for selection of *EGFR* TKI therapy.

Question 7: What Is the Role of KRAS Analysis in Selecting Patients for Targeted Therapy With *EGFR* TKIs?

7.1: Recommendation: KRAS mutation testing is not recommended as a sole determinant of *EGFR* TKI therapy.

Question 8: What Additional Testing Considerations Are Important in the Setting of Secondary or Acquired *EGFR* TKI Resistance?

8.1: Recommendation: If a laboratory performs testing on specimens from patients with acquired resistance to *EGFR* kinase inhibitors, such tests should be able to detect the secondary *EGFR* T790M mutation in as few as 5% of cells.

Section III: How Should *ALK* Testing Be Performed?

Question 9: What methods should be used for *ALK* testing?

9.1: Recommendation: Laboratories should use an *ALK* FISH assay using dual-labeled break-apart probes for selecting patients for *ALK* TKI therapy; *ALK* immunohistochemistry, if carefully validated, may be considered as a screening methodology to select specimens for *ALK* FISH testing.

9.2: Recommendation: RT-PCR is not recommended as an alternative to FISH for selecting patients for *ALK* inhibitor therapy.

9.3: Expert consensus opinion: A pathologist should be involved in the selection of sections for *ALK* FISH testing, by assessing tumor architecture, cytology, and specimen quality.

9.4: Expert consensus opinion: A pathologist should participate in the interpretation of *ALK* FISH slides, either by performing the analysis directly or by reviewing the interpretations of cytogeneticists or technologists with specialized training in solid tumor FISH analysis.

9.5: Expert consensus opinion: Testing for secondary mutations in *ALK* associated with acquired resistance to *ALK* inhibitors is not currently required for clinical management.

Section IV: Should Other Genes Be Routinely Tested in Lung Adenocarcinoma?

Question 10: Are Other Molecular Markers Suitable for Testing in Lung Cancer?

10.1a: Recommendation: Testing for *EGFR* should be prioritized over other molecular markers in lung adenocarcinoma.

10.1b: Suggestion: After *EGFR* testing, testing for *ALK* should be prioritized over other proposed molecular markers in lung adenocarcinoma, for which published evidence is insufficient to support testing guideline development at the present time.

Section V: How Should Molecular Testing of Lung Adenocarcinomas Be Implemented and Operationalized?

Question 11: Must All Adenocarcinomas Be Tested for Both *EGFR* and *ALK*?

11.1: Expert consensus opinion: Laboratories may implement testing algorithms to enhance the efficiency of molecular testing of lung adenocarcinomas, provided the overall turnaround time requirements are met.

Question 12: How Should *EGFR* and *ALK* Results Be Reported?

12.1: Expert consensus opinion: *EGFR* mutation testing reports and *ALK* FISH reports should include a results and interpretation section readily understandable by oncologists and by nonspecialist pathologists.

Question 13: How Should *EGFR* and *ALK* Testing Be Validated?

13.1: Expert consensus opinion: *EGFR* and *ALK* testing validation should follow the same guidelines as for other molecular diagnostics and FISH tests.

Question 14: How Should Quality Assurance Be Maintained?

14.1: Expert consensus opinion: Laboratories should follow similar quality control and quality assurance policies and procedures for *EGFR* and *ALK* testing in lung cancers as for other clinical laboratory assays. In particular, laboratories performing *EGFR* and *ALK* testing for TKI therapy should enroll in proficiency testing, if available.

CISH, chromogenic *in situ* hybridization; EGFR, epidermal growth factor receptor; FISH, fluorescence *in situ* hybridization; PCR, polymerase chain reaction; RT-PCR, reverse transcription–polymerase chain reaction; TKI, tyrosine kinase inhibitor; TNM, tumor, node, metastasis.

Participants.—Three cochairs without conflicts of interest were selected, one from each of the 3 sponsoring professional societies: College of American Pathologists, International Association for the Study of Lung Cancer, and Association for Molecular Pathology. Writing and advisory panels were constituted from additional experts from these societies.

Evidence.—Three unbiased literature searches of electronic databases were performed to capture published articles from January 2004 through February 2012, yielding 1533 articles whose abstracts were screened to identify 521 pertinent articles that were then reviewed in detail for their relevance to the recommendations. Evidence was formally graded for each recommendation.

Consensus Process.—Initial recommendations were formulated by the cochairs and panel members at a public meeting. Each guideline section was assigned to at least 2 panelists. Drafts were circulated to the writing panel (version 1), advisory panel (version 2), and the public (version 3) before submission (version 4).

Conclusions.—The 37 guideline items address 14 subjects, including 15 recommendations (evidence grade A/B). The major recommendations are to use testing for *EGFR* mutations and *ALK* fusions to guide patient selection for therapy with an epidermal growth factor receptor (EGFR) or anaplastic lymphoma kinase (ALK) inhibitor, respectively, in all patients with advanced-stage adenocarcinoma, regardless of sex, race, smoking history, or other clinical risk factors, and to prioritize *EGFR* and *ALK* testing over other molecular predictive tests. As scientific discoveries and clinical practice outpace the completion of randomized clinical trials, evidence-based guidelines developed by expert practitioners are vital for communicating emerging clinical standards. Already, new treatments targeting genetic alterations in other, less common driver oncogenes are being evaluated in lung cancer, and testing for these may be addressed in future versions of these guidelines (Table 3).

▶ Molecular testing is rapidly becoming part of the standard evaluative approach for patients with lung cancer, particularly lung adenocarcinomas. This clinical practice guideline for the approach to molecular testing for lung cancer is a collaborative effort of the College of American Pathologists (CAP), the International Association for the Study of Lung Cancer (IASLC), and the Association for Molecular Pathology (AMP), whose expert panel performed an extensive systematic literature review and analysis to arrive at the evidence-based recommendations outlined in Table 3.

We understand now that a majority of lung adenocarcinomas harbor identifiable driver mutations.[1] Of these, the identification of genetic alterations in epidermal growth factor rector (EGFR) and anaplastic lymphoma kinase (ALK) have had a major impact on therapeutic approaches. For patients with advanced-stage lung adenocarcinoma in whom an activating EGFR mutation or ALK rearrangement is identified, first-line therapy has shifted from conventional chemotherapy to targeted inhibition.[2,3]

For those of us on the diagnostic end of lung cancer evaluation, this raises the important questions of which patients with lung cancer should be tested for EGFR mutations and ALK rearrangements, and more specifically which patient specimens should be sent for molecular testing. The recommendations most relevant to these questions are outlined in Section I of Table 3. To briefly summarize some of the salient points:

- EGFR mutation and ALK rearrangement testing should be ordered for patients with advanced-stage (predominantly Stage IV) lung adenocarcinoma who are suitable for therapy, at the time of diagnosis or at time of recurrence or progression from lower stage to advanced disease.
- Patients with lung adenocarcinoma should not be excluded from molecular testing on the basis of clinical characteristics (eg, smoking history, gender, etc.).
- In settings where adenocarcinoma is completely excluded, specifically lung cancer resection with full excision of the tumor, EGFR and ALK testing are not recommended.
- In settings of limited lung cancer specimens (eg, biopsies or cytology) where an adenocarcinoma component cannot be completely excluded, EGFR and ALK testing may be useful even if the biopsy demonstrates squamous or small cell histology.
- The panel encouraged EGFR mutation and ALK rearrangement testing for patients presenting with Stage I, II, or III disease, but acknowledged that the decision to do so should be made locally by the testing laboratory in collaboration with the oncology team (see article by Leighl et al in this section).
- In settings of limited lung cancer specimens (eg, biopsies or cytology) where an adenocarcinoma component cannot be completely excluded, EGFR and

ALK testing may be useful even if the biopsy demonstrates squamous or small cell histology.

- The panel encouraged EGFR mutation and ALK rearrangement testing for patients presenting with Stage I, II, or III disease, but acknowledged that the decision to do so should be made locally by the testing laboratory in collaboration with the oncology team (see article by Leighl et al in this section).

L. T. Tanoue, MD

References

1. Cancer Genome Atlas Research Network. Comprehensive molecular profiling of lung adenocarcinoma. *Nature.* 2014;511:543-550.
2. Mok TS, Wu YL, Thongprasert S, et al. Gefitinib or carboplatin-paclitaxel in pulmonary adenocarcinoma. *N Engl J Med.* 2009;361:947-957.
3. Solomon BJ, Mok T, Kim DW, et al; PROFILE 1014 Investigators. First-line crizotinib versus chemotherapy in ALK-positive lung cancer. *N Engl J Med.* 2014;371: 2167-2177.

Using Multiplexed Assays of Oncogenic Drivers in Lung Cancers to Select Targeted Drugs

Kris MG, Johnson BE, Berry LD, et al (Memorial Sloan Kettering Cancer Ctr, NY; Dana-Farber Cancer Inst, Boston, MA; Vanderbilt-Ingram Cancer Ctr, Nashville, TN; et al)

JAMA 311:1998-2006, 2014

Importance.—Targeting oncogenic drivers (genomic alterations critical to cancer development and maintenance) has transformed the care of patients with lung adenocarcinomas. The Lung Cancer Mutation Consortium was formed to perform multiplexed assays testing adenocarcinomas of the lung for drivers in 10 genes to enable clinicians to select targeted treatments and enroll patients into clinical trials.

Objectives.—To determine the frequency of oncogenic drivers in patients with lung adenocarcinomas and to use the data to select treatments targeting the identified driver(s) and measure survival.

Design, Setting, and Participants.—From 2009 through 2012, 14 sites in the United States enrolled patients with metastatic lung adenocarcinomas and a performance status of 0 through 2 and tested their tumors for 10 drivers. Information was collected on patients, therapies, and survival.

Interventions.—Tumors were tested for 10 oncogenic drivers, and results were used to select matched targeted therapies.

Main Outcomes and Measures.—Determination of the frequency of oncogenic drivers, the proportion of patients treated with genotype-directed therapy, and survival.

Results.—From 2009 through 2012, tumors from 1007 patients were tested for at least 1 gene and 733 for 10 genes (patients with full genotyping). An oncogenic driver was found in 466 of 733 patients (64%). Among these 733 tumors, 182 tumors (25%) had the *KRAS* driver; sensitizing *EGFR*, 122 (17%); *ALK* rearrangements, 57 (8%); other *EGFR*, 29 (4%); 2 or more genes, 24 (3%); *ERBB2* (formerly *HER2*), 19 (3%); *BRAF*, 16 (2%); *PIK3CA*, 6 (<1%); *MET* amplification, 5 (<1%); *NRAS*, 5 (<1%); *MEK1*, 1 (<1%); *AKT1*, 0. Results were used to select a targeted therapy or trial in 275 of 1007 patients (28%). The median survival was 3.5 years (interquartile range [IQR], 1.96-7.70) for the 260 patients with an oncogenic driver and genotype-directed therapy compared with 2.4 years (IQR, 0.88-6.20) for the 318 patients with any oncogenic driver(s) who did not receive genotype-directed therapy (propensity score–adjusted hazard ratio, 0.69 [95% CI, 0.53-0.9], $P = .006$).

Conclusions and Relevance.—Actionable drivers were detected in 64% of lung adenocarcinomas. Multiplexed testing aided physicians in selecting therapies. Although individuals with drivers receiving a matched targeted agent lived longer, randomized trials are required to determine if targeting therapy based on oncogenic drivers improves survival.

Trial Registration.—clinicaltrials.gov Identifier: NCT01014286

▶ Oncogenic drivers are molecular alterations critical to the development of cancer.[1] The importance of these drivers is that they are potentially actionable by targeted inhibition of downstream effects that initiate or maintain neoplastic processes. The best known of these oncogenic drivers are somatic mutations in the epidermal growth factor receptor gene (EGFR) and rearrangements of the anaplastic lymphoma kinase (ALK), for which effective targeted therapies have been developed and for which testing in patients with advanced lung adenocarcinoma is now routine in many centers.

This multicenter study by Kris and colleagues included 1007 patients with Stage IV or recurrent adenocarcinoma of the lung. The primary objective was to determine the frequency of 10 oncogenic driver mutations. The secondary objectives were to define the co-occurrence of drivers in a single tumor and to document the ability to use the data to select treatment or a clinical trial targeting the identified driver(s) and to measure survival. Of the 1007 patients, 733 had specimens sufficient to test for all 10 genes; of these, 466 (64%) had an oncogene driver. The most common mutations were KRAS (25%), sensitizing EGFR (17%), and ALK rearrangements (8%). Only 3% of tumors had more than 1 oncogenic driver. Fig 2A in the original article demonstrates survival outcomes for patients with an oncogenic driver mutation who received targeted therapy ($n = 260$; median survival 3.5 years), patients with an oncogenic driver mutation who did not receive targeted therapy ($n = 318$; median survival 2.4 years), and patients with no identified driver ($n = 360$; median survival 2.1 years) ($P < .002$). There was a clear survival advantage for patients with an oncogenic driver mutation who received targeted therapy.

The important take-home message is that more than half of patients with advanced adenocarcinoma of the lung have oncogenic driver mutations, an increasing number of which are actionable. In this nonrandomized cohort, patients with targetable oncogenic drivers who underwent genotype-directed therapy had a longer median survival than patients with targetable oncogenic drivers who did not. Because the trial was not randomized, further research on outcomes is needed. These findings highlight the importance of a systematic approach to molecular testing for patients with advanced adenocarcinoma of the lung.[2]

L. T. Tanoue, MD

References

1. Cancer Genome Atlas Research Network. Comprehensive molecular profiling of lung adenocarcinoma. *Nature*. 2014;511:543-550.
2. Lindeman NI, Cagle PT, Beasley MB, et al; College of American Pathologists International Association for the Study of Lung Cancer and Association for Molecular Pathology. Molecular testing guideline for selection of lung cancer patients for EGFR and ALK tyrosine kinase inhibitors: guideline from the College of American Pathologists, International Association for the Study of Lung Cancer, and Association for Molecular Pathology. *J Mol Diagn*. 2013;15:415-453.

4 Pleural, Interstitial Lung, and Pulmonary Vascular Disease

Introduction

In this chapter, we take a look at 10 articles from the literature exploring pleural disease, interstitial lung disease, and pulmonary vascular disease.

Some of the most compelling research in pulmonary disease during the past year involved interstitial lung disease. We first review a study evaluating the role of DNA methylation in IPF by evaluating tissue samples from actual patients. We then review a negative therapeutic study evaluating the role of n-acetyl cysteine, followed by a pair of studies that have paved the way for directed medical therapy in this devastating disease.

We then review diverse publications regarding pleural disease. We start with a comparison of pleural fluid pressure monitoring techniques. We then explore the role of pleural plaques in lung function in a cohort of miners with high levels of asbestos exposure. We finish with a cost analysis comparing tunneled pleural catheters to talc pleurodesis for the management of malignant pleural effusions.

We then shift to pulmonary vascular disease and look into the role of gender in RV function. Next, we take a look at the CHEST PAH treatment guideline and finish the chapter with a look at the controversial role of thrombolysis in intermediate venous thromboembolism.

C. D. Spradley, MD

Interstitial Lung Disease

Relationship of DNA Methylation and Gene Expression in Idiopathic Pulmonary Fibrosis

Yang IV, Pedersen BS, Rabinovich E, et al (Univ of Colorado School of Medicine, Aurora; Univ of Pittsburgh Med Ctr, PA; et al)
Am J Respir Crit Care Med 190:1263-1272, 2014

Rationale.—Idiopathic pulmonary fibrosis (IPF) is an untreatable and often fatal lung disease that is increasing in prevalence and is caused by complex interactions between genetic and environmental factors. Epigenetic mechanisms control gene expression and are likely to regulate the IPF transcriptome.

Objectives.—To identify methylation marks that modify gene expression in IPF lung.

Methods.—We assessed DNA methylation (comprehensive high-throughput arrays for relative methylation arrays [CHARM]) and gene expression (Agilent gene expression arrays) in 94 patients with IPF and 67 control subjects, and performed integrative genomic analyses to define methylation–gene expression relationships in IPF lung. We validated methylation changes by a targeted analysis (Epityper), and performed functional validation of one of the genes identified by our analysis.

Measurements and Main Results.—We identified 2,130 differentially methylated regions (DMRs; <5% false discovery rate), of which 738 are associated with significant changes in gene expression and enriched for expected inverse relationship between methylation and expression ($P < 2.2 \times 10^{-16}$). We validated 13/15 DMRs by targeted analysis of methylation. Methylation–expression quantitative trait loci (methyl-eQTL) identified methylation marks that control *cis* and *trans* gene expression, with an enrichment for *cis* relationships ($P < 2.2 \times 10^{-16}$). We found five *trans* methyl-eQTLs where a methylation change at a single DMR is associated with transcriptional changes in a substantial number of genes; four of these DMRs are near transcription factors (castor zinc finger 1 [CASZ1], FOXC1, MXD4, and ZDHHC4). We studied the *in vitro* effects of change in CASZ1 expression and validated its role in regulation of target genes in the methyl-eQTL.

Conclusions.—These results suggest that DNA methylation may be involved in the pathogenesis of IPF.

► In their study published in the Blue Journal, Yang and colleagues explored the role of DNA methylation in idiopathic pulmonary fibrosis (IPF) lungs. The authors assessed lung tissue from 94 patients with IPF and 67 controls. They identified 2130 differentially methylated regions, of which 738 were associated with regulation of gene expression, specifically reduction in expression.

DNA methylation results in down regulation of gene expression, particularly when it occur in or around promoter regions. Cigarette smoking and environmental factors are known to influence levels of methylation. Previous studies have identified suspect targets but were limited by sample size. This study, as pointed out by the authors, suffers from the limitation that samples were obtained from heterogeneous tissue and not specific cell types.

The authors reported that there were extensive alterations in DNA methylation, some of which were known to have strong associations with IPF. Additional areas of interest were also identified. The authors point out that these may prove promising future targets for therapy in IPF.

C. D. Spradley, MD

Randomized Trial of Acetylcysteine in Idiopathic Pulmonary Fibrosis

The Idiopathic Pulmonary Fibrosis Clinical Research Network (Univ of Michigan, Ann Arbor; Univ of Alabama at Birmingham; Duke Clinical Res Inst, Durham, NC; et al)

N Engl J Med 370:2093-2101, 2014

Background.—Acetylcysteine has been suggested as a beneficial treatment for idiopathic pulmonary fibrosis, although data from placebo-controlled studies are lacking.

Methods.—In our initial double-blind, placebo-controlled trial, we randomly assigned patients who had idiopathic pulmonary fibrosis with mild-to-moderate impairment in pulmonary function to receive a three-drug regimen of prednisone, azathioprine, and acetylcysteine; acetylcysteine alone; or placebo. The study was interrupted owing to safety concerns associated with the three-drug regimen. The trial continued as a two-group study (acetylcysteine vs. placebo) without other changes; 133 and 131 patients were enrolled in the acetylcysteine and placebo groups, respectively. The primary outcome was the change in forced vital capacity (FVC) over a 60-week period.

Results.—At 60 weeks, there was no significant difference in the change in FVC between the acetylcysteine group and the placebo group (−0.18 liters and −0.19 liters, respectively; $P = 0.77$). In addition, there were no significant differences between the acetylcysteine group and the placebo group in the rates of death (4.9% vs. 2.5%, $P = 0.30$ by the log-rank test) or acute exacerbation (2.3% in each group, $P > 0.99$).

Conclusions.—As compared with placebo, acetylcysteine offered no significant benefit with respect to the preservation of FVC in patients with idiopathic pulmonary fibrosis with mild-to-moderate impairment in lung function. (Funded by the National Heart, Lung, and Blood Institute and others; ClinicalTrials.gov number, NCT00650091.)

▶ In 1 of 3 studies published in the May 29 *New England Journal of Medicine*, The Idiopathic Pulmonary Fibrosis Clinical Research Network presented the results of the PANTHER-IPF trial. The original study design compared acetylcysteine alone to acetylcysteine plus prednisone plus azathioprine to placebo in a 1:1:1 randomization. The combination arm was discontinued early at the request of the data safety monitoring board. The resulting 2-arm study was the subject of this publication.

The primary endpoint was reduction in forced vital capacity, and multiple secondary endpoints were prespecified. There was no significant difference between the intervention and placebo arms at 60 weeks, making this a negative study (Fig 2 in the original article). There were trends toward improvement in the treatment arm for a number of secondary endpoints, but the final conclusion drawn was that acetylcysteine was not effective in preventing decline in forced vital capacity at 60 weeks compared with placebo in patients with mild to moderate idiopathic pulmonary fibrosis diagnosed by high-resolution computed tomography or biopsy.

C. D. Spradley, MD

A Phase 3 Trial of Pirfenidone in Patients with Idiopathic Pulmonary Fibrosis

King TE Jr, for the ASCEND Study Group (Univ of California; et al)
N Engl J Med 370:2083-2092, 2014

Background.—In two of three phase 3 trials, pirfenidone, an oral antifibrotic therapy, reduced disease progression, as measured by the decline in forced vital capacity (FVC) or vital capacity, in patients with idiopathic pulmonary fibrosis; in the third trial, this end point was not achieved. We sought to confirm the beneficial effect of pirfenidone on disease progression in such patients.

Methods.—In this phase 3 study, we randomly assigned 555 patients with idiopathic pulmonary fibrosis to receive either oral pirfenidone (2403 mg per day) or placebo for 52 weeks. The primary end point was the change in FVC or death at week 52. Secondary end points were the 6-minute walk distance, progression-free survival, dyspnea, and death from any cause or from idiopathic pulmonary fibrosis.

Results.—In the pirfenidone group, as compared with the placebo group, there was a relative reduction of 47.9% in the proportion of patients who had an absolute decline of 10 percentage points or more in the percentage of the predicted FVC or who died; there was also a relative increase of 132.5% in the proportion of patients with no decline in FVC ($P < 0.001$). Pirfenidone reduced the decline in the 6-minute walk distance ($P = 0.04$) and improved progression-free survival ($P < 0.001$). There was no significant between-group difference in dyspnea scores ($P = 0.16$) or in rates of death from any cause ($P = 0.10$) or from idiopathic pulmonary fibrosis ($P = 0.23$). However, in a prespecified pooled analysis incorporating results from two previous phase 3 trials, the between-group difference favoring pirfenidone was significant for death from any cause ($P = 0.01$) and from idiopathic pulmonary fibrosis ($P = 0.006$). Gastrointestinal and skin-related adverse events were more common in the pirfenidone group than in the placebo group but rarely led to treatment discontinuation.

Conclusions.—Pirfenidone, as compared with placebo, reduced disease progression, as reflected by lung function, exercise tolerance, and progression-free survival, in patients with idiopathic pulmonary fibrosis. Treatment was associated with an acceptable side-effect profile and fewer deaths. (Funded by InterMune; ASCEND ClinicalTrials.gov number, NCT01366209.)

▶ The ASCEND trial is the result of conflicting data from 2 previous randomized double-blind placebo-controlled trials comparing pirfenidone, a novel antifibrotic agent, to placebo for the treatment of mild to moderate idiopathic pulmonary fibrosis. Inclusion criteria were similar to the PANTHER-IPF study (see above), and the study included patients with mild to moderate disease. Unlike PANTHER-IPF, the ASCEND trial was a positive trial with the treatment arm outperforming the placebo arm when comparing the primary and a number of prespecified secondary endpoints (Fig 2 in the original article). Mortality benefit did not reach clinical significance, but pooled data including the 2 previous phase III trials (Table 2 in the original article) did show statistically significant benefit. There was a slight increase in mild to moderate gastrointestinal and skin side effects in the treatment arm, and the study drug was well tolerated.

The year 2014 will go down in history as a big year for lung disease with the Food and Drug Administration approval of 2 new drugs for the treatment of idiopathic pulmonary fibrosis. Patients will benefit from these new options for life-prolonging treatment for what just last year was thought of as an untreatable disease. Intermune, the manufacturer of pirfenidone and the sponsor of the ASCEND trial, will also undoubtedly benefit in light of the hefty reported 6-figure sticker price for a year of therapy.

C. D. Spradley, MD

Efficacy and Safety of Nintedanib in Idiopathic Pulmonary Fibrosis

Richeldi L, for the INPULSIS Trial Investigators (Univ of Southampton, UK; et al)

N Engl J Med 370:2071-2082, 2014

Background.—Nintedanib (formerly known as BIBF 1120) is an intracellular inhibitor that targets multiple tyrosine kinases. A phase 2 trial suggested that treatment with 150 mg of nintedanib twice daily reduced lung-function decline and acute exacerbations in patients with idiopathic pulmonary fibrosis.

Methods.—We conducted two replicate 52-week, randomized, double-blind, phase 3 trials (INPULSIS-1 and INPULSIS-2) to evaluate the efficacy and safety of 150 mg of nintedanib twice daily as compared with placebo in patients with idiopathic pulmonary fibrosis. The primary end point was the annual rate of decline in forced vital capacity (FVC). Key secondary end points were the time to the first acute exacerbation and the change from baseline in the total score on the St. George's Respiratory Questionnaire, both assessed over a 52-week period.

Results.—A total of 1066 patients were randomly assigned in a 3:2 ratio to receive nintedanib or placebo. The adjusted annual rate of change in FVC was −114.7 ml with nintedanib versus −239.9 ml with placebo (difference, 125.3 ml; 95% confidence interval [CI], 77.7 to 172.8; $P < 0.001$) in INPULSIS-1 and −113.6 ml with nintedanib versus −207.3 ml with placebo (difference, 93.7 ml; 95% CI, 44.8 to 142.7; $P < 0.001$) in INPULSIS-2. In INPULSIS-1, there was no significant difference between the nintedanib and placebo groups in the time to the first acute exacerbation (hazard ratio with nintedanib, 1.15; 95% CI, 0.54 to 2.42; $P = 0.67$); in INPULSIS-2, there was a significant benefit with nintedanib versus placebo (hazard ratio, 0.38; 95% CI, 0.19 to 0.77; $P = 0.005$). The most frequent adverse event in the nintedanib groups was diarrhea, with rates of 61.5% and 18.6% in the nintedanib and placebo groups, respectively, in INPULSIS-1 and 63.2% and 18.3% in the two groups, respectively, in INPULSIS-2.

Conclusions.—In patients with idiopathic pulmonary fibrosis, nintedanib reduced the decline in FVC, which is consistent with a slowing of disease progression; nintedanib was frequently associated with diarrhea, which led to discontinuation of the study medication in less than 5% of patients. (Funded by Boehringer Ingelheim; INPULSIS-1 and INPULSIS-2 ClinicalTrials.gov numbers, NCT01335464 and NCT01335477.)

► The tyrosine kinase inhibitor nintedanib acts on multiple targets including vascular endothelia growth factor, fibroblast growth factor, and platelet-derived growth factor. The cell-signaling pathways activated by these tyrosine kinases are believed to play an important role in the pathophysiology of idiopathic pulmonary fibrosis. The results of the industry sponsored INPULSIS-1 and INPULSIS-2 trials were published in the same issue of the *New England Journal of Medicine* with PANTHER-IPF and the ASCEND trial. The result was positive with a reduction in decline of the forced vital capacity attributed to the intervention in both trials (Fig 1 in the original article), resulting in FDA approval of a second drug for the treatment of idiopathic pulmonary fibrosis in the same year.

There were a few issues with the studies that require mentioning: INPULSIS-1 did not demonstrate an increased time to acute exacerbation where INPULSIS-2 did (Fig 2 in the original article). Additionally, there were more myocardial infarctions in both studies in the treatment arms compared with placebo. Additionally, mild to moderate diarrhea was reported in the majority of patients in the treatment arm in both studies, and there were more instances of liver function abnormalities in patients receiving the inhibitor. Additionally, like its newly approved competitor pirfenidone, nintedanib will come with a hefty sticker price.

C. D. Spradley, MD

Pleural Disease

Comparison of Pleural Pressure Measuring Instruments

Lee HJ, Yarmus L, Kidd D, et al (Johns Hopkins Univ, Baltimore, MD; et al)
Chest 146:1007-1012, 2014

Objective.—The objective of this study was to compare the accuracy of a handheld digital manometer (DM) and U-tube (UT) manometer with an electronic transducer (ET) manometer during thoracentesis.

Methods.—Thirty-three consecutive patients undergoing thoracentesis were enrolled in the study. Pleural pressure (Ppl) measurements were made using a handheld DM (Compass; Mirador Biomedical), a UT water manometer, and an ET (reference instrument). End-expiratory Ppl was recorded after catheter insertion, after each aspiration of 240 mL, and prior to catheter removal. Volume of fluid removed, symptoms during thoracentesis, pleural elastance, and pleural fluid chemistry were also evaluated.

Results.—A total of 594 Ppl measurements were made in 30 patients during their thoracenteses. There was a strong linear correlation coefficient between elastance for the DM and ET ($r = 0.9582$, $P < .001$). Correlation was poor between the UT and ET ($r = 0.0448$, $P = .84$). Among the 15 patients who developed cough, recorded ET pressures ranged from −9 to +9 cm H_2O at the time of symptom development, with a mean (SD) of −2.93 (4.89) cm H_2O. ET and DM measurements among those patients with cough had a low correlation between these measurements ($R^2 = 0.104$, $P = .24$). Nine patients developed chest discomfort and had ET pressures that ranged from −26 to +6 cm H_2O, with a mean (SD) of −7.89 (9.97) cm H_2O.

Conclusions.—The handheld DM provided a valid and easy-to-use method to measure Ppl during thoracentesis. Future studies are needed to investigate its usefulness in predicting clinically meaningful outcomes.

▶ In this small, unfunded study out of Johns Hopkins published in *Chest*, the authors compare 3 methods of pleural manometry: electronic transducer (ET), U-tube (UT), and a proprietary handheld digital manometer (DM) (Fig 1 in the original article). The authors performed 594 individual measurements on 30 consecutive patients. A measurement from each device was made at each point in drainage.

The authors found excellent correlation between the standard ET manometer and the DM manometer but not between the ET manometer and the UT manometer (Fig 2 in the original article). The digital manometer correctly predicted nonexpandable lung in 5 of 5 patients with end expiratory pleural pressures less than −20 cm H_2O. UT manometry was not predictive. Cough was associated with a pressure of −2.93 cm H_2O, and pain was associated with a pressure of−7.89.

The study demonstrated good correlation between the DM manometer and the more cumbersome gold standard ET manometer. This lays the groundwork for future studies addressing the clinical implications of manometry during thoracentesis. The authors point out, however, that the device costs about $40 and has no associated common procedural terminology code, thus disincentivizing its widespread use.

C. D. Spradley, MD

Pleural Plaques and Their Effect on Lung Function in Libby Vermiculite Miners

Clark KA, Flynn JJ III, Goodman JE, et al (Univ of South Carolina, Columbia; Health Network America, Tinton Falls, NJ; Gradient Corporation, Cambridge, MA; et al)
Chest 146:786-794, 2014

Background.—Multiple studies have investigated the relationship between asbestos-related pleural plaques (PPs) and lung function, with disparate and inconsistent results. Most use chest radiographs to identify PPs and simple spirometry to measure lung function. High-resolution CT (HRCT) scanning improves the accuracy of PP identification. Complete pulmonary function tests (PFTs), including spirometry, lung volumes, and diffusing capacity of the lung for carbon monoxide, provide a more definitive assessment of lung function. The goal of this study was to determine, using HRCT scanning and complete PFTs, the effect of PPs on lung function in Libby vermiculite miners.

Methods.—The results of HRCT scanning and complete PFTs performed between January 2000 and August 2012 were obtained from the medical records of 166 Libby vermiculite miners. Multivariate regression analyses with Tukey multivariate adjustment were used to assess statistical associations between the presence of PPs and lung function. Adjustments were made for age, BMI, smoking history, duration of employment, and years since last occupational asbestos exposure.

Results.—Nearly 90% of miners ($n = 149$) had evidence of PPs on HRCT scan. No significant differences in spirometry results, lung volumes, or diffusing capacity of the lung for carbon monoxide were found between miners with PPs alone and miners with normal HRCT scans. Miners with both interstitial fibrosis and the presence of PPs had a significantly decreased total lung capacity in comparison with miners with normal

HRCT scans ($P = .02$). Age, cumulative smoking history, and BMI were significant covariates that contributed to abnormal lung function.

Conclusions.—Asbestos-related PPs alone have no significant effect on lung function in Libby vermiculite miners.

► In this retrospective study published in *Chest*, Clark and colleagues set out to answer the question of whether isolated pleural plaques have an impact on lung function in subjects with history of asbestos exposure. The study operates on the premise that previous studies depended on simple chest x-ray, simple spirometry, or both to identify plaques and quantify dysfunction. The authors based their comparison on high-resolution computed tomography (HRCT) data and full pulmonary function testing including lung volumes and diffusion capacity.

In a 12-year sample, the team identified 166 miners with HRCT and full pulmonary function tests (PFTs) and stratified them based on age, body mass index, smoking status, duration of employment, and years since exposure. Pleural plaques were stratified into 3 levels. The sample was divided into 4 groups by HRCT finding: normal, isolated pleural plaques, pleural plaques and fibrosis, and "other CT abnormalities" (Table 2 in the original article).

Findings of fibrosis and "other CT abnormalities" correlated with reduced lung function compared with "normal." As would be expected, age, smoking more than 15 pack-years, and BMI also correlated with decline in lung function. Isolated pleural plaques did not (Table 4 in the original article).

The authors point out that discrepancies in previous studies may be attributed to occult fibrosis that was not apparent on chest radiographs in line with expert opinion.

Author-identified limitations of this study include the variable timing of CT and pulmonary function testing as well as the small size of the reference population. They rightly point out, however, that the study benefited from a uniform study population and methodology that is more robust than previous investigations.

On the basis of the findings of Clark and colleagues, the assumption that pleural plaques have no influence on lung function can be considered sound.

C. D. Spradley, MD

Comparing Cost of Indwelling Pleural Catheter vs Talc Pleurodesis for Malignant Pleural Effusion

Penz ED, Mishra EK, Davies HE, et al (Univ of Saskatchewan, Saskatoon, Canada; Univ of Oxford, England; et al)

Chest 146:991-1000, 2014

Background.—Malignant pleural effusion is associated with short life expectancy and significant morbidity. A randomized controlled trial comparing indwelling pleural catheters (IPCs) with talc pleurodesis found that IPCs reduced in-hospital time and the need for additional procedures but were associated with excess adverse events.

TABLE 4.—Resource Use, Mean Cost, and Mean Cost Difference Between IPC and Talc in US$

Category	IPC		Talc	
	Resources Used	Cost, Mean (SD), $	Resources Used	Cost, Mean (SD), $
Initial intervention				
Intervention procedures	51	797 (36)	53	476 (47)
Mean LOS,[a] d	2.49 (7)	1,147 (2,961)	4.98 (4)	2,461 (1,834)
	N = 51		N = 51	
Day-case visit	32 visits	325 (260)	0 visits	0
Total initial intervention costs, $	2,276 (2,849)		2,939 (1,844)	
Total ongoing drainage costs, $	1,011 (732)		57 (213)	
Adverse events				
Outpatient visits[b]	33	336 (694)	41	401 (1,440)
Inpatient visits[b]	15	1,188 (4,453)	30	871 (2,327)
Procedures[b]	3	19 (76)	46	227 (694)
Diagnostic imaging[c]	34 6	43 (106)	66 2	52 (137)
Total adverse events costs, $	1,653 (4,693)		1,555 (3,737)	
Total cost, $	4,993 (5,529)		4,581 (4,359)	
Difference in costs, $				
Total cost[d]				
Mean difference[e]		401		
95% CI		(− 1,387 to 2,261)		
Adverse events cost[d]				
Mean difference[e]		76		
95% CI		(− 1,524 to 1,786)		
Combined initial intervention and ongoing drainage cost[d]				
Mean difference[e]		316		
95% CI		(− 603 to 1,426)		

See Table 1 and 2 legends for expansion of abbreviations.
[a]Mean LOS associated with insertion of initial intervention (includes those who were not admitted in the IPC group).
[b]Total number of visits or procedures performed in each group.
[c]Total number of chest radiographs (top) and CT scans (bottom) performed in each group
[d]Bootstrap estimate of mean cost difference and 95% CI.
[e]IPC minus Talc.
Reprinted from Penz ED, Mishra EK, Davies HE, et al. Comparing Cost of Indwelling Pleural Catheter vs Talc Pleurodesis for Malignant Pleural Effusion. Chest. 2014; 146:991-1000, © 2014, American College of Chest Physicians.

Methods.—Using data from the clinical trial, we compared costs associated with use of IPCs and with talc pleurodesis. Resource use and adverse events were captured through case report forms over the 1-year trial follow-up. Costs for outpatient and inpatient visits, diagnostic imaging, nursing, and doctor time were obtained from the UK National Health Service reference costs and University of Kent's Unit Costs of Health and Social Care 2011 and inflated to 2013 using the UK Consumer Price Index. Procedure supply costs were obtained from the manufacturer. Difference in mean costs was compared using nonparametric bootstrapping. All costs were converted to US dollars using the Organisation for Economic Co-operation and Development Purchasing Power Parity Index.

Results.—Overall mean cost (SD) for managing patients with IPCs and talc pleurodesis was $4,993 ($5,529) and $4,581 ($4,359), respectively.

The incremental mean cost difference was $401, with 95% CI of –$1,387 to $2,261. The mean cost related to ongoing drainage in the IPC group was $1,011 ($732) vs $57 ($213) in the talc pleurodesis group (P =.001). This included the cost of drainage bottles, dressing changes in the first month, and catheter removal. There was no significant difference in cost of the initial intervention or adverse events between the groups. For patients with survival <14 weeks, IPC is significantly less costly than talc pleurodesis, with mean cost difference of –$1,719 (95% CI, –$3,376 to –$85).

Conclusions.—There is no significant difference in the mean cost of managing patients with IPCs compared with talc pleurodesis. For patients with limited survival, IPC appears less costly.

Trial Registry.—isrctn.org; No.: ISRCTN87514420; URL: www.isrctn.org (Table 4).

▶ In this study published in *Chest*, the authors compare the medical costs associated with indwelling pleural catheters (IPC) vs talc pleurodesis for the management of malignant pleural effusions. In this UK study, cost data from the TIME 2 trial was obtained and compared. This trial found no significant difference between the 2 techniques in terms of symptom management, although more complications were noted in the IPC group.

In the cost analysis (Table 4), on average IPC costs $401 more than talc pleurodesis, which is not significant. The cost analysis actually favors IPC if survival is less than 14 weeks. The difference is made up by drainage-associated costs in the long term in the IPC vs upfront hospital cost in the talc pleurodesis group. If patients require significant weekly nursing support for IPC, the pre-14-week benefit is lost. The authors conclude that, in the end, barring the special situations noted here, choice of procedure should be based on preference after discussion of risks and benefits.

C. D. Spradley, MD

Pulmonary Vascular Disease

The Right Ventricle Explains Sex Differences in Survival in Idiopathic Pulmonary Arterial Hypertension

Jacobs W, van de Veerdonk MC, Trip P, et al (VU Univ Med Centre, Amsterdam, The Netherlands; et al)

Chest 145:1230-1236, 2014

Background.—Male sex is an independent predictor of worse survival in pulmonary arterial hypertension (PAH). This finding might be explained by more severe pulmonary vascular disease, worse right ventricular (RV) function, or different response to therapy. The aim of this study was to investigate the underlying cause of sex differences in survival in patients treated for PAH.

Methods.—This was a retrospective cohort study of 101 patients with PAH (82 idiopathic, 15 heritable, four anorexigen associated) who were diagnosed at VU University Medical Centre between February 1999 and

January 2011 and underwent right-sided heart catheterization and cardiac MRI to assess RV function. Change in pulmonary vascular resistance (PVR) was taken as a measure of treatment response in the pulmonary vasculature, whereas change in RV ejection fraction (RVEF) was used to assess RV response to therapy.

Results.—PVR and RVEF were comparable between men and women at baseline; however, male patients had a worse transplant-free survival compared with female patients ($P = .002$). Although male and female patients showed a similar reduction in PVR after 1 year, RVEF improved in female patients, whereas it deteriorated in male patients. In a mediator analysis, after correcting for confounders, 39.0% of the difference in transplant-free survival between men and women was mediated through changes in RVEF after initiating PAH medical therapies.

Conclusions.—This study suggests that differences in RVEF response with initiation of medical therapy in idiopathic PAH explain a significant portion of the worse survival seen in men.

▶ In this intriguing single-center observational study by Jacobs and colleagues published in *Chest*, the authors explore response to therapy and sex differences in survival in pulmonary arterial hypertension (PAH). The data from the study confirmed the frequent observation that men with PAH have poorer survival than matched female subjects. They chose to explore the "why" by comparing response to therapy in terms of change in pulmonary vascular resistance by right heart catheterization and change in right ventricular ejection fraction (RVEF) by cardiac magnetic resonance.

Men had an 87% 1-year and 57% 5-year survival in the study compared with 100% and 85% in women (Fig 1 in the original article). There was no difference in change in pulmonary vascular resistance between the groups but women had improvement in RVEF, and men demonstrated decline. Fundamentally, the female right ventricle seemed to respond to pharmacotherapy, whereas the male RV did not. This study confirms that men are the weaker sex and hints that it may be the result of women having stronger hearts. Additional studies are needed to evaluate the pathophysiology associated with the difference identified.

C. D. Spradley, MD

Pharmacologic Therapy for Pulmonary Arterial Hypertension in Adults: CHEST Guideline and Expert Panel Report

Taichman DB, Ornelas J, Chung L, et al (Univ of Pennsylvania, Philadelphia; CHEST, Glenview, IL; Stanford Univ and Palo Alto VA Health Care System; et al)

Chest 146:449-475, 2014

Objective.—Choices of pharmacologic therapies for pulmonary arterial hypertension (PAH) are ideally guided by high-level evidence. The objective of this guideline is to provide clinicians advice regarding pharmacologic therapy for adult patients with PAH as informed by available evidence.

Methods.—This guideline was based on systematic reviews of English language evidence published between 1990 and November 2013, identified using the MEDLINE and Cochrane Library databases. The strength of available evidence was graded using the Grades of Recommendations, Assessment, Development, and Evaluation methodology. Guideline recommendations, or consensus statements when available evidence was insufficient to support recommendations, were developed using a modified Delphi technique to achieve consensus.

Results.—Available evidence is limited in its ability to support high-level recommendations. Therefore, we drafted consensus statements to address many clinical questions regarding pharmacotherapy for patients with PAH. A total of 79 recommendations or consensus statements were adopted and graded.

Conclusions.—Clinical decisions regarding pharmacotherapy for PAH should be guided by high-level recommendations when sufficient evidence is available. Absent higher level evidence, consensus statements based upon available information must be used. Further studies are needed to address the gaps in available knowledge regarding optimal pharmacotherapy for PAH.

▶ In August, Taichman and colleagues published the CHEST Guideline and Expert Panel on pharmacologic treatment of pulmonary arterial hypertension (PAH). The guideline provides 79 separate graded recommendations, which are essentially the summary of clinical trial results available to date. It makes for a laborious read but does provide a "one-stop shop" for guidance concerning PAH therapy based on the evidence.

The authors emphasize the importance of early involvement of PAH experts in collaboration with local physicians. They also strongly endorse vasoreactivity testing and calcium-channel blockade in the appropriate patients. They warn against advanced therapy in asymptomatic individuals and endorse the treatment of contributing factors such as sleep-disordered breathing. They advise the use of intravenous prostanoid therapy in patients presenting with class 4 symptoms.

Additional recommendations include the initiation of combination therapy in patients with inadequate clinical response (class III and IV) despite monotherapy, as well as consideration for triple therapy should the same scenario play out in combination. The guideline provides recommendations for most therapies currently available on the US market with the notable singular exception of oral treprostinil.

They endorse pregnancy prevention and referral to high-risk centers for those who get pregnant. The guideline also endorses oxygen supplementation when necessary at altitude, vaccination, and avoidance of elective surgical procedures. When necessary, surgeries should be performed at a PAH center using a multidisciplinary team including cardiac anesthesia.

The guideline provides a thorough and useful (if dry) reference for guiding clinical therapy in PAH.

C. D. Spradley, MD

Fibrinolysis for Patients with Intermediate-Risk Pulmonary Embolism

Meyer G, for the PEITHO Investigators (Université Paris Descartes, France)
N Engl J Med 370:1402-1411, 2014

Background.—The role of fibrinolytic therapy in patients with intermediate-risk pulmonary embolism is controversial.

Methods.—In a randomized, double-blind trial, we compared tenecteplase plus heparin with placebo plus heparin in normotensive patients with intermediate-risk pulmonary embolism. Eligible patients had right ventricular dysfunction on echocardiography or computed tomography, as well as myocardial injury as indicated by a positive test for cardiac troponin I or troponin T. The primary outcome was death or hemodynamic decompensation (or collapse) within 7 days after randomization. The main safety outcomes were major extracranial bleeding and ischemic or hemorrhagic stroke within 7 days after randomization.

Results.—Of 1006 patients who underwent randomization, 1005 were included in the intentionto- treat analysis. Death or hemodynamic decompensation occurred in 13 of 506 patients (2.6%) in the tenecteplase group as compared with 28 of 499 (5.6%) in the placebo group (odds ratio, 0.44; 95% confidence interval, 0.23 to 0.87; $P = 0.02$). Between randomization and day 7, a total of 6 patients (1.2%) in the tenecteplase group and 9 (1.8%) in the placebo group died ($P = 0.42$). Extracranial bleeding occurred in 32 patients (6.3%) in the tenecteplase group and 6 patients (1.2%) in the placebo group ($P < 0.001$). Stroke occurred in 12 patients (2.4%) in the tenecteplase group and was hemorrhagic in 10 patients; 1 patient (0.2%) in the placebo group had a stroke, which was hemorrhagic ($P = 0.003$). By day 30, a total of 12 patients (2.4%) in the tenecteplase group and 16 patients (3.2%) in the placebo group had died ($P = 0.42$).

Conclusions.—In patients with intermediate-risk pulmonary embolism, fibrinolytic therapy prevented hemodynamic decompensation but increased the risk of major hemorrhage and stroke. (Funded by the Programme Hospitalier de Recherche Clinique in France and others; PEITHO EudraCT number, 2006-005328-18; ClinicalTrials.gov number, NCT00639743.)

▶ In the largest study of its kind to date, the PEITHO investigators addressed the role of fibrinolytic therapy in patients with intermediate-risk venous thromboembolism (VTE). Their findings were published in April in the *New England Journal of Medicine*.

Intermediate risk was defined as echocardiographic or computed tomography findings of right ventricular dysfunction and laboratory evidence of myocardial injury. All 1006 patients were hemodynamically stable at randomization. They then received either weight-based tenecteplase plus heparin or heparin plus placebo. By day 7, 13 patients in the treatment arm and 28 patients in the placebo group reached the primary endpoint of death from any cause or hemodynamic decompensation. This was countered, however, by the increased risk of bleeding at day 7 encountered by the intervention group (Fig 1 in the original article).

The authors' conclusion was that, although the primary endpoint favored the use of tenecteplase, it was at the expense of increased major bleeding. This is especially important because the component of the primary endpoint responsible for the majority of the effect way hypotension (systolic blood pressure of < 90 mm Hg), which is of questionable clinical significance. It is important to note that, as was seen in other studies of fibrinolysis, risk of bleeding is significantly higher in patients over 75 years of age.

The bottom line: In patients with intermediate risk VTE, you can choose to use a thrombolytic, but proceed with caution.

C. D. Spradley, MD

5 Community-Acquired Pneumonia

Introduction

Community-acquired pneumonia (CAP) is a very common, serious, and potentially lethal illness across the population. Its incidence increases with age, which means that as the population in the United States ages, the costs of managing CAP will increase dramatically. A recent study of Medicare fee-for-service patients hospitalized with healthcare-associated pneumonia and CAP illustrates the cost of this disease. Medicare patients hospitalized with pneumonia were estimated to have an excess cost over similar patients who did not get pneumonia of at least $7 billion.[1]

The first group of articles this year addresses various risk factor elements for pneumonia admission and readmission. Dang et al followed, prospectively for 5 years, a population-based cohort of hospitalized pneumonia patients to identify risk factors for readmission throughout the 5-year period. A different, but equally important, question was addressed by Prescott et al. They looked at 30-day readmissions to determine the diagnosis for readmission and found that less than half were for pneumonia, thus illustrating the issues around co-morbidities in pneumonia patients. A different, but increasingly common, area of risk is the risk for aspiration. Lee et al analyzed a group of patients hospitalized with aspiration to create a profile of risk for this disease.

Diagnosis is another important area of research, especially since as many as half of CAP cases never receive a definitive diagnosis. This means that treatment is often empiric, an approach that usually works but likely exacerbates the antibiotic resistance problem. In the diagnostic arena, Hakki et al published a study addressing the use of nasopharyngeal swabs to identify viral causes of pneumonia by correlating swab results with bronchoalveolar lavage. The importance of looking for viral etiologies is illustrated in the study by Karhu et al, who found that, with an aggressive search for organism, up to 50% of ventilated patients with pneumonia had a viral etiology. Another important study in diagnostics was published by Lee J et al, whose group identified a model to predict which patients with pneumonia are likely to be bacteremic. This model can be used to identify those who need blood cultures or do not.

Pneumococcal disease remains the most common bacterial cause of CAP even in the era of conjugate vaccines. With the recent introduction of PCV 13, Tam et al looked at whether invasive disease was decreasing across the population as it had with PCV 7. It is still early, but it seems to be happening. However, it is not yet clear whether non-covered strains will increase in prevalence. Most of the strains not covered by the vaccine are considered to be relatively mild in virulence. However, somewhat disturbing is the finding by Syk et al of a mutant in a laboratory train of serotype 1 streptococcus pneumonia that increases the virulence of that serotype 1.

Comorbidities can greatly complicate the management of CAP, especially in older patients. Included are 2 articles addressing cardiovascular events. Mortensen et al attempted to address the literature controversy involving the use of azithromycin and an increase in cardiovascular events. Their study of Veteran's Administration patients concluded that the overall benefit in survival with the use of azithromycin justifies its use. Cardiovascular events have been associated in general with episodes of pneumonia. Cangemi et al have tried to explain this association and found that platelet activation factors are very elevated in those patients with clinical evidence of myocardial infarction, suggesting a possible association between pneumonia and activation of platelets resulting in cardiovascular events.

Other articles that present new information to help in management of CAP include a prospective study community onset of bacteremic acinetobacter pneumonia, a review of the etiology and outcome of community-acquired infections in HIV-infected patients, the use of biologic therapies in Legionellosis, and macrolide/azalide therapy for nodular/bronchiectatic mycobacterium avium complex lung disease.

Finally, I have included an article about a new approach to developing a vaccine against staphylococcus aureus. Spaulding et al have found a vaccine directed against secreted rather than cell surface virulence factors that is having some success in laboratory animals. A vaccine against staphylococcal infections would be a great advance; hopefully, this approach will succeed.

Janet R. Mauer, MD, MBA

Reference

1. Thomas CP, Ryan M, Chapman JD, et al. Incidence and cost of pneumonia in medicare beneficiaries. *Chest*. 2012;172:973-981.

Rates and Risk Factors for Recurrent Pneumonia in Patients Hospitalized With Community-Acquired Pneumonia: Population-Based Prospective Cohort Study With 5 Years of Follow-up

Dang TT, Eurich DT, Weir DL, et al (Univ of Alberta, Edmonton, Canada; et al)
Clin Infect Dis 59:74-80, 2014

Background.—The rates and risk factors for developing *recurrent* pneumonia following hospitalization with community-acquired pneumonia (CAP) are poorly understood.

Methods.—We examined a population-based cohort of patients with CAP who survived hospital admission and who were free of pneumonia for at least 3 months. We collected clinical, functional, and medication-related information and pneumonia severity index (PSI). Using linked databases we followed patients for 5 years and captured any clinical episode of pneumonia 90 days or more post-discharge. We used Cox proportional hazards models (adjusted for age, sex, PSI, functional status, medications) to determine rates and independent correlates of recurrent pneumonia.

Results.—The final cohort included 2709 inpatients; 43% were 75 years or older, 34% were not fully independent, and 56% had severe pneumonia. Over 5 years of follow—up, 245 (9%; 95% confidence interval [CI], 8%—10%) patients developed recurrent pneumonia, and 156 (64%) of these episodes required hospitalization. Rate of recurrence was 3.0/100 person—years and median time to recurrence was 317 days (interquartile range, 177—569); 32 (13%) patients had 2 or more recurrences. In multivariable analyses only age > 75 years (adjusted $P = .047$) and less than fully independent functional status (12% recurrence rate with impaired functional status vs 7% for fully independent; adjusted hazard ratio, 1.7; 95% CI, 1.3—2.2; $P < .001$) were significantly associated with recurrent pneumonia.

Conclusions.—One of 11 patients who survived CAP hospitalization had recurrent pneumonia over 5 years and those with impaired functional status were at particularly high risk. Recurrent pneumonia is common and more attention to preventive strategies at discharge and closer follow-up over the long-term seem warranted (Fig 1).

▶ The problem of recurrent community-acquired pneumonia (CAP) has been sparsely studied. The authors postulated that it would be valuable to have a more complete picture of the rates of and risks for recurrent pneumonia over a

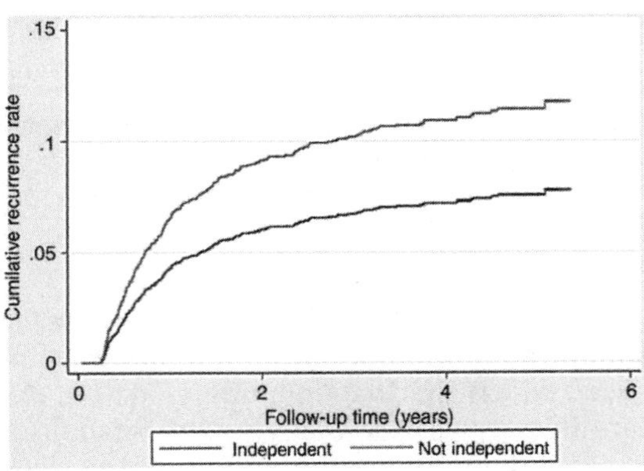

FIGURE 1.—Rates of recurrent pneumonia according to functional status: cumulative incidence curves. (Reprinted from Dang TT, Eurich DT, Weir DL, et al. Rates and risk factors for recurrent pneumonia in patients hospitalized with community-acquired pneumonia: population-based prospective cohort study with 5 years of follow-up. *Clin Infect Dis.* 2014;59:74-80, by permission of the Infectious Diseases Society of America.)

5-year period. Existing studies of recurrent pneumonia were found to have limitations in terms of population size, nonrepresentative populations, lack of clinical detail, and short follow-up periods, among other things. The potential benefit of having a clearer picture of those at risk of recurrent disease would be 2-fold: to apprise patients of the risk and to put into place measures that might help prevent the recurrence. Only age > 75 years and impaired functional status were associated significantly with recurrent disease (Fig 1). Typical risk factors for an initial event of CAP include medical comorbidities or use of certain types of medications, but these were not identified as risks for recurrence. The authors point out that previous research has shown that it is relatively common to identify different risk factors for the recurrence of an event than for the initial episode.[1] An explanation for this is that a high percentage of the cohort would be defined as high risk for the initial event; those developing recurrence would likely fall within a subset of the initial risk factors. The median time to recurrence was almost a year. Within 90 days of discharge, 2% of patients had recurrences or relapses (and were excluded from this study); these tended to be in people with heart failure or chronic obstructive pulmonary disorder. The limitations of this study are that the data documenting recurrences were via an administrative database linked to the original episode's clinical radiographic documentation. Thus, detailed clinical information in reference to the recurrent episode was not used; recurrences could therefore have been miscoded or misclassified as pneumonia when, in fact, they were actually a different clinical condition. Finally, the risk factors were not updated during the 5-year follow-up, so patients may have developed new risks that are not recorded in the study. Nevertheless, this is the most complete study of recurrent CAP to date and will hopefully help physicians better manage their pneumonia patients.

J. R. Maurer, MD

Reference

1. Dahabreh IJ, Kent DM. Index event bias as an explanation for the paradoxes of recurrence risk research. *JAMA*. 2011;305:822-823.

Diagnoses of Early and Late Readmissions after Hospitalization for Pneumonia: A Systematic Review

Prescott HC, Sjoding MW, Iwashyna TJ (Univ of Michigan, Ann Arbor)
Ann Am Thorac Soc 11:1091-1100, 2014

Rationale.—Pneumonia is a frequent cause of hospitalization, yet drivers of post-pneumonia morbidity remain poorly characterized. Causes of hospital readmissions may elucidate important sources of morbidity and are of particular interest given the U.S. Hospital Readmission Reductions Program.

Objectives.—To review the primary diagnoses of early (≤30 d) and late (≥31 d) readmissions after pneumonia hospitalization.

Methods.—Systematic review of MEDLINE, Embase, and CINAHL databases. We identified original research studies of adults aged 18 years or older, hospitalized for pneumonia, and for whom cause-specific readmission rates were reported. Two authors abstracted study results and assessed study quality.

Measurements and Main Results.—Of the 1,243 citations identified, 12 met eligibility criteria. Included studies were conducted in the United States, Spain, Canada, Croatia, and Sweden. All-cause 30-day readmission rates ranged from 16.8 to 20.1% across administrative studies; the weighted average for the studies using chart review was 11.6% (15.6% in United States-based studies). Pneumonia, heart failure/cardiovascular causes, and chronic obstructive pulmonary disease/pulmonary causes are the most common reasons for early readmission after pneumonia hospitalization. Although it was the single most common cause for readmission, pneumonia accounted for only 17.9 to 29.4% of all 30-day readmissions in administrative studies and a weighted average of 23.0% in chart review studies. After accounting for study population, there was no clear difference in findings between claims-based versus chart-review studies. Few studies assessed readmissions beyond 30 days, although the limited available data suggest similar primary diagnoses for early and late readmissions. No studies assessed whether reasons for readmission were similar to patients' reasons for healthcare use before hospitalization.

Conclusions.—Pneumonia, heart failure/cardiovascular disease, and chronic obstructive pulmonary disease/pulmonary disease are the most common readmission diagnoses after pneumonia hospitalization. Although pneumonia was the most common readmission diagnosis, it accounted for only a minority of all readmissions. Late readmission diagnoses are less thoroughly described, and further research is needed to understand how hospitalization for pneumonia fits within the broader context of patients' health trajectory.

▶ The article in this section by Dang et al addresses timing and rates of recurrence of community-acquired pneumonia. This systematic review by Prescott et al asks a similar, but quite different, question: What are the diagnoses for which patients are readmitted after an admission for pneumonia? As has been noted in other studies[1-3] only a minority—less than one-third—of the readmissions either within 30 days of discharge or later after discharge are for recurrent or relapsed pneumonia. Many of the readmissions especially within the first 30 days of discharge are attributed to heart failure or other cardiac issues and preexisting pulmonary disease. In many cases, it is likely the physiological stress and inflammatory milieu of the pneumonia was a major contributor to the considerable worsening of these comorbid conditions that required admissions for management. Interestingly, the major reasons for readmission beyond 30 days was not different from readmissions within 30 days. With the Centers for Medicare and Medicaid Services' keen focus on readmission for any cause within 30 days and current penalties ranging up to $1 million for early readmissions, studies such as this help us better understand the importance of being aware of and addressing as optimally as possible all the patient comorbidities. However, sometimes deterioration is hard to predict, and so instituting early follow-up in patients with underlying heart and lung disease postdischarge is essential.

J. R. Maurer, MD

References

1. Dharmarajan K, Hsieh AF, Lin Z, et al. Diagnoses and timing of 30-day readmissions after hospitalization for heart failure, acute myocardial infarction, or pneumonia. *JAMA*. 2013;309:355-363.
2. Jasti H, Mortensen EM, Obrosky DS, Kapoor WN, Fine MJ. Causes and risk factors for rehospitalization of patients hospitalized with community-acquired pneumonia. *Clin Infect Dis*. 2008;46:550-556.
3. Dang TT, Eurich DT, Weir DL, Marrie TJ, Majumdar SR. Rates and risk factors for recurrent pneumonia in patients hospitalized with community-acquired pneumonia: population-based prospective cohort study with 5 years of follow-up. *Clin Infect Dis*. 2014;59:74-80.

Characteristics and Outcomes of Patients Hospitalized Following Pulmonary Aspiration

Lee A, the United States Critical Illness and Injury Trials Group (Mayo Clinic Florida, Jacksonville; et al)
Chest 146:899-907, 2014

Background.—Pulmonary aspiration is an important recognized cause of ARDS. Better characterization of patients who aspirate may allow identification of potential risks for aspiration that could be used in future studies to mitigate the occurrence of aspiration and its devastating complications.

Methods.—We conducted a secondary analysis of the Lung Injury Prediction Score cohort to better characterize patients with aspiration, including their potential risk factors and related outcomes.

Results.—Of the 5,584 subjects at risk for ARDS and who required hospitalization, 212 (3.8%) presented with aspiration. Subjects who aspirated were likely to be male (66% vs 56%, $P < .007$), slightly older (59 years vs 57 years), white (73% vs 61%, $P = .0004$), admitted from a nursing home (15% vs 5.9%, $P < .0001$), have a history of alcohol abuse (21% vs 8%, $P < .0001$), and have lower Glasgow Coma Scale (median, 13 vs 15; $P < .0001$). Aspiration subjects were sicker (higher APACHE [Acute Physiology and Chronic Health Evaluation] II score), required more mechanical ventilation (54% vs 32%, $P < .0001$), developed more moderate to severe ARDS (12% vs 3.8%, $P < .0001$), and were twofold more likely to die in-hospital, even after adjustment for severity of illness (OR = 2.1; 95% CI, 1.2-3.6). Neither obesity nor gastroesophageal reflux was associated with aspiration.

Conclusions.—Aspiration was more common in men with alcohol abuse history and a lower Glasgow Coma Scale who were admitted from a nursing home. It is independently associated with a significant increase in the risk for ARDS as well as morbidity and mortality. Findings from this study may facilitate the design of future clinical studies of aspiration-induced lung injury.

▶ The Lung Injury Prediction Score (LIPS) is a tool published in 2009 and validated in 2011 in which a number of factors are used to identify patients at high risk of developing acute respiratory distress syndrome (ARDS).[1] The tool includes 14 elements that are scored as either "yes" or "no" depending on whether the patient has that element. If the score is "yes," then a point value is assigned. One of the elements (or risk factors) in the LIPS is aspiration. Because aspiration was identified as a predictor of ARDS when the LIPS was developed, the authors decided to better characterize the patients who fit into this group using the original LIPS cohort patients. The goal was to "identify the burden of illness, consequences of aspiration, and risk factors associated with aspiration." The stated purpose is to use the data to generate hypotheses to support design of future clinical trials on aspiration and eventually to identify potential therapeutic targets aimed at reducing aspiration-related lung injury. Hopefully, the promise of prospective clinical trials in this highly morbid condition will be realized in the near future.

J. R. Maurer, MD

Reference

1. Gajic O, Dabbagh O, Park PK, et al; U.S. Critical Illness and Injury Trials Group, Lung Injury Prevention Study Investigators (USCIITG-LIPS). Early identification of patients at risk of acute lung injury: evaluation of lung injury prediction score in a multicenter cohort study. *Am J Respir Crit Care Med.* 2011;183:462-470.

Predictive Value of Testing Nasopharyngeal Samples for Respiratory Viruses in the Setting of Lower Respiratory Tract Disease

Hakki M, Strasfeld LM, Townes JM (Oregon Health and Science Univ, Portland)
J Clin Microbiol 52:4020-4022, 2014

To determine the predictive value of nasopharyngeal (NP) sample testing for respiratory viruses (RVs) in suspected lower respiratory tract disease, 72 paired NP and bronchoalveolar lavage (BAL) fluid specimen sets, mostly from transplant recipients or patients with hematologic malignancies, were analyzed. Overall, 31.3% of the specimens tested positive for an RV. In 19 sets (26.4%), the NP and BAL fluid specimens were both positive for an RV; in 3 sets (4.2%), the NP specimens were positive but the BAL fluid specimens were negative; and in 3 other sets, the NP specimens were negative but the BAL fluid specimens were positive. The positive and negative predictive values of the NP specimens were 86.4% and 94%, respectively.

▶ Polymerase chain reaction-based testing has made respiratory virus testing easy, accurate, and quick. Virus found in the nasopharynx may correlate with lower respiratory tract disease and can potentially reduce the need for more invasive approaches, such as bronchoscopy, for diagnosis of lower respiratory tract infections. In addition, the diagnosis can be achieved more quickly. The issue is this: How good is the correlation of nasopharyngeal findings with the organism(s) in the lower respiratory tract? Most correlation studies have focused on specific viruses or specific types of patients, and the results probably cannot be generalized to other situations. In this study, the authors retrospectively reviewed a series of patient data in which bronchoscopy was used to collect lavage fluid that was tested for viruses and nasopharyngeal swabs were also performed, although not necessarily at the same time. The correlation was very good. However, the retrospective nature of this study, the nonconcurrent collection of the specimens, and failure to protect against contamination of the lower respiratory tract by nasopharyngeal secretions with nasal passage of the bronchoscope make the data less compelling. A future prospective study would be useful; if these findings are confirmed, many bronchoscopies could be avoided, and patient stress and costs could be decreased.

J. R. Maurer, MD

Lower Respiratory Tract Virus Findings in Mechanically Ventilated Patients With Severe Community-Acquired Pneumonia

Karhu J, Ala-Kokko TI, Vuorinen T, et al (Oulu Univ Hosp, Finland; Univ of Turku, Finland)

Clin Infect Dis 59:62-70, 2014

Background.—The role of viral infections in the etiology of severe community-acquired pneumonia (SCAP) was prospectively evaluated from 2008 to 2012 at a university-level intensive care unit.

Methods.—Clinical data and microbiological tests were assessed: blood cultures, urine pneumococcal and legionella antigens, *Mycoplasma pneumoniae and Chlamydia pneumoniae* antibodies from paired serums, and respiratory virus detection by multiplex, real-time polymerase chain reaction (PCR) from nasopharyngeal swabs and lower tracheal specimens via intubation tube.

Results.—Of 49 mechanically ventilated SCAP patients (21 men and 28 women; median age, 54 years), the etiology was identified in 45 cases (92%). There were 21 pure bacterial infections (43%), 5 probably pure viral infections (10%), and 19 mixed bacterial-viral infections (39%), resulting in viral etiology in 24 patients (49%). Of 26 viruses, 21 (81%) were detected from bronchial specimens and 5 (19%) from nasopharyngeal swabs. Rhinovirus (15 cases, 58%) and adenovirus (4 cases, 15%) were the most common viral findings. The bacterial-viral etiology group had the highest peak C-reactive protein levels (median, 356 [25th-75th percentiles, 294-416], $P = .05$), whereas patients with probably viral etiology had the lowest peak procalcitonin levels (1.7 [25th-75th percentiles, 1.6–1.7]). The clinical characteristics of pure bacterial and mixed bacterial-viral etiologies were comparable. Hospital stay was longest among the bacterial group (17 vs 14 days; $P = .02$).

Conclusions.—Viral findings were demonstrated in almost half of the SCAP patients. Clinical characteristics were similar between the pure bacterial and mixed bacterial-viral infections groups. The frequency of viral detection depends on the availability of PCR techniques and lower respiratory specimens.

▶ Common bacterial pathogens in patients with community-acquired pneumonia (CAP) have been described and incorporated into the accepted guidelines for management of this disease.[1] The most common of these organisms is *Streptococcus* pneumonia. Most initial therapy is directed toward this organism and the organisms are common in younger patients, *Mycoplasma pneumonia* and *Chlamydia pneumonia.* Although viruses are thought to be responsible for a significant percentage of CAP cases, the epidemiology and distribution of these cases is less studied. Unless influenza is suspected, antiviral therapy is rarely used in initial treatment. More than 50% of CAP cases are treated in the outpatient setting, and many of those never receive a specific etiologic diagnosis. The more severe cases that are admitted to hospital—also many without a specific diagnosis—are generally aggressively treated with antibiotics. The assumption is that the vast majority of these are bacterial. In this study, an aggressive approach was taken to determine specific etiologies in the most severe CAP cases, those requiring mechanical ventilation. The surprising finding that up to half of these cases had pure viral or mixed bacterial-viral causes should encourage early use of sophisticated testing, such as molecular diagnostic approaches including polymerase chain reaction tests. Early identification of viral etiologies should help direct more appropriate therapy.

J. R. Maurer, MD

Reference

1. Mandell LA, Wunderink RG, Anzueto A, et al. Infectious Diseases Society of America/American Thoracic Society consensus guidelines on the management of community-acquired pneumonia in adults. *Clin Infect Dis.* 2007;44:S27-S72.

Bacteremia prediction model using a common clinical test in patients with community-acquired pneumonia

Lee J, Hwang SS, Kim K, et al (Seoul Natl Univ Bundang Hosp, Republic of Korea; Inha Univ College of Medicine, Incheon South Korea)
Am J Emerg Med 32:700-704, 2014

Purpose.—The aim of this study was to construct a bacteremia prediction model using commonly available clinical variables in hospitalized patients with community-acquired pneumonia (CAP).

Basic Procedures.—A prospective database including patients who were diagnosed with CAP in the emergency department was analyzed. Independent risk factors were investigated by using multivariable analysis in

60% of the cohort. We assigned a weighted value to predictive factor and made a prediction rule. This model was validated both internally and externally with the remaining 40% of the cohort and a cohort from an independent hospital. The *low-risk group for bacteremia* was defined as patients who have a risk of bacteremia less than 3%.

Main Findings.—A total of 2422 patients were included in this study. The overall rate of bacteremia was 5.7% in the cohort. The significant factors for predicting bacteremia were the following 7 variables: systolic blood pressure less than 90 mm Hg, heart rate greater than 125 beats per minute, body temperature less than 35 °C or greater than 40 °C, white blood cell less than 4000 or 12,000 cells per microliter, platelets less than 130,000 cells per microliter, albumin less than 3.3 g/dL, and C-reactive protein greater than 17 mg/dL. After using our prediction rule for the validation cohorts, 78.7% and 74.8% of the internal and external validation cohorts were classified as low-risk bacteremia groups. The areas under the receiver operating characteristic curves were 0.75 and 0.79 for the internal and external validation cohorts.

Principal Conclusions.—This model could provide guidelines for whether to perform blood cultures for hospitalized CAP patients with the goal of reducing the number of blood cultures.

▶ Blood cultures are usually not performed in patients presenting with community-acquired pneumonia (CAP) because most patients will not be bacteremic and can be effectively treated as outpatients without blood cultures. The decision about whether to draw blood cultures becomes more difficult when the patient is moderately, but not severely, ill. The Infectious Diseases Society of America/American Thoracic Society consensus guidelines on the management of community-acquired pneumonia in adults provides guidelines for identifying risk factors that warrant drawing blood cultures.[1] However, using these guidelines results in many negative blood cultures.[2] The purpose of this study was to produce a more useful model to predict bacteremia in patients with CAP that would further reduce the number of unnecessary blood cultures. Seven variables were identified in a prospective cohort of patients, 60% of whom were used to identify the variables and 40% of whom, along with a cohort from another hospital, were used to validate the model. The model should be validated in other populations in other geographic areas. It may be a useful start to further reducing the number of unnecessary blood cultures in CAP patients in whom the results are rarely used for management and the study is both costly and uncomfortable for the patient.

J. R. Maurer, MD

References

1. Mandell LA, Wunderink RG, Anzueto A, et al. Infectious Diseases Society of America/American Thoracic Society consensus guidelines on the management of community-acquired pneumonia in adults. *Clin Infect Dis*. 2007;44:S27-S72.
2. Falguera M, Trujillano J, Caro S, et al. A prediction rule for estimating the risk of bacteremia in patients with community-acquired pneumonia. *Clin Infect Dis*. 2009;49:409-416.

Invasive Pneumococcal Disease After Implementation of 13-Valent Conjugate Vaccine

Iroh Tam P-Y, Madoff LC, Coombes B, et al (Univ of Minnesota Children's Hosp, Minneapolis; Massachusetts Dept of Public Health, Boston; Univ of Minnesota, Minneapolis; et al)

Pediatrics 134:210-217, 2014

Objective.—To examine whether there is a different clinical profile and severity of invasive pneumococcal disease (IPD) in children caused by non-vaccine types in the era of 13-valent pneumococcal conjugate vaccine (PCV13).

Methods.—Observational study of childhood IPD in Massachusetts based on state public health surveillance data comparing pre-PCV13 (2007–2009) and post-PCV13 (2010–2012) eras.

Results.—There were 168 pre-PCV13 cases of IPD and 85 post-PCV13 cases of IPD in Massachusetts children ≤5 years of age. PCV13 serotypes declined by 18% in the first 2 years after PCV13 use ($P = .011$). In the post-PCV13 phase, a higher proportion of children were hospitalized (57.6% vs 50.6%), and a higher proportion of children had comorbidity (23.5% vs 19.6%). Neither difference was statistically significant, nor were comparisons of IPD caused by vaccine and nonvaccine types. Children with comorbidities had higher rates of IPD caused by a nonvaccine type (27.6% vs 17.2%; $P = .085$), were more likely to be hospitalized (80.4% vs 50%; $P < .0001$), and were more likely to have a longer hospital stay (median of 3 days vs 0.5 days; $P = .0001$).

Conclusions.—Initial data suggest that nonvaccine serotypes are more common in children with underlying conditions, who have greater morbidity from disease. In the post-PCV13 era, a larger proportion of patients are hospitalized, but mortality rates are unchanged. Routine vaccination with PCV13 may not be enough to reduce the risk in patients with comorbidity.

▶ When 7-valent conjugate vaccine against *Streptococcus* pneumonia (PCV7) was introduced in 2000, the numbers of invasive pneumococcal disease decreased considerably in the United States. It decreased specifically, not only with respect to the 7 vaccine serotypes, but also overall. Even though it was only given to young children, invasive disease also decreased in adults. However, subsequently, invasive disease from nonvaccine serotypes increased, and the population at risk shifted to include a greater proportion of children with chronic illness. Subsequently in 2010, 13-valent conjugate vaccine (PCV13) was introduced to cover both the initial 7 serotypes included in PCV7 as well as 6 additional clinically relevant serotypes that had become more prevalent after the widespread uptake of PCV7. The most important of the included serotypes were 19A, 7F, and 6A. A number of serotypes are not covered by PCV13 and are thought to be less virulent. It is expected that less invasive pneumococcal disease will be seen in the era of PCV13, but it is not known whether some of the not-covered serotypes will "fill the void" and cause more invasive disease, as happened after the introduction of PCV7. So the objective of this study was both to look at the clinical picture and outcomes of invasive pneumococcal disease in young children in Massachusetts and to examine the epidemiology of invasive disease and differences before and after PCV13. Although the data in this study are from early after the introduction of the new vaccine, it does not show nearly the impact of the initiation of PCV7 as might be expected. What it does show is a higher rate of invasive disease in patients with comorbidities and who received PCV13 and a high requirement for hospitalization. The authors recommend administering 23-valent polysaccharide vaccine to these higher risk children in addition to the PCV13. The behavior and impact of PCV13 noncovered serotypes in the post-PCV13 era is not yet clearly defined.

J. R. Maurer, MD

Emergence of Hypervirulent Mutants Resistant to Early Clearance During Systemic Serotype 1 Pneumococcal Infection in Mice and Humans

Syk A, Norman M, Fernebro J, et al (Karolinska Univ Hosp, Stockholm, Sweden)

J Infect Dis 210:4-13, 2014

Background.—Streptococcus pneumoniae serotype 1 has a high likelihood of causing invasive disease. Serotype 1 isolates belonging to CC228 are associated with low mortality, while CC217 isolates exhibit high mortality in patients.

Methods.—Clinical pneumococcal isolates and mutants were evaluated in wild-type C57BL/6 mice, macrophagedepleted mice, neutrophil-depleted mice, and SIGN-R1 knockout mice. In vitro models included binding and phagocytosis by THP-1 cells, capsule measurements, hydrogen peroxide production, and viability assays.

Results.—During early systemic infection in mice with serotype 1, large-colony variants appeared in blood. Similar large colonies were found in blood specimens from patients with invasive disease. Large morphotypes contained higher numbers of viable bacteria, grew faster, produced no or little hydrogen peroxide, and contained mutations in the *spxB* gene. *spxB* mutants were considerably more virulent in wild-type mice, less susceptible to early host clearance than wild-type strains after intravenous infection, but impaired in colonization. *spxB* mutants were less efficiently phagocytosed by macrophages than wild-type bacteria, which, in contrast to *spxB* mutants, caused more-severe disease when macrophages or SIGN-R1 were depleted.

Conclusions.—Hypervirulent *spxB* mutants are selected in both mice and patients and are resistant to early macrophage-mediated clearance.

► Serotype 1 *Streptococcus* pneumonia has a high invasive disease potential in humans and can cause infections in otherwise healthy individuals. In many parts of the world, it is among the top 5 disease-causing serotypes. However, infections with this serotype have generally been reported to be relatively mild and to cause few or no fatalities. Most *Streptococcus* pneumonia have a spxB gene that encodes a pyruvate oxidase and results in endogenous production of hydrogen peroxide, which is potentially suicidal and limits the invasiveness of the bacteria. Mutations in this gene result in bacterial colonies unable to produce hydrogen peroxide and that are potentially larger and more virulent to the host. This type of bacteria has been shown to be more difficult for macrophages to clear. The authors identified this mutation in serotype 1 *Streptococcus* pneumonia. Although the mutation occurs in only a portion of the bacteria and may even be a small number, the mutant bacteria have the potential to be much more virulent or invasive than wild-type bacteria. The potential could be for a change to more aggressive invasive behavior by serotype 1 infections in areas in which this hypervirulent mutant exists and proliferates.

J. R. Maurer, MD

Association of Azithromycin With Mortality and Cardiovascular Events Among Older Patients Hospitalized With Pneumonia

Mortensen EM, Halm EA, Pugh MJ, et al (VA North Texas Health Care System, Dallas, TX; Univ of Texas Southwestern Med Ctr, Dallas; South Texas Veterans Health Care System, San Antonio, TX; et al)

JAMA 311:2199-2208, 2014

Importance.—Although clinical practice guidelines recommend combination therapy with macrolides, including azithromycin, as first-line therapy for patients hospitalized with pneumonia, recent research suggests that azithromycin may be associated with increased cardiovascular events.

Objective.—To examine the association of azithromycin use with all-cause mortality and cardiovascular events for patients hospitalized with pneumonia.

Design.—Retrospective cohort study comparing older patients hospitalized with pneumonia from fiscal years 2002 through 2012 prescribed azithromycin therapy and patients receiving other guideline-concordant antibiotic therapy.

Setting.—This study was conducted using national Department of Veterans Affairs administrative data of patients hospitalized at any Veterans Administration acute care hospital.

Participants.—Patients were included if they were aged 65 years or older, were hospitalized with pneumonia, and received antibiotic therapy concordant with national clinical practice guidelines.

Main Outcomes and Measures.—Outcomes included 30- and 90-day all-cause mortality and 90-day cardiac arrhythmias, heart failure, myocardial infarction, and any cardiac event. Propensity score matching was used to control for the possible effects of known confounders with conditional logistic regression.

Results.—Of 73,690 patients from 118 hospitals identified, propensity-matched groups were composed of 31,863 patients exposed to azithromycin and 31,863 matched patients who were not exposed. There were no significant differences in potential confounders between groups after matching. Ninety-day mortality was significantly lower in those who received azithromycin (exposed, 17.4%, vs unexposed, 22.3%; odds ratio [OR], 0.73; 95% CI, 0.70-0.76). However, we found significantly increased odds of myocardial infarction (5.1% vs 4.4%; OR, 1.17; 95% CI, 1.08-1.25) but not any cardiac event (43.0% vs 42.7%; OR, 1.01; 95% CI, 0.98-1.05), cardiac arrhythmias (25.8% vs 26.0%; OR, 0.99; 95% CI, 0.95-1.02), or heart failure (26.3% vs 26.2%; OR, 1.01; 95% CI, 0.97-1.04).

Conclusions and Relevance.—Among older patients hospitalized with pneumonia, treatment that included azithromycin compared with other antibiotics was associated with a lower risk of 90-day mortality and a smaller increased risk of myocardial infarction. These findings are consistent with a net benefit associated with azithromycin use.

▶ Current guidelines for both outpatient-treated and more severe in-hospital treated community-acquired pneumonia (CAP) recommend macrolides either as single-drug therapy or in combination with other drugs.[1] However, the *New England Journal of Medicine* in 2012 published an article suggesting that azithromycin treatment compared with amoxicillin or ciprofloxacin in a Medicaid population resulted in a higher risk of cardiovascular and all-cause mortality.[2] However, other studies have shown no such association between azithromycin and cardiac mortality.[3,4] The purpose of the study reported here was to "assess the association of azithromycin use and outcomes within 90 days of hospital admission, including cardiovascular events... and mortality, for patients 65 and older who were hospitalized with pneumonia." The authors were particularly interested in trying to determine whether the potential benefits of azithromycin outweighed the potential harms. To do this, they used the Veterans Administration health care administrative and clinical databases of patients hospitalized with pneumonia between October 1, 2001, and September 30, 2012. This provided almost 64 000 almost entirely male patients (98%) over age 65 years, half of whom received azithromycin for their pneumonia and half of whom did not. The authors concluded that the significant survival benefit of azithromycin was a greater benefit than the potential harm of a small increased risk of myocardial infarction that was observed in azithromycin-treated patients. This study does not support the initial 2012 *New England Journal of Medicine* Medicaid study conclusions. However, although this study population was large, it was completely retrospective and therefore should be considered only a starting point for a more definitive randomized prospective study that will put this issue to rest. That study should include a more gender-balanced population that uses clinical data and does not rely solely on *International Classification of Diseases, Ninth Revision,* diagnoses, which are notoriously unreliable.

J. R. Maurer, MD

References

1. Mandell LA, Wunderink RG, Anzueto A, et al. Infectious Diseases Society of America/American Thoracic Society consensus guidelines on the management of community-acquired pneumonia in adults. *Clin Infect Dis.* 2007;44:S27-S72.
2. Ray WA, Murray KT, Hall K, Arbogast PG, Stein CM. Azithromycin and the risk of cardiovascular death. *N Engl J Med.* 2012;366:1881-1890.
3. Svanström H, Pasternak B, Hviid A. Use of azithromycin and death from cardiovascular causes. *N Engl J Med.* 2013;368:1704-1712.
4. O'Connor CM, Dunne MW, Pfeffer MA, et al; Investigators in the WIZARD Study. Azithromycin for the secondary prevention of coronary heart disease events: the WIZARD study: a randomized controlled trial. *JAMA.* 2003;290:1459-1466.

Platelet Activation Is Associated With Myocardial Infarction in Patients With Pneumonia

Cangemi R, in collaboration with the SIXTUS Study Group (Sapienza Univ of Rome, Italy)

J Am Coll Cardiol 64:1917-1925, 2014

Background.—Troponins may be elevated in patients with pneumonia, but associations with myocardial infarction (MI) and with platelet activation are still undefined.

Objectives.—The aim of this study was to investigate the relationship between troponin elevation and in vivo markers of platelet activation in the early phase of hospitalization of patients affected by community-acquired pneumonia.

Methods.—A total of 278 consecutive patients hospitalized for community-acquired pneumonia, who were followed up until discharge, were included. At admission, platelet activation markers such as plasma soluble P-selectin, soluble CD40 ligand, and serum thromboxane B_2 (TxB_2) were measured. Serum high-sensitivity cardiac troponin T levels and electrocardiograms were obtained every 12 and 24 h, respectively.

Results.—Among 144 patients with elevated high-sensitivity cardiac troponin T, 31 had signs of MI and 113 did not. Baseline plasma levels of soluble P-selectin and soluble CD40 ligand and serum TxB_2 were significantly higher in patients who developed signs of MI. Logistic regression analysis showed plasma soluble CD40 ligand ($p < 0.001$) and soluble P-selectin ($p < 0.001$), serum TxB_2 ($p = 0.030$), mean platelet volume ($p = 0.037$), Pneumonia Severity Index score ($p = 0.030$), and ejection fraction ($p = 0.001$) to be independent predictors of MI. There were no significant differences in MI rate between the 123 patients (45%) taking aspirin (100 mg/day) and those who were not aspirin treated (12% vs. 10%; $p = 0.649$). Aspirin-treated patients with MIs had higher serum TxB_2 compared with those without MIs ($p = 0.005$).

Conclusions.—MI is an early complication of pneumonia and is associated with in vivo platelet activation and serum TxB_2 overproduction; aspirin 100 mg/day seems insufficient to inhibit thromboxane biosynthesis.

(MACCE in Hospitalized Patients With Community-acquired Pneumonia; NCT01773863)

▶ A number of recent reports have highlighted a relationship between cardiovascular events and pneumonia.[1,2] One prospective study showed an association of elevated cardiac enzymes in association with pneumonia, but that study did not clarify any relationship with myocardial infarction. The authors of the current prospective study speculated that the increased rate of cardiovascular events in patients with pneumonia might be related to the inflammatory milieu that exists in patients with severe, acute illness. In particular, in acute infections, platelet activation biomarkers are elevated. Activated platelets are essential components of the series of events that occur, which result in coronary artery occlusion and myocardial infarction (MI). Thus, in the setting of acute inflammation, platelet overactivation might result not only in an appropriate inflammatory response but also in an untoward cardiac event. The study consisted of measuring both troponin and platelet activation biomarkers in patients with pneumonia and correlating with the clinical picture. In the study population, 52% of patients with pneumonia had troponin elevations, and of those 22% had clinical signs of MI (electrocardiographic findings). Platelet activation markers were significantly higher in those with clinical MI. Of note, chest pain was not a common feature of MI; however, severity of pneumonia was associated with higher rate of MI, and MIs typically occurred within 48 hours of presentation. Both platelet hyperaggregation and nonresponse to aspirin were seen in this group. What is not clear from this study is the meaning of elevated troponins in the 113 patients who did not have electrocardiographic evidence of MI. However, isolated elevated troponin is a marker of cardiac ischemia and may have some as yet undetermined prognostic value. It seems appropriate to monitor patients with severe pneumonia who have elevated troponins on admission for signs of MI.

J. R. Maurer, MD

References

1. Corrales-Medina VF, Musher DM, Wells GA, Chirinos JA, Chen L, Fine MJ. Cardiac complications in patients with community-acquired pneumonia: incidence, timing, risk factors, and association with short-term mortality. *Circulation.* 2012;125:773-781.
2. Chang CL, Mills GD, Karalus NC, et al. Biomarkers of cardiac dysfunction and mortality from Community-acquired pneumonia in adults. *PLoS One.* 2013;8:e62612.

A 16-Year Prospective Study of Community-Onset Bacteremic *Acinetobacter* Pneumonia: Low Mortality With Appropriate Initial Empirical Antibiotic Protocols

Davis JS, McMillan M, Swaminathan A, et al (Charles Darwin Univ, Northern Territory, Australia; Royal Darwin Hosp, Darwin, Northern Territory, Australia)
Chest 146:1038-1045, 2014

Background.—The genus *Acinetobacter*, well known as a nosocomial pathogen, can also cause severe community-onset pneumonia. Previous small case series have suggested fulminant disease and a pooled hospital mortality of >60%.

Methods.—We conducted a prospective observational study of all episodes of bacteremic, community-onset, and radiologically confirmed pneumonia due to *Acinetobacter* species at a tertiary referral hospital in tropical Australia from 1997 to 2012 following the introduction of routine empirical treatment protocols covering *Acinetobacter.* Demographic, clinical, microbiologic, and outcome data were collected.

Results.—There were 41 episodes of bacteremic community-onset *Acinetobacter* pneumonia, of which 36 had no indicators suggesting healthcare-associated infection. Of these, 38 (93%) were Indigenous Australians, one-half were men, the average age was 44.1 years, and 36 episodes (88%) occurred during the rainy season. All patients had at least one risk factor, with hazardous alcohol intake in 82%. Of the 37 isolates available for molecular speciation, 35 were *Acinetobacter baumannii* and two were *Acinetobacter nosocomialis.* All isolates were susceptible in vitro to gentamicin, meropenem, and ciprofloxacin, but only one was fully susceptible to ceftriaxone. ICU admission was required in 80%. All 41 patients received appropriate antibiotics within the first 24 h of admission, and 28- and 90-day mortality were both low at 11%.

Conclusions.—Community-acquired *Acinetobacter* pneumonia is a severe disease, with the majority of patients requiring ICU admission. Most patients have risk factors, particularly hazardous alcohol use. Despite this severity, correct initial empirical antibiotic therapy in all patients was associated with low mortality.

► *Acinetobacter* species are not exactly at the top of most physicians' list when they see a patient in the emergency department with community-acquired pneumonia (CAP). Even in a patient with multiple medical issues, it would probably not make the differential diagnosis list. However, *Acinetobacter*, like other previously only nosocomially acquired infections such as methicillin-resistant *Staphylococcus aureus*, are now presenting as CAP, particularly in tropical and subtropical regions and in the wake of natural disasters.[1,2] *Acinetobacter* is a feared organism in the nosocomial setting in which generally very compromised patients acquire it and often die from it. Because of its association with the hospital setting, one might expect that those in the community acquiring this organism also have some intimate relationship with healthcare facilities; however, in the present ambitious 16-year prospective study, only 5 of 41 patients had that connection. All patients had at least 1 risk factor; more than 80% were smokers and/or high alcohol users, and 41% has chronic lung disease. The disease developed rapidly and often presented with lobar consolidation and severe sepsis requiring intensive care unit admission. Despite this, and unlike nosocomially acquired *Acinetobacter* infections and previously reported *Acinetobacter* series of community-acquired disease, only 11% died.[3,4] The authors speculate that the low mortality rate is likely due to early diagnosis and adherence to pneumonia treatment protocols, the young age (mean 44 years) of patients, and aggressive supportive care. Probably the most important factor in the better survival is that *Acinetobacter* was in the differential diagnosis when antibiotics were started. The message here is that physicians in high-risk geographic areas should consider *Acinetobacter* when treating rapid-onset, severe pneumonia presenting during the warm, wet season.

J. R. Maurer, MD

References

1. Leung WS, Chu CM, Tsang KY, Lo FH, Lo KF, Ho PL. Fulminant community-acquired *Acinetobacter baumannii* pneumonia as a distinct clinical syndrome. *Chest*. 2006;129:102-109.
2. Chen MZ, Hsueh PR, Lee LN, Yu CJ, Yang PC, Luh KT. Severe community-acquired pneumonia due to *Acinetobacter baumannii*. *Chest*. 2001;120:1072-1077.
3. Kang SJ, Kang CI, Park SY, et al. Epidemiology and clinical features of community-onset *Acinetobacter baumannii* infections. *Infect Control Hosp Epidemiol*. 2012;33:1053-1055.
4. Ong CW, Lye DC, Khoo KL, et al. Severe community-acquired *Acinetobacter baumannii* pneumonia: an emerging highly lethal infectious disease in the Asia-Pacific. *Respirology*. 2009;14:1200-1205.

Community-acquired lung respiratory infections in HIV-infected patients: microbial aetiology and outcome

Cilloniz C, Torres A, Polverino E, et al (Univ of Barcelona, Spain)

Eur Respir J 43:1698-1708, 2014

We describe the aetiology of community-acquired pneumonia (CAP) in HIV-infected patients, risk factors for bacterial or *Pneumocystis jirovecii* CAP and prognostic factors of 30-day mortality. This was a prospective observational study of 331 consecutive adult CAP cases in HIV-infected patients (January 2007 to July 2012). 128 (39%) patients had $CD4^+$ cell counts <200 per mm^3 and 99 (43%) had HIV RNA levels <200 copies per mL on antiretroviral therapy. *Streptococcus pneumoniae* was the most frequent microorganism in the group with $CD4^+$ cell counts ≥ 200 per mm^3; *P. jirovecii* was the most frequent microorganism in the group with $CD4^+$ cell counts <200 per mm^3 and in patients with HIV RNA ≥ 200 copies per mL. Predictors of bacterial CAP were: time with symptoms ≤ 5 days (OR 2.6, 95% CI 1.5-4.4), C-reactive protein level ≥ 22 $mg\,dL^{-1}$ (OR 4.3, 95% CI 2.3-8.2) and hepatitis C virus co-infection (OR 2.3, 95% CI 1.4-3.9). White blood cell count ≤ 4×10^{12} per L (OR 3.7, 95% CI 1.2-11.5), lactate dehydrogenase (LDH) level ≥ 598 $U{\cdot}L^{-1}$ (OR 12.9, 95% CI 4.2-39.7) and multilobar infiltration (OR 5.8, 95% CI 1.9-19.5) were predictors of *P. jirovecii*. Overall 30-day mortality was 7%. Appropriate antibiotic treatment (OR 0.1, 95% CI 0.03-0.4), LDH ≥ 598 $U{\cdot}L^{-1}$ (OR 6.2, 95% CI 1.8-21.8) and mechanical ventilation (OR 22.0, 95% CI 6.2-78.6) were the variables independently associated with 30-day mortality. The described predictors may help clinicians to distinguish between bacterial and *P. jirovecii* pneumonia in patients with suspected or confirmed HIV infection.

▶ Patients infected with HIV, even those on highly active antiretroviral treatment (HAART), have a risk of developing community-acquired pneumonia (CAP) that approaches 25 times that of the population without HIV. Those patients who have a $CD4^+$ lymphocyte count $< 200\ mm^3$ are at particular risk and have additional susceptibility to *Pneumocystis jirovecii* (PCP) pneumonia. It may be difficult in patients infected with HIV to distinguish between bacterial pneumonia (CAP) and PCP. The investigators in this report performed a prospective study aimed at describing the clinical and microbial characteristics in HIV patients with CAP to identify the risk factors associated with CAP and PCP and to identify 30-day mortality prognostic factors. In addition to using $CD4^+$ counts to identify patients at high risk for PCP, they measured HIV RNA to determine whether it is a helpful parameter in discriminating between PCP and CAP. There are not a lot of surprises in the authors' findings. Of note, HIV RNA analysis with a cutoff of 200 copies/mL identified approximately the same risk groups as the $CD4^+$ cutoff. Bacterial pneumonia was most common in patients on adequate HAART therapy and PCP in those not on HAART. It was surprising that half of the patients presenting were not on HAART therapy and that 37% had low $CD4^+$ counts. This was attributed to late presenters and failure to adhere to therapy. The best predictors of bacterial pneumonia, other than adequate antiviral treatment, were short clinical course, cotrimoxazole prophylaxis, high C-reactive protein, and hepatitis C virus coinfection. Mortality in 30 days was under 10% and related to severity of illness and PCP diagnosis. This study serves to emphasize that even in the era of widespread HAART use, many patients are untreated or undertreated, and PCP should remain a part of the differential diagnosis when treating HIV patients with pneumonia.

J. R. Maurer, MD

Legionellosis and biologic therapies

Bodro M, Carratalà J, Paterson DL (Univ of Barcelona, Spain; Univ of Queensland Centre for Clinical Res, Brisbane, Australia)

Respir Med 108:1223-1228, 2014

Background.—Biologic therapies are widely used in inflammatory diseases, and they are associated to an increased infection risk, especially to granulomatous and intracellular infections such as *Legionella*.

Results.—A review of the literature revealed 105 cases of *Legionella* pneumonia in patients taking biologic therapies. Sixty-four patients (65.3%) were treated with infliximab, 23 (23.5%) with adalimumab, 5 (5%) with etanercept and 3 (3%) with rituximab. Seventy-one per cent of the patients were treated for rheumatologic diseases and 16% for inflammatory bowel diseases. The majority of the patients received one or more concomitant immunosuppressive drugs, especially steroids (43%). Overall mortality was 19%. *Legionella* pneumonia might complicate therapy with biologic therapies, especially in patients being treated with infliximab or adalimumab given concomitantly with other immunosuppressive medications during their first 6 months of treatment.

Conclusion.—Physicians should be aware of this potentially severe association. Early recognition and treatment would likely result in reduced morbidity and mortality.

► A large number of biologic agents are now available to treat a variety of conditions. Many of these are monoclonal antibodies directed against specific cell surface antigens, but others are receptor antagonists or blockers with specific targets. Originally designed for treating malignancies, the therapeutic spectrum has greatly increased to include autoimmune and other inflammatory diseases. Most of these agents are considered to be mildly to significantly immunosuppressive (and some are even used in transplant immunosuppression), and their use may predispose the patient to opportunistic infection. Reports of tuberculosis in particular, as well as other intracellular infections, listeriosis and legionellosis, have led the U.S. Food and Drug Administration to require a black box warning. The authors of this study focus on *Legionella* with the aim of analyzing the association of *Legionella* pneumonia with these biologic agents and to "characterize the clinical presentation, duration of biologic treatment at onset of infection, the use of concomitant immunosuppressive medication, and outcomes of the *Legionella* infection cases in patients treated with biologics." Of the reported cases of *Legionella* infection in this setting, 2 important points deserve emphasis: first, infliximab and adalimumab, both tumor necrosis factor-alpha inhibitors, appear to be the biologics most often associated with *Legionella* infection, and second, the risk for infection occurs early in treatment.

J. R. Maurer, MD

Macrolide/Azalide Therapy for Nodular/Bronchiectatic *Mycobacterium Avium* Complex Lung Disease

Wallace RJ Jr, Brown-Elliott BA, McNulty S, et al (Univ of Texas Health Science Ctr at Tyler)
Chest 146:276-282, 2014

Background.—There is no large study validating the appropriateness of current treatment guidelines for *Mycobacterium avium* complex (MAC) lung disease. This is a retrospective single-center review evaluating the efficacy of macrolide/azalide-containing regimens for nodular/bronchiectatic (NB) MAC lung disease.

Methods.—Patients were treated according to contemporary guidelines with evaluation of microbiologic responses. Macrolide susceptibility of MAC isolates was done at initiation of therapy, 6 to 12 months during therapy, and on the first microbiologic recurrence isolate. Microbiologic recurrence isolates also underwent genotyping for comparison with the original isolates.

Results.—One hundred eighty patients completed > 12 months of macrolide/azalide multidrug therapy. Sputum conversion to culture negative occurred in 154 of 180 patients (86%). There were no differences in response between clarithromycin or azithromycin regimens. Treatment regimen modification occurred more frequently with daily (24 of 30 [80%]) vs intermittent (2 of 180 [1%]) therapy (P =.0001). No patient developed macrolide resistance during treatment. Microbiologic recurrences during therapy occurred in 14% of patients: 73% with reinfection MAC isolates, 27% with true relapse isolates (P =.03). Overall, treatment success (ie, sputum conversion without true microbiologic relapse) was achieved in 84% of patients. Microbiologic recurrences occurred in 74 of 155 patients (48%) after completion of therapy: 75% reinfection isolates, 25% true relapse isolates.

Conclusions.—Current guidelines for macrolide/azalide-based therapies for NB MAC lung disease result in favorable microbiologic outcomes for most patients without promotion of macrolide resistance. Intermittent therapy is effective and significantly better tolerated than daily therapy. Microbiologic recurrences during or after therapy are common and most often due to reinfection MAC genotypes.

► Antimycobacterial regimens containing either clarithromycin or azithromycin have been used for a number of years to treat *Mycobacterium avium* complex (MAC) lung disease. Use of one of these drugs in combination with more traditional antimycobacterials have been reported to result in good responses.[1,2] However, the variability of the regimens used, the type and distribution of the disease, the emergence of multiple MAC genotypes in the same patient (confusing definitions of relapse vs reinfection), and the length of treatment have made study results difficult to interpret. Thus, the focus of this report is to provide data on patient outcomes over a population of 180 patients with the same pathophysiology of their MAC infection in which the same additional drug regimen was used with either azithromycin or clarithromycin for the same minimum treatment period with the same definitions for sputum conversion, treatment failure, relapse, and reinfection. Even though it details a single-center and retrospective study, the value of this report is that it provides the most useful (consistent) data to date to determine whether the current guidelines for treatment of this disease are appropriate. The guidelines are not based on prospective randomized trials because this is an uncommon disease that is not well studied; thus, the type of validation provided here is extremely useful to reassure practitioners treating 1 or 2 of these patients.

J. R. Maurer, MD

References

1. Wallace RJ Jr, Brown BA, Griffith DE, Girard WM, Murphy DT. Clarithromycin regimens for pulmonary Mycobacterium avium complex. The fi rst 50 patients. *Am J Respir Crit Care Med.* 1996;153:1766-1772.

2. Griffith DE, Brown BA, Murphy DT, Girard WM, Couch L, Wallace RJ Jr. Initial (6-month) results of three-times-weekly azithromycin in treatment regimens for Mycobacterium avium complex lung disease in human immunodeficiency virus-negative patients. *J Infect Dis.* 1998;178:121-126.

Inhaled antibiotics for stable non-cystic fibrosis bronchiectasis: a systematic review

Brodt AM, Stovold E, Zhang L (Federal Univ of Rio Grande, Brazil; St George's Univ of London, UK)

Eur Respir J 44:382-393, 2014

We conducted a meta-analysis of randomised trials to evaluate the efficacy and safety of inhaled antibiotics in patients with stable non-cystic fibrosis (CF) bronchiectasis.

We searched the Cochrane Airways Group Register of Trials from inception until March 2014. 12 trials with 1264 adult patients were included, of which five were unpublished studies. Eight trials on 590 patients contributed data to the meta-analysis. Amikacin, aztreonam, ciprofloxacin, gentamicin, colistin or tobramycin were used for 4 weeks to 12 months. Inhaled antibiotics were more effective than placebo or symptomatic treatment in reducing sputum bacterial load (five trials; weighted mean difference $-2.65 \log_{10} \text{CFU}\cdot\text{g}^{-1}$, 95% CI -4.38–$-0.92 \log_{10} \text{CFU}\cdot\text{g}^{-1}$), eradicating the bacteria from sputum (six trials; risk ratio 4.2, 95% CI 1.66–10.64) and reducing the risk of acute exacerbations (five trials; risk ratio 0.72, 95% CI 0.55–0.94). Bronchospasm occurred in 10% of patients treated with inhaled antibiotics compared with 2.3% in the control group (seven trials; risk ratio 2.96, 95% CI 1.30–6.73), but the two groups had the same withdrawal rate due to adverse events (12.2%).

Inhaled antibiotics may provide an effective suppressive antibiotic therapy with an acceptable safety profile in adult patients with stable non-CF bronchiectasis and chronic bronchial infection.

▶ Non-cystic fibrosis (CF) bronchiectasis treatment is much less studied than treatments for CF; however, in many geographic regions, it remains an important and debilitating disease. Sputum production and other symptoms result in ongoing pulmonary damage and impair the patient's ability to work and be productive. Recently, bacterial load has been identified as directly related to systemic and airway inflammation and correlates with more severe respiratory symptoms, exacerbations, and hospitalizations.[1] Both intravenous antibiotics and nebulized gentamicin in this study significantly improved markers of inflammation. This was in direct contrast to a 2007 Cochrane systematic review that showed no benefit to prolonged antibiotics to reducing exacerbations.[2] This review did not separately assess the impact of systemic versus nebulized antibiotics. Because of the advantages of using inhaled over systemic antibiotics, the authors of the current systematic review specifically assessed studies using nebulized antibiotics in this disease. Twelve randomized trials were selected for the review, but only 8 were included in the analysis. In general, some trials (but not all) showed improvement in each of the parameters: reduced bacteria load, eradication of bacteria from sputum, and reduced exacerbations. The conclusions state that nebulized antibiotics may be helpful; however, the conclusion is based on somewhat mixed results, and a more definitive statement requires robust data from further primary studies to be convincing.

J. R. Maurer, MD

References

1. Chalmers JD, Smith MP, McHugh BJ, Doherty C, Govan JR, Hill AT. Short- and long-term antibiotic treatment reduces airway and systemic inflammation in non-cystic fibrosis bronchiectasis. *Am J Respir Crit Care Med.* 2012;186:657-665.
2. Evans DJ, Bara AI, Greenstone M. Prolonged antibiotics for purulent bronchiectasis in children and adults. *Cochrane Database Syst Rev.* 2007;(2):CD001392.

Vaccination Against *Staphylococcus aureus* Pneumonia

Spaulding AR, Salgado-Pabón W, Merriman JA, et al (Univ of Iowa; et al)
J Infect Dis 209:1955-1962, 2014

Background.—*Staphylococcus aureus* causes serious infections in both hospital and community settings. Attempts have been made to prevent human infection through vaccination against bacterial cell-surface antigens; thus far all have failed. Here we show that superantigens and cytolysins, when used in vaccine cocktails, provide protection from *S. aureus* USA100-USA400 intrapulmonary challenge.

Methods.—Rabbits were actively vaccinated (wild-type toxins or toxoids) or passively immunized (hyperimmune serum) against combinations of superantigens (toxic shock syndrome toxin 1, enterotoxins B and C, and enterotoxin-like X) and cytolysins (α-, β-, and γ-toxins) and challenged intrapulmonarily with multiple strains of *S. aureus*, both methicillin-sensitive and methicillin-resistant.

Results.—Active vaccination against a cocktail containing bacterial cell-surface antigens enhanced disease severity as tested by infective endocarditis. Active vaccination against secreted superantigens and cytolysins resulted in protection of 86 of 88 rabbits when challenged intrapulmonarily with 9 different *S. aureus* strains, compared to only 1 of 88 nonvaccinated animals. Passive immunization studies demonstrated that production of neutralizing antibodies was an important mechanism of protection.

Conclusions.—The data suggest that vaccination against bacterial cell-surface antigens increases disease severity, but vaccination against secreted virulence factors provides protection against *S. aureus*. These results advance our understanding of *S. aureus* pathogenesis and have important implications in disease prevention.

▶ *Staphylococcus aureus* causes a wide variety of infections, including life-threatening cavitary pneumonia, disfiguring soft-tissue abscesses, infective endocarditis, and sepsis. This wide array of human infections reflects the bacteria's many cell surface and secreted virulence factors. Exotoxins such as cytolysin account for the high morbidity and mortality associated with staph. In addition to antibiotic treatment, complete resolution of infections often requires surgical drainage and long hospitalizations. Because of the impact of these bacteria, a number of attempts have been made to develop a vaccine against it. To date, however, these attempts have not been successful. It is not entirely clear why they have failed, but some evidence in animals suggests that the vaccines directed against surface virulence factors actually worsened the infection rather than reduced it. The authors postulated that a vaccine directed against secreted virulence factors, rather than cell surface virulence factors, might be more effective. They were able to clearly demonstrate the effectiveness of this approach in a rabbit model, thus setting the stage for development of a human vaccine. An antistaphylococcal vaccine would be of great value, particularly to populations in whom staphylococcal disease is a lethal threat.

J. R. Maurer, MD

6 Lung Transplantation

Introduction

This year's articles on lung transplantation begin with a look at the pre-transplant period both from the patient and the donor perspective. Over the last decade or so, many advances have been made in extending donor criteria and assessing or managing donor organs that have made it possible for the number of lung transplants performed per year worldwide to grow by nearly 50 percent. Two significant developments that fueled this increase were the use of non-heart beating donors and the ability to manage potentially marginal organs extracorporeally for extended periods to determine and improve viability. I have included an article describing reasonable outcomes in patients in which the donor lungs have come from drowning victims. "Drowned" lungs typically have disruption of surfactant regardless of the type of drowning and may have a host of other issues depending on the type of water involved. The new donor management techniques help assess lungs like these that were not previously eligible for donation.

On the potential recipient side, increased concern about outcomes of transplant recipients has focused attention on risk factors of transplant candidates. Articles included here address issues such as the level of renal function and the body mass index necessary to ensure a good post-transplant outcome, particularly important issues as both the age of transplant recipients and the severity of their lung disease has increased over the past 10 years. In addition, technological improvements in measuring anti-HLA and other antibodies pre-transplant, as well as sophisticated genetic testing, allow the identification of high-risk candidates. Two articles in these areas illustrate this progress.

The last article involving pre-transplant patients is a description of a number of patients with pulmonary veno-occlusive disease who were placed on the transplant waitlist. This is the first good description of the clinical picture of these patients with a very rare disease and a reminder of how rapidly they can deteriorate despite drug therapy.

Despite lung transplantation's 30-year history, long-term survival remains despite mild improvement in the last decade, one of the lowest of the solid organ transplants. A key feature is chronic lung allograft dysfunction, primarily but not exclusively due to small airway (bronchiolitis obliterans) and vascular disease. Early acute rejection, gastroesophageal reflux with aspiration, various pulmonary infections, as well as tissue HLA mismatching, are among the risk factors that have been identified. We have included several reports that try to further define risks or course or management of this issue. Jaksch et al report in a single-center study that using Alemtuzumab, an extremely immunosuppressive anti-CD 25 antibody, dramatically reduced the rate of acute rejection, one of the primary risk factors for chronic lung allograft dysfunction (CLAD). Air pollution is identified in a separate report as a newer risk factor for the development of CLAD. A new internal risk factor may be related to long-term use of corticosteroids in maintenance immunosuppressive regimens. Hodge et al report that downregulation of glucocorticoid receptors with chronic prednisone use may allow an increase in cytokines and influx of immune cells into the lung, resulting in lower levels of immunosuppression and potentially a risk for chronic rejection. In terms of treatment, Azithromycin continues to be studied as a potential modifier, if not prevention, of the course of chronic lung allograft dysfunction, as reported by Vos et al.

Other articles of interest include a report on a new, more specific means of identifying the replication of cytomegalovirus in bronchoalveolar lavage fluid, a characterization of post-transplant patients that require a return to the intensive care unit and their outcomes, a report on the early development—and often difficult diagnosis—of diverticulitis in post-transplant patients, and a report on the long-term outcome of living donor transplants.

Janet R. Mauer, MD, MBA

Use of the Donor Lung After Asphyxiation or Drowning: Effect on Lung Transplant Recipients

Whitson BA, Hertz MI, Kelly RF, et al (The Univ of Minnesota, Minneapolis; The Ohio State Univ Wexner Med Ctr, Columbus; The Univ of Pittsburgh Med Ctr, PA)

Ann Thorac Surg 98:1145-1151, 2014

Background.—With the relative paucity of acceptable donors for lung transplantation, criteria for extended donor consideration are being explored. We sought to evaluate the suitability of donors whose cause of death was asphyxiation or drowning (A/D) as a potential option to enlarge the donor pool.

Methods.—We queried the United Network for Organ Sharing (UNOS) Standard Transplant Analysis and Research registry for lung transplantation from 1987 to 2010 to assess associations between cause of death and recipient survival using the Kaplan-Meier method. To adjust for potential confounders, we used a Cox proportional hazards model and a logistic regression model to evaluate incidence of rejection within the first year.

Results.—There were 18,250 adult primary lung transplantations performed, with 309 A/D donors. There was no difference in survival between groups (log-rank, $p = 0.52$). There were no differences in demographics, length of stay, airway dehiscence, lung allocation score (LAS), or ischemic time in univariate analysis (all $p > 0.05$). The A/D lung recipients had fewer deaths from pulmonary causes (5.8% versus 9.5%; $p = 0.02$).

Proportional hazards analysis was significant for double lung transplantation (hazard ratio [HR], 0.85; 95% confidence interval [CI], 0.8–0.9), height difference (HR, 1.002; 95% CI, 1.00–1.003), donor age greater than 50 years (HR, 0.89; 95% CI, 0.83–0.96), and recipient age greater than 55 years (HR, 0.8; 95% CI, 0.76–0.84). A/D cause of death did not impact survival in multivariate analysis.

Conclusions.—A/D as a donor cause of death was not associated with poor long-term survival or incidence of rejection in the first year after transplantation. Donor cause of death by A/D, when carefully evaluated and selected, should not automatically exclude the organ from transplant consideration. These results provide important justification for potentially broadening the donor pool safely.

▶ Even with recent developments in salvaging and optimizing donor organs by extended donor criteria, postcardiac death retrieval, and ex vivo perfusion, the number of patients awaiting lung transplant far outnumbers the number of available donor organs. In this study, the authors sought to determine whether potential donors traditionally excluded because of the cause of death might actually provide viable organs. The usual causes of death of lung donors include intracranial events (36.4%), blunt trauma to the head (27%), and gunshot wound/stabbing (22.9%). Of the remaining 14%, approximately 1.5% comes from drowning and asphyxiation victims. That is because the lungs of these patients have traditionally been thought to be unsuitable. The authors used retrospective data from the United Network for Organ Sharing to study the outcomes of patients receiving 309 organs from drowning and asphyxiation donors and found no increased risk of death or rejection during the first posttransplant year. These data are retrospective, so the specific selection criteria of the donors dying from these causes are unknown. Drowning victims, who often die of profound hypoxemia and acidosis, can be particularly problematic. Although by different mechanisms, both fresh and salt water cause impairments of the surfactant and integrity of the alveolar-capillary membrane. Salt water also can cause influx of protein-rich fluid into the alveoli, creating a noncardiac pulmonary edema picture. In addition, waterborne pathogenic organisms may be inhaled. Newer mechanisms of maintaining and optimizing organs for extended time periods may help to recover more of these organs in which the pathophysiologic impact of the drowning may not be immediately apparent.

J. R. Maurer, MD

Assessment of Different Threshold Preoperative Glomerular Filtration Rates as Markers of Outcomes in Lung Transplantation

Osho AA, Castleberry AW, Snyder LD, et al (Duke Univ Med Ctr, Durham, NC)

Ann Thorac Surg 98:283-290, 2014

Background.—The evidence behind the widely used pre-lung transplant glomerular filtration rate (GFR) cutoff of 50 mL/min per 1.73 m^2 is limited. This study reviews data from a large cohort to assess outcomes associated with this historical cutoff and to estimate other possible cutoffs that might be appropriate in lung transplantation.

Methods.—We conducted a retrospective cohort analysis of lung recipients at a single center. Recursive partitioning and receiver operating characteristics analysis were used to estimate other potential GFR cutoffs with 1-year mortality as the outcome. Postoperative outcomes around the various cutoffs, including survival, acute kidney injury, and dialysis, were assessed using χ^2, Kaplan-Meier, and Cox regression methods.

Results.—A total of 794 lung recipients met study inclusion criteria. Compared with 778 patients with GFR 50 mL/min per 1.73 m^2 or greater at time of transplant, 16 patients with GFR below this cutoff were older and more likely to have restrictive disease. One-year mortality below the cutoff was 31.3% compared with 15.1% above the cutoff ($p = 0.021$). Recursive partitioning estimated potential GFR cutoff values between 46 and 61 mL/min per 1.73 m^2. Patients with GFR below these cutoffs were at significantly higher risk for adverse outcomes ($p < 0.05$). Receiver operating characteristics analysis was less successful at identifying meaningful cutoff values with areas under the curve approximately 0.5.

Conclusions.—Study results support the practice of requiring candidate GFR 50 mL/min per 1.73 m^2 or greater for lung transplantation. Future work should focus on reproducing the analysis in a larger cohort of patients including more individuals with low GFR.

▶ One component of the selection criteria for potential lung transplant recipients has been their renal function. The reason this has been considered important is that the major immunosuppressive groups used for maintenance immunosuppression, both calcineurin drugs and cytotoxic drugs, have known short- and long-term impacts on renal function. In fact, as many as 15% of patients will have creatinine levels >2.5 mg/dL within 5 years of transplant, and almost 5% will be on renal dialysis or have received a renal transplant.[1] Despite these statistics, the rigor around requiring relatively normal renal function in potential candidates has been relaxed considerably. For example, many of the patients now being transplanted for pulmonary fibrosis are older than 60 years and have age-related lower glomerular filtration rates than younger candidates. But is this relaxation of medical nonpulmonary criteria a wise move? In this study, the authors found that patients with creatinine clearances <50 mL/min had significantly worse early death rates than those with better renal function, although the deaths were not necessarily related to their renal function. This suggests that lower levels of renal function may be a more general indicator of health and portend a poor prognosis. A larger study with more patients is required to confirm these findings; however, transplant centers should be mindful of these findings and should advise patients that poor renal function may be a negative prognostic factor.

J. R. Maurer, MD

Reference

1. Registries. The International Society for Heart & Lung Transplantation. https://www.ishlt.org/registries/slides.asp?slides=heartLungRegistry. Accessed December 27, 2014.

Body Mass Index in Lung Transplant Candidates: A Contra-indication to Transplant or Not?

Ruttens D, Verleden SE, Vandermeulen E, et al (Univ Hosp Gasthuisberg Leuven, Belgium)

Transplant Proc 46:1506-1510, 2014

Background.—According to International Society of Heart and Lung Transplantation criteria, high body mass index (BMI; ≥30 kg/m^2) is a relative contraindication for lung transplantation (LT). On the other hand, low BMI may be associated with worse outcome. We investigated the influence of pre-LT BMI on survival after LT in a single-center study.

Methods.—Patients were divided according to the World Health Organization criteria into 4 groups: BMI <18.5 kg/m^2 (underweight), BMI 18.5–24.9 kg/m^2 (normal weight), BMI 25–29.9 kg/m^2 (overweight), and BMI ≥30 kg/m^2 (obesity). An additional analysis was made per underlying disease.

Results.—BMI was determined in a cohort of 546 LT recipients, of which 28% had BMI <18.5 kg/m^2. Underweight resulted in similar survival (P =.28) compared with the normal weight group. Significantly higher mortality was found in overweight (P =.016) and obese patients (P =.031) compared with the normal-weight group. Subanalysis of either underweight (P =.19) or obese COPD patients (P =.50) did not reveal worse survival. In patients with interstitial lung disease, obesity was associated with increased mortality (P =.031) compared with the normal-weight group. In cystic fibrosis patients, underweight was not associated with a higher mortality rate (P =.12) compared with the normal-weight group.

Conclusions.—Low pre-LT BMI did not influence survival rate in our cohort, independently from underlying disease.

▶ Body mass index (BMI) has always been a factor in the selection of patients for lung transplant, with both underweight and overweight (particularly obese) patients considered relative risks or contraindications to the procedure. This has been problematic for candidate selection because many potential recipients do not fall in the normal BMI range. Several studies have reported on outcomes for both low and high BMIs and report contradictory findings. Probably the most definitive, although retrospective, review was one that looked at the United Network for Organ Sharing database. (1) It supported the "relative contraindication" selection criteria for both low BMI (< 18.5 kg/m^2) and high BMI (> 25 kg/m^2). However, it seems this issue remains controversial because at the end stages of lung disease, certain diseases, such as cystic fibrosis and chronic obstructive pulmonary disease, are often accompanied by significant weight loss. This study aims to make a case for removing bias against selection of low-BMI patients by showing basically equivalent outcomes in underweight patients independent of the underlying disease. BMI is a difficult and soft criterion to use in determining eligibility for transplant. This study, like most of its predecessors, is retrospective and, therefore, subject to all the limitations of that type of study. It would be useful to study prospectively the specific challenges faced by transplant recipient who is over- or underweight with a view to implementing specific interventions that might improve outcomes in those groups.

J. R. Maurer, MD

Pre-transplant donor HLA-specific antibodies: Characteristics causing detrimental effects on survival after lung transplantation

Smith JD, Ibrahim MW, Newell H, et al (Harefield Hosp, Middlesex, UK)

J Heart Lung Transplant 33:1074-1082, 2014

Background.—The impact of Luminex-detected HLA antibodies on outcomes after lung transplantation is unclear. Herein we have undertaken a retrospective study of pre-transplant sera from 425 lung transplants performed between 1991 and 2003.

Methods.—Pre-transplant sera, originally screened by complement-dependent cytotoxicity (CDC) assays, were retrospectively tested for the presence of HLA-specific antibodies using HLA-coated Luminex beads and C4d deposition on Luminex beads. The results were correlated with graft survival at 1 year.

Results.—Twenty-seven patients were retrospectively identified as having been transplanted against donor-specific HLA antibodies (DSA) and 36 patients against non–donor-specific HLA antibodies (NDSA). DSA-positive patients had 1-year survival of 51.9% compared with 77.8% for NDSA and 71.8% for antibody-negative patients ($p = 0.029$). One-year survival of patients with complement-fixing DSA was 12.5% compared with 62.5% for non–complement-fixing DSA, 75.8% for non-complement-fixing NDSA and 71.8% for antibody-negative patients ($p < 0.0001$). DSA-positive patients with mean fluorescence intensity (MFI) >5,000 had 1-year survival of 33.3% compared with 71.4% for MFI 2,000 to 5000 and 62.5% for MFI <2,000 ($p = 0.0046$). Multivariable analysis revealed DSA to be an independent predictor of poor patient survival within 1 year ($p = 0.0010$, hazard ratio [HR] = 3.569) as well as complement-fixing DSA ($p < 0.0001$, HR = 11.083) and DSA with MFI >5,000 ($p = 0.0001$, HR = 5.512).

Conclusions.—Pre-formed DSA, particularly complement-fixing DSA, and high MFI are associated with poor survival within the first year after lung transplantation. Risk stratification according to complement fixation or MFI levels may allow for increased transplantation in sensitized patients.

▶ Preformed donor-specific anti-human leukocyte antigen (HLA) antibodies have long been a known threat to the survival of lung and other solid organ transplants. Potential recipients have always been routinely checked for the existence of these antibodies and carefully screened against potential donors if they have significant antibody titers. Traditionally, the method used to measure these antibodies was a serologically based complement-dependent cytotoxicity assay. In the past few years, the introduction of a solid-phase, bead-based assay (Luminex system) has proven much more sensitive in detecting anti-HLA antibodies.[1] In light of this, transplant centers have begun to explore the impact of these antibodies by retesting the stored pretransplant sera of posttransplant patients against their donors. In this early article that reports on a relatively small population, the number of recipients transplanted with donor organs to which they had antibodies was surprisingly high. Better matching with these sensitive assays may improve survival, although this remains to be seen. As well, photopheresis or anti-antibody drugs can be used to remove these anti-HLA donor-specific and other types of antibodies to improve survival.[2] The key is the increased ability to identify the antibodies.

J. R. Maurer, MD

References

1. Tait BD, Hudson F, Cantwell L, et al. Review article: luminex technology for HLA antibody detection in organ transplantation. *Nephrology (Carlton)*. 2009;14:247-254.
2. Baskaran G, Tiriveedhi V, Ramachandran S, et al. Efficacy of extracorporeal photopheresis in clearance of antibodies to donor-specific and lung-specific antigens in lung transplant recipients. *J Heart Lung Transplant*. 2014;33:950-956.

Genetic Variation in Caveolin-1 Affects Survival After Lung Transplantation

Vandermeulen E, Ruttens D, Verleden SE, et al (Katholieke Universiteit Leuven and UZ Leuven, Belgium; et al)

Transplantation 98:354-359, 2014

Background.—Caveolin-1 (*CAV-1*), a structural protein of the cell membrane, is involved in tissue homeostasis, inflammation, oxidative stress, microbial clearance, and fibrosis.

Methods.—We investigated a genetic predisposition of the *CAV-1* gene on survival, acute and chronic rejection, lymphocytic bronchiolitis (LB), and respiratory infection after lung transplantation (LTx).

Results.—In 503 of 568 patients, the *CAV-1* (rs3807989) polymorphism was successfully determined; 92 had the AA, 234 the AG, and 177 the GG genotype. Patients with the GG genotype had a decreased mortality with a adjusted hazard ratio of 0.72 (CI = 0.53-0.98; $P = 0.034$), but no association was found with chronic rejection, LB, acute rejection, or respiratory infections, although significantly less patients with the GG genotype died of infections ($P = 0.029$). Airway neutrophilia ($P = 0.047$) and systemic C-reactive protein (CRP, $P = 0.034$) were decreased over time in the GG carriers compared to carriers of the A allele.

Conclusion.—We conclude that the GG genotype of CAV-1 is protective, associated with a decreased overall mortality but not with acute or chronic rejection, LB, and respiratory infections after LTx. The decreased mortality was linked with less infections of any kind and also lower systemic CRP, and airway neutrophils were observed, suggesting an overall decreased susceptibility for infectious complications in carriers of the GG genotype.

▶ Genetic characteristics of individuals have been studied primarily with respect to susceptibility to chronic lung allograft dysfunction based on genetic variants that encode for certain cytokines or other inflammatory markers that have been associated with loss of lung function. This study looks more generally at genetic variants that might be associated with better or worse survival after transplantation. The caveolae are invaginations in cell membranes that carry 3 small proteins, caveolin-1 (CAV-1), caveolin-2, or caveolin-3. Of most interest with respect to potential transplant survival is CAV-1, expressed in endothelial, epithelial, fibroblast, and inflammatory cells, and known to have anti-inflammatory, anti-proliferative, and anti-oxidative properties. In addition, it appears to promote clearance of microbes. This same group has also recently investigated genetic variants in immunoglobulin (Ig)G receptors looking for "a specific genetic variant of the low-affinity IgG Fc region receptor II-a (FCGR2A) [that] is a single nucleotide polymorphism (SNP; rs12746613) 13 kb away from a missense SNP (nonsynonymous mutation)."[1] This specific variant is associated with autoimmune diseases that have similar immunological pathways to that of lung transplant rejection. In this study, the group showed that the TT variant had worse survival, but not more chronic lung airway dysfunction. The positive side of this research is that as the genetic understanding of "good" and "bad" outcomes improves, patients, families, and physicians may be able to better appreciate posttransplant risks and have more realistic expectations.

J. R. Maurer, MD

Reference

1. Ruttens D, Verleden SE, Goeminne PC, et al. Genetic variation in immunoglobulin G receptor affects survival after lung transplantation. *Am J Transplant*. 2014;14:1672-1677.

Characteristics of Patients with Pulmonary Venoocclusive Disease Awaiting Transplantation

Wille KM, Sharma NS, Kulkarni T, et al (Univ of Alabama at Birmingham; et al)
Ann Am Thorac Soc 11:1411-1418, 2014

Rationale.—Pulmonary venoocclusive disease (PVOD) is an uncommon cause of pulmonary arterial hypertension (PAH). However, unlike PAH, treatment options for PVOD are usually quite limited. The impact of the lung allocation score on access to transplantation for patients with PVOD and the clinical course of these patients have not been well-described.

Objectives.—To examine the association between the diagnosis of PVOD and lung transplantation for patients on the transplant waiting list.

Methods.—Patients with a diagnosis of PVOD and PAH registered on the United Network for Organ Sharing wait list for transplantation from May 4, 2005 to May 3, 2013 were included. Lung transplantation was the primary outcome measure. Multivariable analyses were performed to determine the odds of dying or receiving a lung transplant after listing. Survival was compared using Kaplan-Meier and competing risks methods.

Results.—Of 12,251 patients listed for lung transplantation, 49 with PVOD and 647 with PAH were identified. There were no significant differences in the lung allocation score between patients with PVOD and PAH at listing, transplant, or wait list removal for death/too sick for transplant. By 6 months, 22.6% of patients with PVOD had been removed from the wait list due to death, compared with 11.0% of patients with PAH (Chi-square $P = 0.03$). Patients with PVOD who died or were considered too sick for transplant were removed from the waiting list sooner after listing (22 vs. 105 d, $P = 0.08$). There was no difference in the proportion of patients with PVOD and PAH transplanted (50.0 vs. 47.6%, $P = 0.60$).

Conclusions.—In the lung allocation score era, patients with PVOD may be at higher risk for death while on the transplant waiting list. After wait list registration, close monitoring for disease progression is advised.

▶ An uncommon cause of pulmonary hypertension is pulmonary venoocclusive disease (PVOD). Often misdiagnosed initially as primary pulmonary hypertension (PPH), it can be distinguished from the much more common PPH by the finding of pulmonary edema on x-ray. Unlike PPH, the response to vasodilator therapy can be deleterious because dilation of the pulmonary arterioles without ability to increase the venous capacity can result in increased transcapillary hydrostatic pressure and increasing pulmonary edema.[1] Thus, it is critical that a correct diagnosis is made in these patients early so they are not put at increased risk by treatment for PPH. No pharmacological treatment has been shown to be effective in this disease, and patients are usually referred immediately for transplant consideration if they meet other transplant criteria. In this study, the authors looked at whether the allocation of donor organs fairly assessed the severity of PVOD compared with PPH patients on the wait list because little is known about how PVOD patients fare on the transplant wait list. In 2005, the Lung Allocation Score (LAS) system was implemented.[2] It exchanged the older first-come, first-served approach to donor allocation with a sickest-first approach. In this system, waiting list patients are regularly reassessed and scored according to the following parameters: presence of diabetes, predicted FVC, supplemental oxygen requirement, pulmonary artery pressures/capillary wedge mean, blood gases, 6-minute walk distance, and serum creatinine. Candidates with higher scores move up the list. Some studies have suggested that the LAS might overestimate the survival times for patients with PPH, making them at higher risk for death on the wait list compared to other diagnoses.[3] This may be particularly true for patients with pulmonary hypertension due to PVOD because this study found that after controlling for age, sex, race, region, diabetes, allocation score at listing, thoracic diagnosis, and mean pulmonary artery pressure, PVOD patients had a higher risk of death or removal because they were too sick to transplant than patients with PPH, who themselves may have a higher wait-list mortality than predicted by the current LAS. The authors caution, appropriately, that PVOD patients need close follow-up to be moved up the wait list and avoid becoming too sick to transplant; it may also be that the LAS needs some revision to more accurately assess the sickest patients with pulmonary hypertension so that they can receive higher scores as they become sicker.

J. R. Maurer, MD

References

1. Palmer SM, Robinson LJ, Wang A, Gossage JR, Bashore T, Tapson VF. Massive pulmonary edema and death after prostacyclin infusion in a patient with pulmonary veno-occlusive disease. *Chest*. 1998;113:237-240.
2. Takahashi SM, Garrity ER. The impact of the lung allocation score. *Semin Respir Crit Care Med*. 2010;31:108-114.
3. Gomberg-Maitland M, Glassner-Kolmin C, Watson S, et al. Survival in pulmonary arterial hypertension patients awaiting lung transplantation. *J Heart Lung Transplant*. 2013;32:1179-1186.

Alemtuzumab in Lung Transplantation: An Open-Label, Randomized, Prospective Single Center Study

Jaksch P, Ankersmit J, Scheed A, et al (Med Univ of Vienna, Wien, Austrian)

Am J Transplant 14:1839-1845, 2014

Induction therapy with alemtuzumab followed by lower maintenance immunosuppression (IS) has been associated with reduced morbidity and mortality in abdominal and heart transplantation (TX). In the current study, alemtuzumab, in combination with reduced levels of maintenance IS, was compared to thymoglobulin in combination with standard IS. Sixty consecutive patients who underwent lung transplantation (LUTX) at a single center were prospectively randomized in two groups: group A received alemtuzumab in conjunction with reduced doses of tacrolimus, steroids and mycophenolate mofetil. Group B received thymoglobulin in association with standard dose IS. Patient and graft survival, freedom from acute cellular rejection (ACR), lymphocytic bronchiolitis, bronchiolitis obliterans syndrome, kidney function, infectious complications and posttransplant lymphoproliferative disorder were analyzed. Alemtuzumab induction therapy resulted in complete the absence of ACR episodes ≥ A2 within the first year post-TX. The difference to thymoglobulin was significant (alemtuzumab 0 vs. ATG 0.33; $p = 0.019$). All other factors studied did not show any differences between the two groups. Alemtuzumab induction therapy after LUTX in combination with reduced maintenance IS significantly reduces higher-grade rejection rates. This novel therapeutic agent had no impact on survival, infections rates, kidney function and incidence of malignancies.

► Alemtuzumab is an anti-CD-52 antibody that is intensely immunosuppressive because it effectively depletes mature lymphocytes with the CD-52 protein. It has been used in treatment of T-cell lymphomas, chronic lymphocytic leukemia, and as part of a conditioning regimen for bone marrow transplantation. It was recently approved for use in multiple sclerosis after being taken off the market in 2012. Occasionally, it has been used for solid organ transplant, but the degree of depletion of lymphocytes is usually problematic in that it exposes the recipient to opportunistic infection, especially cytomegaloviral infection. In this study, antithymocyte globulin was compared with alemtuzumab as induction therapy; the authors found no increased risk of infection with alemtuzumab despite its greater potency as an antilymphocyte drug. The anti-infective prophylaxis was fairly standard. The primary finding was that alemtuzumab-induced patients appeared to have almost no acute rejection in the first year, which ought to result in lower rates of chronic lung allograft dysfunction ultimately. The study findings support earlier studies by Shyu S et al.[1] It is, however, hard to imagine that the rates of infection (in the face of both alemtuzumab and traditional immunosuppressives) are not increased. Larger, multicenter studies with follow-up to determine the long-term impact of the drug are needed before alemtuzumab, which is off-label, gains widespread use.

J. R. Maurer, MD

Reference

1. Shyu S, Dew MA, Pilewski JM, et al. Five-year outcomes with alemtuzumab induction after lung transplantation. *J Heart LungTransplant.* 2011;30:743-754.

Air Pollution and the Development of Posttransplant Chronic Lung Allograft Dysfunction

Bhinder S, Chen H, Sato M, et al (Univ of Toronto, Ontario, Canada; Public Health Ontario, Toronto, Canada; Kyoto Univ, Japan)

Am J Transplant 14:2749-2757, 2014

Chronic lung allograft dysfunction (CLAD) is the leading cause of mortality following lung transplantation. We conducted a retrospective cohort study including 397 bilateral lung recipients transplanted in from 1996 to 2009 to determine the association between ambient air pollution, CLAD and mortality. Pollution exposure was assessed using satellite-based estimates of nitrogen dioxide, distance to major roadway and total length of roadways around a patient's home. Cumulative exposures to ozone and particulate matter were estimated from concentrations measured at fixed-site stations near patients' homes using inverse distance weighted interpolation. Cox proportional hazards models were used to estimate the associations of CLAD with air pollution exposure, adjusting for various individual and neighborhood characteristics. During the follow-up, 185 patients developed CLAD (47%) and 101 patients died (25%). Fifty-four deaths (53%) were due to CLAD. We observed an association between CLAD development and road density within 200 m of a patient's home (HR 1.30 [95% CI 1.07–1.58]). Although based on a subgroup of 14 patients, living within 100 m of a highway was associated with a high risk for developing CLAD (HR 4.91 [95% CI 2.22, 10.87]). These data suggest that exposure to traffic-related air pollution is associated with development of CLAD among lung transplant recipients.

▶ Chronic lung allograft dysfunction (CLAD), thought to be a form of chronic rejection, occurs in at least half of lung-transplant patients by 5 years posttransplant. CLAD, characterized primarily by a progressive obstructive process, is a major cause of death and the primary reason for lower rates of long-term survival in lung recipients compared with other solid organ recipients. Despite much research, no single specific precipitant has been identified for the development of CLAD; identified risk factors include numbers and severity of acute rejection episodes, the presence of gastroesophageal reflux, primary graft dysfunction, and infections. It has also long been speculated that the unique direct exposure of the lung to an environment filled with varying amounts of polluting substances could increase the risk of precipitation of airway inflammation resulting in CLAD. A previous European study showed that exposure to traffic-related air pollution increased the morbidity and mortality of lung transplant recipients.[1] The current Canadian study identifies a similar risk and confirms the greater risk in areas in which there is heavy traffic air pollution. These findings, although in small populations, are not surprising given that the presence of high levels of traffic-related air pollution are known to be associated with more severe pulmonary symptoms in patients with existing lung disease and to contribute to pulmonary symptoms in the general population. It is appropriate to counsel candidates for lung transplantation about the potentially higher risks of failure of their graft if they live in a high-pollution environment.

J. R. Maurer, MD

Reference

1. Nawrot TS, Vos R, Jacobs L, et al. The impact of traffic air pollution on bronchiolitis obliterans syndrome and mortality after lung transplantation. *Thorax*. 2011; 66:748-754.

Loss of glucocorticoid receptor from pro-inflammatory T cells after lung transplant

Hodge G, Hodge S, Holmes-Liew CL, et al (Royal Adelaide Hosp, South Australia)

J Heart Lung Transplant 33:957-962, 2014

Background.—Pro-inflammatory cytokines in T and natural killer T (NKT)-like cells increase with time post-transplant in otherwise stable patients, suggesting that some patients become relatively resistant to immunosuppressants such as glucocorticoids (GC). We hypothesized that GC receptor (GCR) would be down-regulated in peripheral blood pro-inflammatory T and NKT-like cells after lung transplantation and loss of GCR would correlate with time post-transplant.

Methods.—Blood was collected from 17 stable lung transplant patients and 17 healthy, aged-matched controls. Intracellular GCR expression and pro-inflammatory cytokines were determined using flow cytometry.

Results.—There was a loss of GCR in $CD8^+$ and $CD8^-$ T and NKT-like cells in transplant patients compared with control subjects (transplants 37 ± 9%, controls 47 ± 12%; GCR^+CD8^+ and $CD8^-$ T cells: transplants 39 ± 13%, controls 58 ± 13%). Loss of GCR was associated with a greater percentage of T cells producing interferon-gamma (IFN-γ) and tumor necrosis factor-alpha (TNF-α) but not NKT-like cells. There was a correlation between the percentage of GCR-negative T cells with months post-transplant ($R = 0.519$, $p = 0.033$) and dose of prednisolone ($R = 0.775$, $p = 0.038$).

Conclusions.—Time post-transplant and prednisolone dose correlate with loss of GCR in pro-inflammatory T cells in stable transplant patients, suggesting the need for reassessment of the long-term use of steroids after lung transplant in view of their attendant significant side effects.

▶ Prednisone remains a common part of long-term maintenance immunosuppression in lung-transplant recipients, albeit in small amounts. Based on data showing chronic use of glucocorticoids can down-regulate glucocorticoid receptors,[1] the authors postulated that this phenomenon happens in survivors of lung transplantation because they were able to demonstrate that proinflammatory cytokines increase in some posttransplant patients. This increase in proinflammatory cytokines accompanied by the presence of natural killer-like T cells suggests a possible functional decrease in the immunosuppression. These findings have potential practical applications for patients. Periodic monitoring of proinflammatory cytokines in stable posttransplant patients may help to identify those in which chronic prednisone use has down-regulated the glucocorticoid receptors and the prednisone is no longer providing immunosuppression. Temporary interruption of steroid treatment may help reduce steroid side effects and allow glucocorticoid receptors to normalize; alternatively, replacement of prednisone with an alternative drug may be an appropriate choice. The potential risk of not identifying a fall in functional immunosuppression, of course, is a risk of late acute rejection and graft compromise.

J. R. Maurer, MD

Reference

1. Berki T, Tavakoli A, Kalmar Nagy KK, Nagy G, Nemeth P. Alterations of glucocorticoid receptor expression during glucocorticoid hormone therapy in renal transplant patients. *Transpl Int.* 2002;15:132-138.

Azithromycin and the Treatment of Lymphocytic Airway Inflammation After Lung Transplantation

Vos R, Verleden SE, Ruttens D, et al (Katholieke Universiteit Leuven and Univ Hosp Gasthuisberg, Belgium; et al)
Am J Transplant 14:2736-2748, 2014

Lymphocytic airway inflammation is a major risk factor for chronic lung allograft dysfunction, for which there is no established treatment. We investigated whether azithromycin could control lymphocytic airway inflammation and improve allograft function. Fifteen lung transplant recipients demonstrating acute allograft dysfunction due to isolated lymphocytic airway inflammation were prospectively treated with azithromycin for at least 6 months (NCT01109160). Spirometry (FVC, FEV_1, FEF_{25-75}, Tiffeneau index) and FeNO were assessed before and up to 12 months after initiation of azithromycin. Radiologic features, local inflammation assessed on airway biopsy (rejection score, IL-17^+ cells/mm^2 lamina propria) and broncho-alveolar lavage fluid (total and differential cell counts, chemokine and cytokine levels); as well as systemic C-reactive protein levels were compared between baseline and after 3 months of treatment. Airflow improved and FeNO decreased to baseline levels after 1 month of azithromycin and were sustained thereafter. After 3 months of treatment, radiologic abnormalities, submucosal cellular inflammation, lavage protein levels of IL-1β, IL-8/ CXCL-8, IP-10/ CXCL-10, RANTES/CCL5, MIP1-α/CCL3, MIP-1β/CCL4, Eotaxin, PDGF-BB, total cell count, neutrophils and eosinophils, as well as plasma C-reactive protein levels all significantly decreased compared to baseline ($p < 0.05$). Administration of azithromycin was associated with suppression of posttransplant lymphocytic airway inflammation and clinical improvement in lung allograft function.

► One of the primary risk factors for (or precursors to) chronic lung allograft dysfunction is lymphocytic bronchial infiltration identified on bronchial biopsies. This inflammatory infiltrate is typically peribronchiolar or peribronchial submucosal infiltrate and consists primarily of $CD8^+$ T lymphocytes. Interleukin (IL)-17-producing lymphocytes (both CD4 and CD8 varieties) with the appropriate cytokines present are thought to be able to induce the evolution of acute to chronic rejection by enabling pro-fibrotic changes that can result in small airway obstruction with chronic lung allograft dysfunction. The authors postulated that if lymphocytic bronchiolitic and bronchial inflammation can be diagnosed early and treated effectively, the ultimate fibrosis and loss of lung function could be avoided. They were able to show that azithromycin significantly decreased the IL-17-mediated lymphocytic inflammation both by repeat biopsy and by measuring decreases in multiple biomarkers of the inflammatory process. Because this type of inflammation precedes the loss of lung function in up to half of patients who develop chronic lung allograft dysfunction, azithromycin could potentially be a preventative treatment. To further clarify its role, a large prospective and randomized trial will be needed to confirm these exciting findings.

J. R. Maurer, MD

High CXCL-16 Levels Correlate With Symptomatic Disease in Lung Transplant Recipients With Human Cytomegalovirus Replication in the Allograft

Weseslindtner L, Görzer I, Küng E, et al (Med Univ of Vienna, Austria)
Am J Transplant 14:2406-2411, 2014

Human cytomegalovirus (HCMV) is an important pathogen in lung transplant recipients (LTRs). In LTRs, HCMV may replicate in the transplanted lung, and this is indicated by HCMV DNA detection in the bronchoalveolar lavage fluid (BALF). Local replication may occur without causing clinical symptoms or, in some patients, it may lead to symptomatic HCMV disease. In the present study, we analyzed whether HCMV replication in the allograft induces CXCL-16, a chemokine that may play a key role in the regulation of mucosal immunity, and investigated whether CXCL-16 levels in BALF can be used to differentiate LTRs with asymptomatic HCMV replication from patients who simultaneously develop disease. In total, BALF samples from 57 LTRs, of whom 8 developed HCMV disease, were assessed for CXCL-16 levels using a quantitative enzyme-linked immunosorbent assay. We found that HCMV replication in the lung triggered a significant rise in CXCL-16 levels in the BALF ($p < 0.001$, Wilcoxon signed-rank test). Furthermore, the CXCL-16 increase, induced by HCMV, was significantly lower in LTRs who did not develop HCMV disease ($p < 0.001$, Mann–Whitney U-test). Thus, CXCL-16 is a potential marker that may contribute to identify those LTRs in whom local HCMV replication in the lung remains asymptomatic.

▶ Despite aggressive chemoprophylaxis and the ability to detect increasing levels of virus by polymerase chain reaction analysis of DNA in bronchoalveolar lavage (BAL) fluid in asymptomatic patients, cytomegalovirus (CMV) detected in infection and tissue invasion remain important risks to lung transplant recipients. When CMV replication is detected in BAL, it may be difficult to determine whether therapeutic interventions for the infection are required. Typically, an arbitrary cutoff of number of viral copies is used to make a management decision. CXCL-16 is a chemokine secreted mainly by macrophages and dendritic cells and is a key attractor of T cells. Its receptor CXCR-6 exists primarily on activated $CD4^+$ T helper cells and $CD8^+$ cytotoxic T cells. The authors studied levels of CXCL-16 in BAL fluid of patients with replicating CMV to see if they could identify a more discriminating means of differentiating those patients who will and those who will not develop clinical CMV disease. In this small study, it appears that pathogenic replication of CMV incites a much larger CXCL-16 response. Although this article reports only preliminary data, if confirmed, the findings could allow more discriminate use of anti-CMV treatment and reduce both the cost and complications of posttransplant management.

J. R. Maurer, MD

Characteristics and Outcomes of Patients With Lung Transplantation Requiring Admission to the Medical ICU

Banga A, Sahoo D, Lane CR, et al (Cleveland Clinic Foundation, OH)
Chest 146:590-599, 2014

Background.—There are few data on characteristics and outcomes among patients with lung transplantation (LT) requiring admission to the medical ICU (MICU) beyond the perioperative period.

Methods.—We interrogated the registry database of all admissions to the MICU at Cleveland Clinic (a 53-bed closed unit) to identify patients with history of LT done >30 days ago (n = 101; mean age, 55.4 ± 12.6 years; 53 men, 48 women). We collected data regarding demographics, history of bronchiolitis obliterans syndrome, preadmission FEV_1, clinical and laboratory variables at admission, MICU course, length of stay, hospital survival, and 6-month survival.

Results.—The most common indication for MICU admission was acute respiratory failure (n = 51, 50.5%). Infections were most frequently responsible for respiratory failure, whereas acute rejection (cellular or humoral) was less likely (16%). Nearly one-fourth of the patients required hemodialysis (24.1%), and more than one-half required invasive mechanical ventilation (53.5%). Despite excellent hospital survival (88 of 101), 6-month survival was modest (56.4%). APACHE (Acute Physiology and Chronic Health Evaluation) III score at admission and single LT were independent predictors of hospital survival but did not predict outcome at 6 months. Functional status at discharge was the only independent predictor of 6-month survival (adjusted OR, 5.1; 95% CI, 1.1-22.7; P = .035).

Conclusions.—Acute rejection is an infrequent cause of decompensation among patients with LT requiring MICU admission. For patients admitted to the MICU, 6-month survival is modest. Functional status at the time of discharge is an independent predictor of survival at 6 months.

► This report from the large lung transplant population looks at the need for readmission to the intensive care unit (ICU) of patients more than 30 days after transplant. This is the largest report of ICU readmission for lung transplant recipients to date. Of note, 90% of the admissions described were patients who had been discharged from hospital posttransplant and were readmissions. Half the patients were in their first year posttransplant; however, 16 of 101 were more than 5 years posttransplant. Acute respiratory failure was the most common admitting diagnosis, and infection was found in about half of these with acute rejection in a handful. What is not noted is whether antibody-mediated rejection was looked for or documented as a cause of the acute respiratory failure, particularly in the patients who were not found to have infections. Also, were the causes of respiratory failure different in those more remote from the time of initial transplant? Poor functional status was the best predictor of 6-month outcomes, which were poor. What would have been interesting to know is what contributed to the poor functional status at discharge. Was it general debilitation, ongoing lung dysfunction, or ongoing need for dialysis? Although this article adds interesting information about the course of lung transplant recipients, it leaves a number of open questions that hopefully future analysis of those who become critically ill after their initial recovery will be able to answer.

J. R. Maurer, MD

Diverticulitis occurs early after lung transplantation

Larson ES, Khalil HA, Lin AY, et al (UCLA; et al)

J Surg Res 190:667-671, 2014

Background.—Lung transplantation recipients are at an increased risk for developing diverticulitis. However, the incidence and natural history of diverticulitis have not been well characterized. Our objective was to identify patient and transplant-related factors that may be associated with an increased risk of developing diverticulitis in this patient population.

Materials and Methods.—This is a retrospective single institution study. All patients who received a lung transplant between May 2008 and July 2013 were evaluated using an existing lung transplantation database. Patient-related factors, the incidence and timing of diverticulitis, and outcomes of medical and surgical management were measured.

Results.—Of the 314 patients who received a lung transplant, 14 patients (4.5%) developed diverticulitis. All episodes (100%) of diverticulitis occurred within the first 2 y after transplantation. Eight patients (57%) required surgery with a mortality rate of 12.5%. Six patients (43%) were managed medically and did not require surgery with a mean follow-up period of 442 d.

Conclusions.—Diverticulitis is common after lung transplantation and occurs with a higher incidence compared with the general population. Diverticulitis occurs early in the posttransplant period, and the majority of patients require surgery. Patients who respond promptly to medical treatment may not require elective resection. A greater awareness of the risk of diverticulitis in the early posttransplant period may allow for earlier diagnosis and treatment.

▶ Abdominal catastrophes are not uncommon after lung transplant and often require rapid and definitive management. In patients with intra-abdominal sepsis, perforation, ischemia, or other issues, the presentation can be indolent and much less dramatic than occurs with the same conditions in patients who are not immunosuppressed. This applies to the signs, laboratory values, and symptoms of the disease. By the time the patient looks very sick, he or she may be moribund. This requires that those caring for these patients must always maintain a high index of suspicion and order the appropriate studies early to establish a definitive diagnosis. This report of diverticulitis following lung transplantation reminds us that this is often a relatively early complication that must be considered within the first week after surgery when the patient is not progressing as expected. More than 50% of the patients in this series, not unlike that of other reports, required surgical treatment.

J. R. Maurer, MD

Morbidity and Mortality of Live Lung Donation: Results From the RELIVE Study

Yusen RD, for the RELIVE Study Group (Washington Univ School of Medicine, St Louis, MO; et al)

Am J Transplant 14:1846-1852, 2014

The Renal and Lung Living Donors Evaluation Study assesses outcomes of live lung (lobectomy) donors. This is a retrospective cohort study at University of Southern California (USC) and Washington University (WASHU) Medical Centers (1993–2006), using medical records to assess morbidity and national databases to ascertain postdonation survival and lung transplantation. Serious complications were defined as those that required significant treatment, were potentially life-threatening or led to prolonged hospitalization. The 369 live lung donors (287 USC, 82 WASHU) were predominantly white, non-Hispanic and male; 72% had a biological relationship to the recipient, and 30% were recipient parents. Serious complications occurred in 18% of donors; 2.2% underwent reoperation and 6.5% had an early rehospitalization. The two centers had significantly different incidences of serious complications ($p < 0.001$). No deaths occurred and no donors underwent lung transplantation during 4000+ person-years of follow-up (death: minimum 4, maximum 17 years; transplant: minimum 5, maximum 19). Live lung donation remains a potential option for recipients when using deceased donor lungs lacks feasibility. However, the use of two live donors for each recipient and the risk of morbidity associated with live lung donation do not justify this approach when deceased lung donors remain available. Center effects and long-term live donor outcomes require further evaluation.

▶ Since the beginning of living donation with the transplantation of a kidney from one identical twin to another in 1954, the option of living donation has become common in kidney transplantation. Less common, but still an option for some patients in selected transplant centers, is living lung and living liver donation. Outcomes of the recipients of these organs (or parts of organs in the case of living liver and living lung recipients) have been generally similar or slightly better than that of patients who receive cadaveric donors. Until recently, however, the long-term outcomes of the donors have not been well documented. This article reports the living lung donor results of a 2006 study called RELIVE (Renal and Lung Living Donors Evaluation Study) that was undertaken to assess these long-term donor outcomes. Unfortunately, because these patients were not prospectively followed, only the perioperative medical records and the Social Security Death Master File were available to follow the outcomes. The report documents a high rate (18%) of serious complications in donors, which is probably underestimated because of limitations of the data available. Although living lung donation is still an option in some centers, changes in the allocation of cadaveric donors since 2005 that has focused on moving the sickest patients to the head of the list has resulted in a decrease in the numbers of living donor lung transplants. This has both positive and negative implications: positive in that the complication rate in donors is almost unacceptably high and negative in that for those few situations in which living lung donation may be the only option, the existing surgical expertise for this operation will be minimal.

J. R. Maurer, MD

7 Sleep Disorders

Introduction

This year's selection of sleep articles highlights the increased focus on non-pulmonary sleep medicine. While there are still a number of articles in this edition on sleep apnea, many investigators are driven toward research where sleep may be a biomarker of disease. I recommend that you read Maglione JE et al's article entitled "Subjective and objective sleep disturbance and longitudinal risk of depression in a cohort of older women." Investigators reported a longitudinal change in depressive symptoms from baseline to 5 years in women who had objective measures of sleep fragmentation at baseline. I also recommend reading the article by Palesh et al, who reported that sleep efficiencies of 85% or higher predicted greater survival in women with breast cancer. It is not clear why poor sleep is associated with poorer outcome, but I do feel this area is drawing greater research interest.

This year, I have selected more articles that focus on insomnia. For a long time, insomnia has taken a backseat to sleep-disordered breathing. Many of us are familiar with cognitive behavioral therapy as a mainstay of treatment for insomnia. However, the paucity of cognitive behavioral therapy practitioners leaves many patients without treatment. There has been increased interest in finding alternative treatments for insomnia. Mindfulness mediation appears to be a promising form of therapy for chronic insomnia. I expect to hear a lot more about mindfulness mediation in the future.

Making this year's picks are also significant articles on sleep-disordered breathing. Many of us see patients with complex sleep apnea syndrome in our practices. Complicating this area is the lack of guidelines on best treatment modality (CPAP, Bilevel, or ASV) and when to treat. Morgenthaler et al's article "The Complex Sleep Apnea Resolution Study: A Prospective Randomized Controlled Trial of Continuous Positive Airway Pressure Versus Adaptive Servoventilation Therapy" reveals that CPAP therapy adequately treats the majority of patients with this disorder and that jumping immediately to ASV is probably not needed. Unfortunately, we still do not know which patients will benefit from CPAP and which will experience CPAP failure.

Finally, I encourage you to read "Risk of Sleep Apnea in Hospitalized Older Patients." I think research examining sleep and its impact on patient-centered outcomes of readmission is only in its infancy. As someone whose practice includes inpatient medicine, I know firsthand that many hospitalized patients are undiagnosed and untreated for sleep-disordered breathing. I think shifting the paradigm to include/expand the practice of sleep medicine to the inpatient setting is on the horizon.

I hope you enjoy this year's selections. Happy reading.

Shirley F. Jones, MD, FCCP, DABSAM

Consequences of Sleep-Disordered Breathing

Obstructive Sleep Apnea and Severe Maternal-Infant Morbidity/Mortality in the United States, 1998-2009

Louis JM, Mogos MF, Salemi JL, et al (Univ of South Florida, Tampa, FL; et al)
Sleep 37:843-849, 2014

Study Objectives.—A recent trend in increasing rates of severe maternal morbidity and mortality despite quality improvements has been noted. The goal of this study is to estimate the national prevalence of obstructive sleep apnea (OSA) in pregnant women and examine associations between OSA and pregnancy-related morbidities, including in-hospital maternal mortality.

Design.—A retrospective, cross-sectional analysis.

Setting.—A nationally representative sample of maternal hospital discharges from 1998-2009.

Patients or Participants.—The analytic sample included 55,781,965 pregnancy-related inpatient hospital discharges.

Interventions.—N/A.

Measurements and Results.—The Nationwide Inpatient Sample (NIS) database was used to identify hospital stays for women who were pregnant or gave birth. Among these women, we determined length of hospital stay, in-hospital mortality, and used International Classification of Diseases, Ninth Revision, Clinical Modification (ICD-9-CM) codes to identify OSA and other outcome measures. Multivariable logistic regression modeling was used to calculate adjusted odds ratios (OR) and 95% confidence intervals (CI) for the associations between OSA and each outcome. The overall rate of OSA was 3.0 per 10,000; however, the rate climbed substantially from 0.7 in 1998 to 7.3 in 2009, with an average annual increase of 24%. After controlling for obesity and other potential confounders, OSA was associated with increased odds of pregnancy-related morbidities including preeclampsia (OR, 2.5; 95% CI, 2.2–2.9), eclampsia (OR, 5.4; 95% CI, 3.3–8.9), cardiomyopathy (OR, 9.0; 95% CI, 7.5–10.9), and pulmonary embolism (OR, 4.5; 95% CI, 2.3–8.9). Women with OSA experienced a more than fivefold increased odds of in-hospital mortality (95% CI, 2.4–11.5). The adverse effects of OSA on selected outcomes were exacerbated by obesity.

Conclusions.—Obstructive sleep apnea is associated with severe maternal morbidity, cardiovascular morbidity, and in-hospital death. Targeted interventions may improve pregnancy outcomes in this group.

▶ Previous studies have shown an association between obstructive sleep apnea (OSA) and gestational diabetes, hypertension, and preeclampsia.[1] This study adds to the literature by examining the largest dataset of more than 55 million pregnancy-related hospital discharges. OSA is associated with increased odds of cardiomyopathy, pulmonary embolism, eclampsia, and in-hospital mortality. The odds risk range from 5.4 to 9 and was independent of comorbid obesity. The investigators noted an increased diagnosis of OSA and obesity over the course of the timeline, which is not surprising given that the rates of obesity are climbing. Women with OSA were more likely to be older, smoke, drink, and use illicit drugs along with being of lower socioeconomic status.

There are obvious limitations to doing research using datasets based on billing codes. However, the high odds ratio in this study should trigger providers and hospitals to focus on increased awareness of OSA in the pregnant women and goals to reduce the adverse outcomes to both mother and baby.

S. F. Jones, MD, FCCP, DABSM

Reference

1. Chen YH, Kang JH, Lin CC, Wang IT, Keller JJ, Lin HC. Obstructive sleep apnea and the risk of adverse pregnancy outcomes. *Am J Obstet Gynecol.* 2012;206: 136.e1-136.e5.

Role of Sleep Apnea and Continuous Positive Airway Pressure Therapy in the Incidence of Stroke or Coronary Heart Disease in Women

Campos-Rodriguez F, Martinez-Garcia MA, Reyes-Nuñez N, et al (Hospital Universitario de Valme, Seville, Spain; Hospital Universitario y Politecnico La Fe, Valencia, Spain; et al)

Am J Respir Crit Care Med 189:1544-1550, 2014

Rationale.—It is unknown whether obstructive sleep apnea (OSA) may be a risk factor for incident cardiovascular events in women.

Objectives.—We sought to investigate whether OSA increases the incidence of a composite of stroke or coronary heart disease (CHD) in women, and the role of continuous positive airway pressure (CPAP) treatment on this association.

Methods.—This was a prospective, observational study conducted in two Spanish teaching hospitals between 1998 and 2007. Consecutive women referred for suspected OSA and free of previous stroke and CHD were analyzed. Women with an apnea–hypopnea index (AHI) less than 10 comprised the control group, and those with an AHI greater than or equal to 10 were diagnosed with OSA and classified as CPAP-treated (adherence $\geq$ 4 h/d) or untreated (adherence $<$ 4 h/d or not prescribed). The follow-up ended in December 2010.

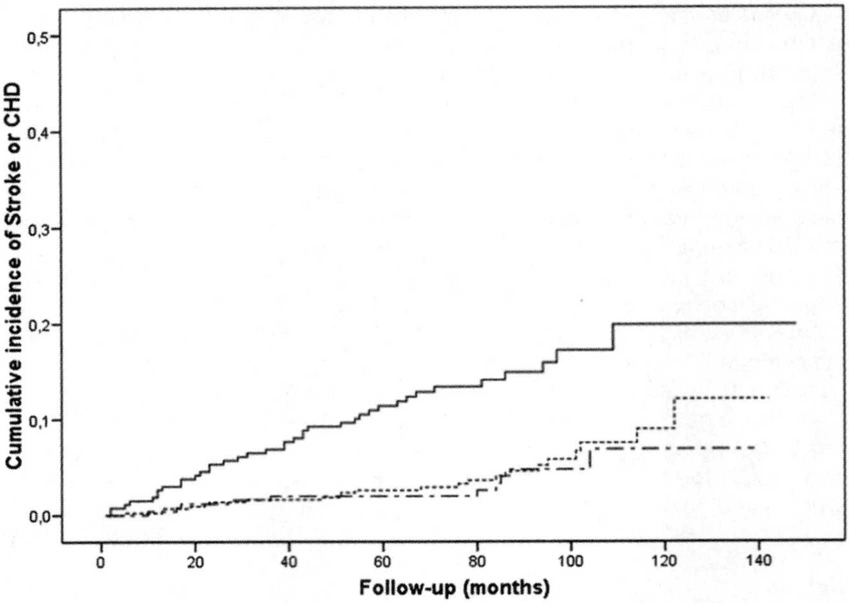

FIGURE 2.—Kaplan-Meier cardiovascular cumulative incidence curves for study groups. AHI = apnea–hypopnea index; CHD = coronary heart disease. *Dashed line*, AHI less than 10 (control group). *Dotted line*, AHI greater than or equal to 10 treated with continuous positive airway pressure. *Straight line*, AHI greater than or equal to 10 untreated. The cumulative incidence of stroke or CHD was significantly higher in the group of women with AHI greater than or equal to 10 and untreated compared with the control group (AHI < 10): $P < 0.0005$. (Reprinted from Campos-Rodriguez F, Martinez-Garcia MA, Reyes-Nuñez N, et al. Role of sleep apnea and continuous positive airway pressure therapy in the incidence of stroke or coronary heart disease in women. *Am J Respir Crit Care Med.* 2014;189:1544-1550, Official Journal of the American Thoracic Society. © 2014, American Thoracic Society, http://www.ajrccm.org.)

Measurements and Main Results.—A total of 967 women were studied (median follow-up, 6.8 yr; interquartile range, 5.2–8.2). The untreated OSA group showed a greater incidence rate of the composite outcome than the control group (2.19 vs. 0.54 per 100 person-years; $P < 0.0005$). Compared with the control group, the fully adjusted hazard ratios for the composite outcome incidence were 2.76 (95% confidence interval [CI], 1.35–5.62) for the untreated OSA group, and 0.91 (95% CI, 0.43–1.95) for the CPAP-treated group. When the type of cardiovascular event was separately assessed, untreated OSA showed a stronger association with incident stroke (adjusted hazard ratio, 6.44; 95% CI, 1.46–28.3) than with CHD (adjusted hazard ratio, 1.77; 95% CI, 0.76–4.09).

Conclusions.—In women, untreated OSA is associated with increased incidence of serious cardiovascular outcomes, particularly incident stroke. Adequate CPAP treatment seems to reduce this risk (Fig 2).

▶ Much of the known literature about the association between increased risk of cardiovascular events and stroke are from studies with little representation from women. For this reason, we do not know if untreated obstructive sleep apnea (OSA) is associated with similar risk in women.

In this prospective observational clinical cohort study of nearly 1000 women conducted over a median follow-up of 82 months, investigators examined the role of OSA and positive airway pressure treatment on the incidence of stroke or coronary heart disease in women. Untreated sleep apnea is associated with increased risk of either first-time stroke or coronary heart disease, but a stronger association was found with stroke. Use of continuous positive airway pressure (CPAP) seems to mitigate the risk (Fig 2).

A major strength in this study is the duration of follow-up and that CPAP compliance was measured objectively using the download data. The limitation of this study is its observational nonrandomized design and its potential for selection bias. The authors address the limitations thoroughly.

The major impact of this study is that there is clearly an association between OSA and stroke or coronary heart disease in women (which is the number 1 leading cause of death in women). The results of this study shed light on the fact that OSA does not have gender bias. Education about the benefits of CPAP treatment is important and should be emphasized.

S. F. Jones, MD, FCCP, DABSM

Nocturnal intermittent hypoxia predicts prevalent hypertension in the European Sleep Apnoea Database cohort study

Tkacova R, on behalf of the European Sleep Apnoea Database study collaborators (P.J. Safarik Univ, Kosice, Slovakia; et al)

Eur Respir J 44:931-941, 2014

Systemic hypertension is associated with obstructive sleep apnoea syndrome (OSAS) but the pathophysiological mechanisms are incompletely understood. A collaborative European network of 24 sleep centres established a European Sleep Apnoea Database to evaluate cardiovascular morbidity associated with OSAS.

11 911 adults referred with suspected OSAS between March 2007 and September 2013 underwent overnight sleep studies, either cardiorespiratory polygraphy or polysomnography. We compared the predictive value of the apnoea–hypopnoea index (AHI) and 4% oxygen desaturation index (ODI) for prevalent hypertension, adjusting for relevant covariates including age, smoking, obesity, dyslipidaemia and diabetes.

Among patients (70% male, mean ± SD age 52 ± 12 years), 78% had AHI > 5 events$\cdot h^{-1}$ and 41% systemic hypertension. Both AHI and ODI independently related to prevalent hypertension after adjustment for relevant covariates ($p < 0.0001$ for linear trend across quartiles (Q) of severity for both variables). However, in multiple regression analysis with both ODI and AHI in the model, ODI was, whereas AHI was not, independently associated with prevalent hypertension: odds ratios (95% CI) for Q4 *versus* Q1 regarding ODI were 2.01 (1.61–2.51) and regarding AHI were 0.92 (0.74–1.15) ($p < 0.0001$ and $p = 0.3054$, respectively).

This cross sectional study suggests that chronic intermittent hypoxia plays an important role in OSAS-related hypertension.

▶ The Wisconsin Sleep Cohort Study showed a dose–response relationship between apnea hypopnea index (AHI) and hypertension after adjusting for confounders.[1] The European Sleep Apnoea Database cohort study similarly evaluated cross-sectional data from nearly 12 000 adults. Although it too noted an independent relationship between the AHI and the oxygen desaturation index (ODI) to prevalent hypertension, after a multiple regression analysis, only the ODI was independently associated with hypertension.

The authors suggested that it is chronic intermittent hypoxia that plays a significant mechanism in the development of hypertension. This is in contrast to other studies that suggest a role of sympathetic activation and arousal in the mechanism.[2]

One of the limitations (and strengths) of the study is the varying methods of diagnosis OSA in this study, which uses both in laboratory and ambulatory methods. Although this obviously led to the study's large sample size, which is nearly 12 times the size of the Wisconsin Sleep Cohort Study, it also led to varying ways of scoring respiratory events. This could have generated the less than robust relationship between AHI and hypertension.

One of the implications of this study is the impact that only ODI carries a significant association with hypertension. If this is true, then scoring sleep studies becomes much more objective and simpler.

S. F. Jones, MD, FCCP, DABSM

References

1. Young T, Peppard P, Palta M, et al. Population-based study of sleep-disordered breathing as a risk factor for hypertension. *Arch Intern Med.* 1997;157: 1746-1752.
2. Prabhakar NR, Kumar GK. Mechanisms of sympathetic activation and blood pressure elevation by intermittent hypoxia. *Respir Physiol Neurobiol.* 2010;174: 156-161.

Diabetes Mellitus Prevalence and Control in Sleep-Disordered Breathing: The European Sleep Apnea Cohort (ESADA) Study

Kent BD, on behalf of the ESADA collaborators (St. Vincent's Univ Hosp, Dublin, Ireland; et al)
Chest 146:982-990, 2014

Background.—OSA is associated with an increased risk of cardiovascular morbidity. A driver of this is metabolic dysfunction and in particular type 2 diabetes mellitus (T2DM). Prior studies identifying a link between OSA and T2DM have excluded subjects with undiagnosed T2DM, and there is a lack of population-level data on the interaction between OSA and glycemic control among patients with diabetes. We assessed the relationship between OSA severity and T2DM prevalence and control in a large multinational population.

Methods.—We performed a cross-sectional analysis of 6,616 participants in the European Sleep Apnea Cohort (ESADA) study, using multivariate regression analysis to assess T2DM prevalence according to OSA severity, as measured by the oxyhemoglobin desaturation index. Patients with diabetes were identified by previous history and medication prescription, and by screening for undiagnosed diabetes with glycosylated hemoglobin (HbA1c) measurement. The relationship of OSA severity with glycemic control was assessed in diabetic subjects.

Results.—T2DM prevalence increased with OSA severity, from 6.6% in subjects without OSA to 28.9% in those with severe OSA. Despite adjustment for obesity and other confounding factors, in comparison with subjects free of OSA, patients with mild, moderate, or severe disease had an OR (95% CI) of 1.33 (1.04-1.72), 1.73 (1.33-2.25), and 1.87 (1.45-2.42) ($P < .001$), respectively, for prevalent T2DM. Diabetic subjects with more severe OSA had worse glycemic control, with adjusted mean HbA1c levels 0.72% higher in patients with severe OSA than in those without sleep-disordered breathing (analysis of covariance, $P < .001$).

Conclusions.—Increasing OSA severity is associated with increased likelihood of concomitant T2DM and worse diabetic control in patients with T2DM (Fig 2).

▶ This is the largest study to date aiming to examine the relationship between obstructive sleep apnea (OSA) severity and type 2 diabetes mellitus (T2DM) prevalence. The study used the European Sleep Apnea Cohort (ESADA)

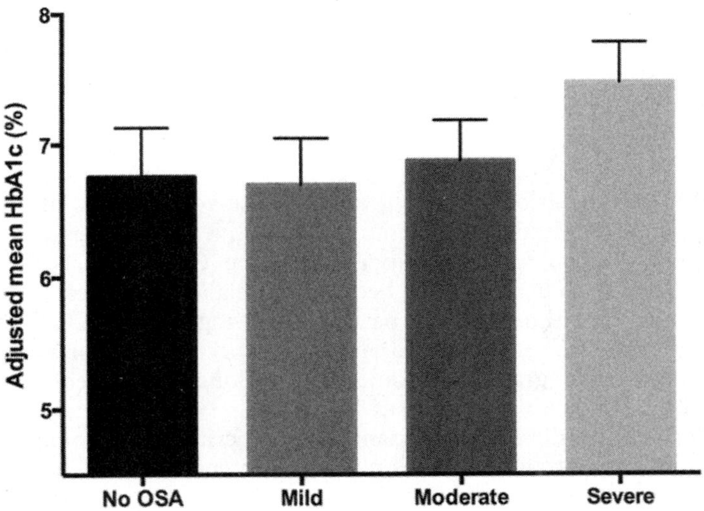

FIGURE 2.—Adjusted mean HbA1c levels among diabetic subjects stratified by OSA severity. Analysis adjusted for age, sex, race, study site, smoking history, alcohol use, average sleep length, BMI, neck circumference, coronary artery disease, congestive heart failure, hyperlipidemia, COPD, psychiatric disease, and medication use. Analysis of covariance, $P < .001$. See Figure 1 legend for expansion of abbreviations. (Reprinted from Kent BD, on behalf of the ESADA collaborators. Diabetes mellitus prevalence and control in sleep-disordered breathing: the European Sleep Apnea Cohort (ESADA) study. *Chest.* 2014;146:982-990, © 2014, American College of Chest Physicians.)

study, which is a prospective multicenter European study. Both full polysomnography or limited cardiopulmonary polygraphy was used in the study population and hemoglobin A1C was used instead of fasting glucose.

The study found a dose responsive curve between OSA severity and prevalence of T2DM with unadjusted odds ratio ranging from 1.85 to 7.12 for mild to severe OSA. There was still an independent relationship even after adjustment for confounders. Another interesting finding was that increasing severity of OSA predicted increased likelihood of suboptimal glycemic control (higher hemoglobin A1C values) (Fig 2).

One of the major strengths of this study is the sample size of more than 6500 participants. The investigators reported severity of OSA based on the oxygen desaturation index, which is more objective and not subject to bias in the scoring of apneas and hypopneas. This is particularly important because different study types were used (full polysomnography vs cardiopulmonary polygraphy). One of the limitations is the cross-sectional nature of the study, which fails to draw cause-and-effect relationship.

Nevertheless, I find this study an important product from the ESADA collaborators. Being able to conduct large multicenter population-based studies from diverse backgrounds will help us understand impact of OSA on a global level.

S. F. Jones, MD, FCCP, DABSM

Non-CPAP Treatment of Sleep-Disordered Breathing

The Complex Sleep Apnea Resolution Study: A Prospective Randomized Controlled Trial of Continuous Positive Airway Pressure Versus Adaptive Servoventilation Therapy

Morgenthaler TI, Kuzniar TJ, Wolfe LF, et al (Mayo Clinic, Rochester, MN; NorthShore Univ HealthSystem, Evanston, IL; Northwestern Univ Feinberg School of Medicine, Chicago, IL; et al)
Sleep 37:927-934, 2014

Introduction.—Prior studies show that adaptive servoventilation (ASV) is initially more effective than continuous positive airway pressure (CPAP) for patients with complex sleep apnea syndrome (CompSAS), but choosing therapies has been controversial because residual central breathing events may resolve over time in many patients receiving chronic CPAP therapy. We conducted a multicenter, randomized, prospective trial comparing clinical and polysomnographic outcomes over prolonged treatment of patients with CompSAS, with CPAP versus ASV.

Methods.—Qualifying participants meeting criteria for CompSAS were randomized to optimized CPAP or ASV treatment. Clinical and polysomnographic data were obtained at baseline and after 90 days of therapy.

Results.—We randomized 66 participants (33 to each treatment). At baseline, the diagnostic apnea-hypopnea index (AHI) was 37.7 ± 27.8 (central apnea index [CAI] = 3.2 ± 5.8) and best CPAP AHI was 37.0 ± 24.9 (CAI 29.7 ± 25.0). After second-night treatment titration, the AHI was 4.7 ± 8.1 (CAI = 1.1 ± 3.7) on ASV and 14.1 ± 20.7

(CAI = 8.8 ± 16.3) on CPAP ($P \leq 0.0003$). At 90 days, the ASV versus CPAP AHI was 4.4 ± 9.6 versus 9.9 ± 11.1 ($P = 0.0024$) and CAI was 0.7 ± 3.4 versus 4.8 ± 6.4 ($P < 0.0001$), respectively. In the intention-to-treat analysis, success (AHI < 10) at 90 days of therapy was achieved in 89.7% versus 64.5% of participants treated with ASV and CPAP, respectively ($P = 0.0214$). Compliance and changes in Epworth Sleepiness Scale and Sleep Apnea Quality of Life Index were not significantly different between treatment groups.

Conclusion.—Adaptive servoventilation (ASV) was more reliably effective than CPAP in relieving complex sleep apnea syndrome. While two thirds of participants experienced success with CPAP, approximately 90% experienced success with ASV. Because both methods produced similar symptomatic changes, it is unclear if this polysomnographic effectiveness may translate into other desired outcomes.

Clinical Trials.—Clinicaltrials.Gov NCT00915499 (Fig 4).

▶ Providers are routinely challenged when it comes to initial management of patients with complex sleep apnea. We are familiar with the knowledge that the use of adaptive servoventilation (ASV) therapy is more effective initially over continuous positive airway pressure (CPAP) but that in some patients, central breathing events may resolve over time. The decision to use CPAP translates into allowing a symptomatic patient to potentially struggle to adapt to

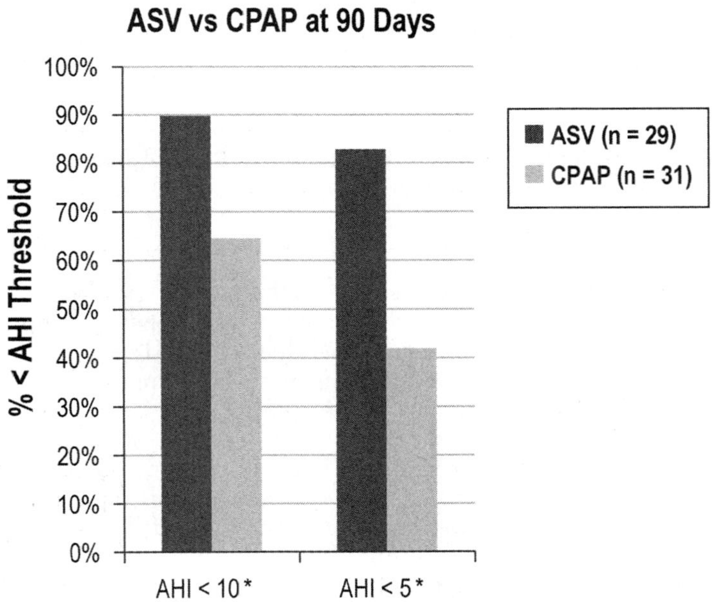

FIGURE 4.—Total AHI at 90 days in participants randomized to adaptive servoventilation (ASV) and continuous positive airway pressure (CPAP). AHI, apnea-hypopnea index. *$P < 0.05$. (Reprinted from Morgenthaler TI, Kuzniar TJ, Wolfe LF, et al. The complex sleep apnea resolution study: a prospective randomized controlled trial of continuous positive airway pressure versus adaptive servoventilation therapy. *Sleep*. 2014;37:927-934, © 2014, American Academy of Sleep Medicine.)

CPAP and the provider's acceptance of higher residual apnea hypopnea indices (due to increased number of centrals) during the initial period. This initial period is also a key period for which patients adapt to PAP therapy and hence permitting use of a device for which AHI is still high and hence less than optimal may affect patient adherence to therapy. The opposing argument is that early use of ASV is a less cost-effective strategy compared with CPAP, especially when dealing with the cost of the machine and cost of potential life-long treatment. Earlier studies comparing the effect of CPAP vs ASV did not include long-term data nor patient-centered outcomes.

Morgenthaler et al conducted a prospective randomized single-blind multi-center trial comparing the efficacy of ASV to CPAP in resolving complex sleep apnea over a 90-day period. Patient-centered outcomes of Epworth sleepiness scale (ESS) and Calgary Sleep Apnea Quality of Life Index were measured. Investigators were not able to identify clinical predictors of adequate response to CPAP defined as AHI <10. Hence, it is not possible to identify which patients' complex sleep apnea will improve (and hence which central breathing events will resolve) with CPAP and which will not. The investigators did report that 90% of patients treated with ASV were able to achieve AHI <10 compared with 64.5% of patients treated with CPAP. This was significant; however, there was no difference in patient-centered outcomes of ESS or CAQOLI at 90 days. I believe this study confirms that providers do not need to use ASV initially and that with follow-up, the majority of patients with complex sleep apnea can be managed with CPAP. We should definitely follow carefully and will still reserve ASV for some patients. Unfortunately, the challenge of identifying which patients will not respond to CPAP remains a mystery.

S. F. Jones, MD, FCCP, DABSM

Tongue Fat and its Relationship to Obstructive Sleep Apnea

Kim AM, Keenan BT, Jackson N, et al (Univ of Pennsylvania, Philadelphia)
Sleep 37:1639-1648, 2014

Study Objectives.—The objective of this study was to determine whether tongue fat is increased in obese sleep apneics compared to obese subjects without sleep apnea. We hypothesized that excess fat is deposited in the tongue in obese patients with sleep apnea.

Design.—Case-control design.

Setting.—Academic medical center.

Patients.—We examined tongue fat in 31 obese controls (apnea-hypopnea index, 4.1 ± 2.7 events/h) and 90 obese apneics (apnea-hypopnea index, 43.2 ± 27.3 events/h). Analyses were repeated in a subsample of 18 gender-, race-, age-, and BMI-matched case-control pairs.

Interventions.—All subjects underwent a MRI with three-point Dixon magnetic resonance imaging. We used sophisticated volumetric reconstruction algorithms to study the size and distribution of upper airway fat deposits in the tongue and masseter muscles within apneics and obese controls.

Measurements and Results.—The data supported our a priori hypotheses that after adjustment for age, BMI, gender, and race, the tongue in apneics was significantly larger ($P = 0.001$) and had an increased amount of fat ($P = 0.002$) compared to controls. Similar results were seen in our matched sample. Our data also demonstrate that within the apneic and normal tongue, there are regional differences in fat distribution, with larger fat deposits at the base of the tongue.

Conclusions.—There is increased tongue volume and deposition of fat at the base of tongue in apneics compared to controls. Increased tongue fat may begin to explain the relationship between obesity and obstructive sleep apnea.

▶ Obesity is a well-known risk factor for obstructive sleep apnea (OSA), but the pathogenesis is not fully understood. In this case-control study of 31 obese controls and 90 obese patients with OSA, tongue fat was measured using magnetic resonance imaging (MRI). Tongue fat was measured in the retropalatal and retroglossal regions. Investigators found that tongues are larger and there is more tongue fat in obese patients with OSA after controlling for age, body mass index, gender, and race compared with obese controls (Table 2 in the original article). Tongue volume and tongue fat correlated with apnea hypopnea index, particularly with measures in the retroglossal area, which could explain why an increase in tongue fat and volume could affect breathing because of its location in the upper airway. The investigators hypothesize that there may be a genetic susceptibility to OSA that is mediated through fat deposition in the tongue. The changes in the tongue may explain the effect of tongue base surgeries in OSA. However, tongue surgeries are usually done in conjunction with other procedures for OSA.

One of the strengths of this study is the group of investigators. They have a long and established track record of studying the upper airway structure using MRI, and this work draws on that experience. Additional studies need to be done, specifically whether weight loss leads to changes in tongue fat.

S. F. Jones, MD, FCCP, DABSM

Non-Pulmonary Sleep

Sleep Restriction Therapy for Insomnia is Associated with Reduced Objective Total Sleep Time, Increased Daytime Somnolence, and Objectively Impaired Vigilance: Implications for the Clinical Management of Insomnia Disorder

Kyle SD, Miller CB, Rogers Z, et al (Univ of Manchester, UK; Univ of Sydney, Australia; et al)
Sleep 37:229-237, 2014

Study Objectives.—To investigate whether sleep restriction therapy (SRT) is associated with reduced objective total sleep time (TST), increased daytime somnolence, and impaired vigilance.

Design.—Within-subject, noncontrolled treatment investigation.

Setting.—Sleep research laboratory.

Participants.—Sixteen patients [10 female, mean age = 47.1 (10.8) y] with well-defined psychophysiological insomnia (PI), reporting TST ≤ 6 h.

Interventions.—Patients were treated with single-component SRT over a 4-w protocol, sleeping in the laboratory for 2 nights prior to treatment initiation and for 3 nights (SRT night 1, 8, 22) during the acute interventional phase. The psychomotor vigilance task (PVT) was completed at seven defined time points [day 0 (baseline), day 1,7,8,21,22 (acute treatment) and day 84 (3 mo)]. The Epworth Sleepiness Scale (ESS) was completed at baseline, w 1-4, and 3 mo.

Measurement and Results.—Subjective sleep outcomes and global insomnia severity significantly improved before and after SRT. There was, however, a robust decrease in PSG-defined TST during acute implementation of SRT, by an average of 91 min on night 1, 78 min on night 8, and 69 min on night 22, relative to baseline ($P < 0.001$; effect size range = 1.60-1.80). During SRT, PVT lapses were significantly increased from baseline (at three of five assessment points, all $P < 0.05$; effect size range = 0.69-0.78), returning to baseline levels by 3 mo ($P = 0.43$). A similar pattern was observed for RT, with RTs slowing during acute treatment (at four of five assessment points, all $P < 0.05$; effect size range = 0.57-0.89) and returning to pretreatment levels at 3 mo ($P = 0.78$). ESS scores were increased at w 1, 2, and 3 (relative to baseline; all $P < 0.05$); by 3 mo, sleepiness had returned to baseline (normative) levels ($P = 0.65$).

Conclusion.—For the first time we show that acute sleep restriction therapy is associated with reduced objective total sleep time, increased daytime sleepiness, and objective performance impairment. Our data have important implications for implementation guidelines around the safe and effective delivery of cognitive behavioral therapy for insomnia.

▶ Cognitive behavioral therapy for insomnia (CBTI) is an effective treatment of insomnia with improvements in sleep that are similar to hypnotics but with long-term efficacy. Fundamental in CBTI is the practice of sleep restriction, which includes no napping, and serves to increase the sleep pressure and address the circadian rhythm component of sleep. As the name implies, sleep restriction is less sleep. The minimal amount of sleep prescribed depends on a number of factors but are centered around patient sleep diaries and can vary among practitioners. Using objective measures of polysomnography and psychomotor vigilance testing, the investigators examined the effect of sleep restriction on the early course of CBTI and found increased self-reported sleepiness and impaired performance on the psychomotor vigilance test.

I think this study is interesting with regard to the short-term effects of sleep restriction in CBTI, particularly for the objective approach the authors used. But I also think that their methods may serve as limitations—specifically incongruencies between psychomotor vigilance testing and actual real-life performance. Overall, I think the literature supporting CBTI for insomnia is robust, and CBTI is an effective therapy; I will continue to recommend it to my patients. There may definitely be a "necessary pain to achieve gain" as the authors simply put it, and patients undergoing CBTI need to be aware of this; however, there is also "light at the end of the tunnel," and we need to express that to our patients as well.

S. F. Jones, MD, FCCP, DABSM

Actigraphy-Measured Sleep Disruption as a Predictor of Survival among Women with Advanced Breast Cancer

Palesh O, Aldridge-Gerry A, Zeitzer JM, et al (Stanford Univ School of Medicine)

Sleep 37:837-842, 2014

Background.—Poor sleep, prevalent among cancer survivors, is associated with disrupted hormonal circadian rhythms and poor quality of life. Using a prospective research design, this study aimed to clarify the relationship between objective measures of sleep efficiency and sleep disruption with survival among women with advanced breast cancer.

Method.—We examined sleep quality and duration via wrist-worn actigraphy and sleep diaries for 3 days among 97 women in whom advanced breast cancer was diagnosed (age = 54.6 ± 9.8 years). Sleep efficiency was operationalized using actigraphy as the ratio of total sleep time to total sleep time plus wake after sleep onset.

Results.—As hypothesized, better sleep efficiency was found to predict a significant reduction in overall mortality (hazard ratio [HR], 0.96; 95% confidence interval [CI], 0.94–0.98; $P < 0.001$) at median 6 y follow-up. This relationship remained significant (HR, 0.94; 95% CI, 0.91–0.97; $P < 0.001$) even after adjusting for other known prognostic factors (age, estrogen receptor status, cancer treatment, metastatic spread, cortisol levels, and depression). Secondary hypotheses were also supported (after adjusting for baseline prognostic factors) showing that less wake after sleep onset (HR, 0.41; 95% CI, 0.25–0.67; $P < 0.001$), fewer wake episodes, (HR, 0.93; 95% CI, 0.88–0.98; $P = 0.007$); and shorter wake episode duration (HR, 0.29; 95% CI, 0.14–0.58; $P < 0.001$) also contributed to reductions in overall mortality.

Conclusions.—These findings show that better sleep efficiency and less sleep disruption are significant independent prognostic factors in women with advanced breast cancer. Further research is needed to determine whether treating sleep disruption with cognitive behavioral and/or pharmacologic therapy could improve survival in women with advanced breast cancer.

▶ Little is known about the relationship between sleep and cancer. Recently, Campos-Rodriguez reported increased hazard ratio for cancer incidence in patients with greater time spent with oxygen saturation <90%, suggesting that longer periods of hypoxia may have an impact on development of cancer.[1] In this article, investigators hypothesized that less sleep disturbance among women with advanced breast cancer would lead to longer overall survival.

The investigators used both sleep diaries and actigraphy to measure sleep. Patients with sleep efficiencies of 85% or greater, lower wake after sleep onset, less wake episodes, and shorter duration of wake episode had greater survival during a 6-year period. The findings of this study imply that markers of sleep may be a prognostic indicator of survival in patients with advanced breast cancer. It is interesting that the same findings were not seen with sleep duration. The explanation for this is unknown. I believe that the study will need to be repeated in a larger cohort and in patients with other types of malignancy to confirm the findings; however, the study is interesting indeed. Providers caring for cancer patients should perhaps consider asking patients about their sleep.

S. F. Jones, MD, FCCP, DABSM

Reference

1. Campos-Rodriguez F, Martinez-Garcia MA, Martinez M, et al; Spanish Sleep Network. Association between obstructive sleep apnea and cancer incidence in a large multicenter Spanish cohort. *Am J Respir Crit Care Med.* 2013;187:99-105.

Rapid Eye Movement Sleep Behavioral Events: A New Marker for Neurodegeneration in Early Parkinson Disease?

Sixel-Döring F, Trautmann E, Mollenhauer B, et al (Paracelsus-Elena-Klinik, Kassel, Germany)

Sleep 37:431-438, 2014

Objective.—To analyze potential markers in sleep for early recognition of neurodegenerative disease in newly diagnosed, unmedicated patients with Parkinson disease (PD) compared to controls.

Methods.—Videopolysomnography (vPSG) was available in 158 newly diagnosed, unmedicated patients with PD and 110 age-, sex-, and education matched healthy controls (HC). Rapid eye movement (REM) sleep was analyzed for REM without atonia (RWA) and studied by review of time-synchronized video. Motor behaviors and/or vocalizations in REM sleep with a purposeful component other than comfort moves were identified as REM sleep behavioral events (RBE). Two or more events had to be present to be classified as "RBE positive." RBE subjects included rapid eye movement sleep behavior disorder (RBD) and non-RBD subjects based on the presence or absence of RWA > 18.2%.

Results.—RBE were detected in 81 of 158 patients with *de novo* PD (51%) and 17 of 110 HC (15%) ($P < 0.001$). RBD was identified in 40/81 RBE-positive patients with PD (25% of all PD patients) and 2 of 17 RBE-positive HC (2% of all controls). RBE-positive patients showed no specific motor or neuropsychological features compared to RBE-negative patients. Patients with PD and HC with RBE had more REM sleep ($P = 0.002$) and a higher periodic leg movements in sleep index ($P = 0.022$) compared to subjects without RBE.

Conclusion.—This first description of REM sleep behavioral events (RBE) shows it occurs more frequently in patients with *de novo* Parkinson disease (PD) than in healthy controls and may be an early sign of neurodegeneration and precede rapid eye movement sleep behavior disorder (RBD). There is no specific phenotype of PD associated with newly defined RBE or RBD at this early stage.

▶ Many of us already know that REM Behavior Disorder (RBD) is common in patients with Parkinson disease and that patients with idiopathic REM Behavior Disorder are at risk for Parkinson disease. Eighty-one percent of patients with idiopathic REM Behavior Disorder develop neurodegeneration after 14 years on average.[1] Violent or exaggerated behaviors such as falling out of the bed are typically what are recognized in these patients on sleep study or by the history. But what about movements that are less violent or exaggerative? Could these represent a milder or earlier presentation of motor problems or early RBD in a vulnerable population?

This study looks at the presence of REM sleep behavioral events (RBE) and REM without atonia (RWA) in patients with clinical diagnosis of Parkinson disease who were not treated with medications and compared the polysomnographic findings with those of healthy controls. RBE and RWA criteria were clearly defined in this study. The findings show a greater number of Parkinson disease patients with polysomnographic findings of RBE and RWA compared with the healthy controls (51% vs 15%). The findings in this study show that findings of RBE may be an early marker of neurodegeneration and early marker of RBD. Interesting is that 15% of healthy controls also had evidence of RBE. What could this mean? Could they also develop neurodegeneration? I believe longitudinal studies are being conducted.

S. F. Jones, MD, FCCP, DABSM

Reference

1. Chokroverty S. Sleep and degenerative neurologic disorders. *Neurol Clin..* 1996; 14:807-826.

Insufficient Sleep in Adolescents and Young Adults: An Update on Causes and Consequences

Owens J, Adolescent Sleep Working Group, and Committee on Adolescence ()
Pediatrics 134:e921-e932, 2014

Chronic sleep loss and associated sleepiness and daytime impairments in adolescence are a serious threat to the academic success, health, and safety of our nation's youth and an important public health issue. Understanding the extent and potential short- and long-term repercussions of sleep restriction, as well as the unhealthy sleep practices and environmental factors that contribute to sleep loss in adolescents, is key in setting public policies to mitigate these effects and in counseling patients and families in the clinical setting.

This report reviews the current literature on sleep patterns in adolescents, factors contributing to chronic sleep loss (ie, electronic media use, caffeine consumption), and health-related consequences, such as depression, increased obesity risk, and higher rates of drowsy driving accidents. The report also discusses the potential role of later school start times as a means of reducing adolescent sleepiness.

▶ This article provides updated information since the 2005 report on excessive sleepiness in adolescents[1] and includes a review of more literature relevant to adolescents today, including the impact of electronic devices, later school start times, obesity risk, and mood disturbances.

Did you know that 75% of US students get less than 8 hours of sleep by the 12th grade?[2] Those with low socioeconomic status may be affected more often, and this could lead to public health implications.

Did you know that in the United States, two-thirds of adolescents have phones in their bedroom?[2] Besides the impact on daytime sleepiness and sleep loss, such devices also emit low levels of light that could impact circadian rhythms.

The article also argues for a change in school start times, highlighting the improvements in symptoms, sleep time, and academic performance. I wonder how many school districts are adopting such a change. With the evidence that US schools lag behind in educational measures compared with other developed countries, delaying school start times may be a means to lessen the gap.[3]

In summary, this article highlights the multiple ways that sleep loss can affect adolescents and young adults. It serves as a nice review and provides information so that pediatricians and sleep specialists can open the discussion about sleep loss and overall health.

S. F. Jones, MD, FCCP, DABSM

References

1. Millman RP, Working group on sleepiness in adolescents/young adults, AAP Committee on Adolescence. Excessive sleepiness in adolescents and young adults: causes, consequences, and treatment strategies. *Pediatrics*. 2005;115:1774-1786.
2. National Sleep Foundation. *2006 Teens and Sleep. Sleep in America Polls*. Washington, DC: National Sleep Foundation; 2006.
3. Brown A. How do students in the United States compare to those around the world? *PBS Newshour.* 2013, http://www.pbs.org/newshour/updates/education-july-dec13-pisaresults_12—02/. Accessed January 22, 2015.

Subjective and Objective Sleep Disturbance and Longitudinal Risk of Depression in a Cohort of Older Women

Maglione JE, Ancoli-Israel S, Peters KW, et al (Univ of California San Diego; California Pacific Med Ctr Res Inst, San Francisco; et al)
Sleep 37:1179-1187, 2014

Objective.—To investigate the longitudinal relationship between subjective and objective sleep disturbance and depressive symptoms.

Design.—Longitudinal.

Setting.—Three US clinical centers.

Participants.—Nine hundred fifty-two community-dwelling older women (70 y or older).

Measurements.—At baseline, subjective sleep quality was assessed using the Pittsburgh Sleep Quality Index (PSQI) and objective sleep measures were assessed with wrist actigraphy. Depressive symptoms were assessed with the Geriatric Depression Scale (GDS) at baseline and approximately 5 y later. The analysis was restricted to women with few (GDS 0-2) depressive symptoms at baseline.

Results.—There was an independent association between greater PSQI score (per standard deviation increase, indicating worse subjective sleep quality) at baseline and greater odds of worsening depressive symptoms (≥2-point increase in GDS) (Multivariate Odds Ratio [MOR] 1.19, confidence interval [CI] 1.01-1.40, $P = 0.036$). Higher scores specifically on the sleep quality (MOR 1.41, CI 1.13-1.77, $P < 0.003$) and sleep latency (MOR 1.21, CI 1.03-1.41, $P = 0.018$) PSQI subscales were also associated with greater odds for worsening depressive symptoms. Objective assessments revealed an association between baseline prolonged wake after sleep onset (WASO ≥60 min) and worsening depressive symptoms at follow-up (MOR 1.36, CI 1.01-1.84, $P = 0.046$). There were no associations between other objectively assessed sleep measures and worsening depressive symptoms.

Conclusions.—In older women with few or no depressive symptoms at baseline, those with more subjectively reported sleep disturbance and more objectively assessed fragmentation of sleep at baseline had greater odds of worsening depressive symptoms 5 y later. Future studies investigating this relationship in more detail are indicated.

▶ Depression in older adults is common, and its presence is associated with negative outcomes.[1,2] Sleep disturbances are common in patients with depression. This longitudinal study of 952 older women aimed to investigate the relationship between baseline subjective and objective sleep and future symptoms of depression. This study draws from a larger study of community-dwelling participants enrolled for a study of osteoporosis. Investigators used actigraphy and questionnaires, both validated tools of outcome measurement. The finding of a longitudinal change in depressive symptoms from baseline to 5 years was reported in women who had objective measures of sleep fragmentation at baseline.

Further research is needed in the area to clarify this relationship and, importantly, to understand ways to mitigate the risk of depression in older women. The strengths of this study is the large sample size and that the investigators in this study have experience with the use of actigraphy and the methods. However, the study is drawn from a larger study whose primary aim was not specific to this research, and the applicability of the findings to other populations is not known. Nevertheless, I think this study is the first to report the relationship between sleep fragmentation at baseline and future depressive symptoms. The findings are worth additional investigation in the field of study.

S. F. Jones, MD, FCCP, DABSM

References

1. Frasure-Smith N, Lesperance F. Depression—a cardiac risk factor in search of a treatment. *JAMA*. 2003;289:3171-3173.
2. Whooley MA, Browner WS. Association between depressive symptoms and mortality in older women. Study of Osteoporotic Fractures Research Group. *Arch Intern Med*. 1998;158:2129-2135.

Risk of Sleep Apnea in Hospitalized Older Patients

Shear TC, Balachandran JS, Mokhlesi B, et al (Univ of Chicago, IL)
J Clin Sleep Med 10:1061-1066, 2014

Background/Objectives.—To assess the prevalence of undiagnosed obstructive sleep apnea (OSA) among general medical inpatients and to investigate whether OSA risk is associated with in-hospital sleep quantity and quality.

Design.—Prospective cohort study.

Setting.—General medicine ward in academic medical center.

Participants.—424 hospitalized adult patients ≥ 50 years old without a sleep disorder diagnosis (mean age 65 years, 57% female, 72% African American).

Main Measures.—The Berlin questionnaire, a validated screen for determining risk of OSA, was administered to hospitalized medical patients. Sleep duration and efficiency were measured via wrist actigraphy. Self-reported sleep quality was evaluated using Karolinska Sleep Quality Index (KSQI).

Key Results.—Two of every 5 inpatients ≥ 50 years old (39.5%, n = 168) were found to be at high risk for OSA. Mean in-hospital sleep duration was ~ 5 h and mean sleep efficiency was 70%. Using random effects linear regression models, we found that patients who screened at high risk for OSA obtained ~ 40 min less sleep per night (−39.6 min [−66.5, −12.8], $p = 0.004$). These findings remained significant after controlling for African American race, sex, and age quartiles. In similar models, those patients who screened at high risk had ~ 5.5% less sleep efficiency per night (−5.50 [−9.96, −1.05], $p = 0.015$). In multivariate analysis, patients at high risk for OSA also had lower self-reported sleep quality on KSQI (−0.101 [−0.164, −0.037], $p = 0.002$).

Conclusion.—Two of every 5 inpatients older than 50 years screened at high risk for OSA. Those screening at high risk have worse in-hospital sleep quantity and quality.

▶ Anyone who sees patients in a hospitalized setting would probably agree that there are a lot of inpatients with obstructive sleep apnea (OSA). Providers would probably also agree with me in that there are many with undiagnosed sleep-disordered breathing. One must wonder in patients admitted with coronary artery disease, myocardial infarction, congestive heart failure if OSA had an integral role in advancement of their disease.

In this article, the primary aim of the study was to better understand the prevalence of undiagnosed OSA in hospitalized patients. Secondary aims were to assess the quality and quantity of sleep using actigraphy and to assess physician knowledge and practices among resident physicians. The investigators used the Berlin questionnaire to assess OSA risk. Subjective sleep quality was assessed using the Pittsburgh Sleep Quality Index, Epworth sleepiness scale, and Karolinska Sleep Log.

There are several limitations to this study, which are nicely addressed by the authors. The gold standard polysomnography was not used, so prevalence of OSA in hospitalized patients is not known. The prevalence of OSA RISK is reported because the Berlin questionnaire was used. Although the Berlin questionnaire is validated and used predominantly in an outpatient setting, I do not see much issue with it being used in this study because eligible patients were ambulatory and community dwelling, and it was conducted within the first 3 days of the hospitalization. Quality and quantity of sleep was measured with actigraphy, which may or may not accurately assess these values. Actigraphy has been used to measure sleep but only in a few studies of intensive care unit patients and selected populations.

I think the take-home points to this study. The inpatient setting is an understudied area for sleep-disordered breathing. We have yet to really understand how many patients have undiagnosed OSA and what is the best way to identify such patients; taken further, we need to determine whether treatment in the inpatient setting has an impact on patient-centered outcomes (readmissions, mortality, length of stay, treatment adherence, etc). I suggest you read article by Kauta et al,[1] whose paradigm to diagnosing central sleep apnea and early treatment resulted in reduction in 30-day hospitalization.

S. F. Jones, MD, FCCP, DABSM

Reference

1. Kauta SR, Keenan BT, Goldberg L, Schwab RJ. Diagnosis and treatment of sleep disordered breathing in hospitalized cardiac patients: a reduction in 30-day hospital readmission rates. *J Clin Sleep Med.* 2014;10:1051-1059.

A Randomized Controlled Trial of Mindfulness Meditation for Chronic Insomnia

Ong JC, Manber R, Segal Z, et al (Rush Univ Med Ctr, Chicago, IL; Stanford Univ Med Ctr, Palo Alto, CA; Univ of Toronto, Ontario, Canada; et al)
Sleep 37:1553-1563, 2014

Study Objectives.—To evaluate the efficacy of mindfulness meditation for the treatment of chronic insomnia.

Design.—Three-arm, single-site, randomized controlled trial.
Setting.—Academic medical center.
Participants.—Fifty-four adults with chronic insomnia.
Interventions.—Participants were randomized to either mindfulness-based stress reduction (MBSR), mindfulness-based therapy for insomnia (MBTI), or an eight-week self-monitoring (SM) condition.
Measurements and Results.—Patient-reported outcome measures were total wake time (TWT) from sleep diaries, the pre-sleep arousal scale (PSAS), measuring a prominent waking correlate of insomnia, and the Insomnia Severity Index (ISI) to determine remission and response as clinical endpoints. Objective sleep measures were derived from laboratory polysomnography and wrist actigraphy. Linear mixed models showed that those receiving a meditation-based intervention (MBSR or MBTI) had significantly greater reductions on TWT minutes (43.75 vs 1.09), PSAS (7.13 vs 0.16), and ISI (4.56 vs 0.06) from baseline-to-post compared to SM. Post hoc analyses revealed that each intervention was superior to SM on each of the patient-reported measures, but no significant differences were found when comparing MBSR to MBTI from baseline-to-post. From baseline to 6-month follow-up, MBTI had greater reductions in ISI scores than MBSR ($P < 0.05$), with the largest difference occurring at the 3-month follow-up. Remission and response rates in MBTI and MBSR were sustained from post-treatment through follow-up, with MBTI showing the highest rates of treatment remission (50%) and response (78.6%) at the 6-month follow-up.
Conclusions.—Mindfulness meditation appears to be a viable treatment option for adults with chronic insomnia and could provide an alternative to traditional treatments for insomnia.
Trial Registration.—Mindfulness-Based Approaches to Insomnia: clinicaltrials.gov, identifier: NCT00768781 (Fig 2).

▶ Insomnia is a widely prevalent problem in the United States with significant personal health and public impact. Sleeping pills and cognitive behavioral therapy for insomnia are both forms of treatment. Sleeping pills carry significant side effects, as well as the development of tolerance and dependence. Cognitive behavioral therapy for insomnia (CBTI) is not widely available. Many of our patients seek complementary and alternative medicine whether providers know it or not. Techniques that are used in complementary and alternative medicine may be useful in patients with insomnia.

This was a randomized controlled trial to evaluate the efficacy of meditation-based therapies on sleep measures. Two meditation-based therapies were used: mindfulness-based stress reduction (MBSR) and mindfulness-based therapy for insomnia (MBTI), which includes meditation but also principles of sleep restriction. Both of these therapies were compared with self-monitoring of sleep diaries (controls).

Both meditation-based approaches reduced total wake time and presleep arousal scale and improved the insomnia severity index compared with self-monitoring (Fig 2). It is important to note that significant improvements were

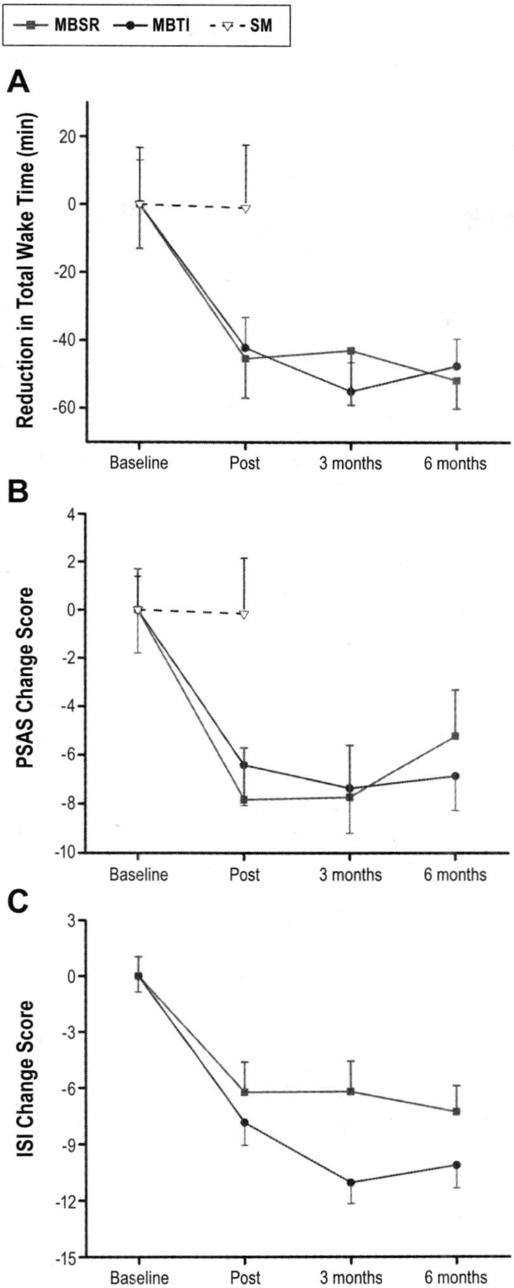

FIGURE 2.—Patient-reported outcomes. (**A**) Total wake time (in minutes; with standard error of the mean) across study arms as reported on sleep diaries. Data presented are change scores from baseline to each assessment point. Raw data (mean, standard deviation, effect sizes) for each arm are reported in Table 2. (**B**) Pre-sleep arousal scale (PSAS) total scores (with standard error of the mean) across study arms. Data presented are change scores from baseline to each assessment point. Raw data (mean, standard deviation, effect sizes) for each arm are reported in Table 2. (**C**) Insomnia Severity Index (ISI) total scores (with standard error of the mean) across the MBSR and MBTI arms. Data presented are change scores from baseline to each assessment point. Raw data (mean, standard deviation, effect sizes) for each arm are reported in Table 2. MBSR, mindfulness-based stress reduction; MBTI, mindfulness-based therapy for insomnia; SM, self-monitoring. (Reprinted from Ong JC, Manber R, Segal Z, et al. A randomized controlled trial of mindfulness meditation for chronic insomnia. *Sleep*. 2014;37:1553-1563, © 2014, American Academy of Sleep Medicine.)

seen only on self-reported measures (sleep diaries) and not on objective measures (PSG and actigraphy). Nevertheless, treatment effects were sustained in the meditation groups with those patients who received MBTI greater that MBSR, which may be due to the addition of the behavioral component of MBTI such as sleep restriction, etc.

Although I am not ready to prescribe mindfulness meditation to all my insomnia patients yet, I do think that this opens the doors to additional research in the field. More questions need to be answered, including applicability, comparative effectiveness research with hypnotics, and with CBTI, for example. Nevertheless, if additional research does show that mindfulness mediation is an effective treatment for chronic insomnia, I think many more patients could be reached and treated.

S. F. Jones, MD, FCCP, DABSM

A Randomized, Double Crossover Study to Investigate the Influence of Saline Infusion on Sleep Apnea Severity in Men

Yadollahi A, Gabriel JM, White LH, et al (Univ Health Network, Toronto, Canada; et al)

Sleep 37:1699-1705, 2014

Study Objectives.—Obstructive sleep apnea (OSA) is commoner in patients with fluid-retaining states than in those without fluid retention, in men than in women, and worsens with aging. In men, OSA severity is related to the amount of fluid shifting out of the legs overnight, but a cause-effect relationship is not established. Our objective was to test the hypothesis that mimicking fluid overload during sleep would increase severity of OSA more in older (≥ 40 years) than in younger men (< 40 years).

Design.—Randomized, single-blind, double crossover study.

Setting.—Research sleep laboratory.

Patients or Participants.—Seven older and 10 younger men with non-severe or no sleep apnea, matched for body mass index.

Interventions.—During the control arm, normal saline was infused to keep the vein open. During intervention, subjects received an intravenous bolus of normal saline (22 mL/kg body weight) after sleep onset while they were wearing compression stockings to prevent fluid accumulation in the legs.

Measurements and Results.—Compared to younger men, infusion of similar amounts of saline in older men caused a greater increase in neck circumference ($P < 0.05$) and in the AHI (32.2 ± 22.1 vs. 2.2 ± 7.1, $P = 0.002$).

Conclusions.—Older men are more susceptible to the adverse effects of intravenous fluid loading on obstructive sleep apnea severity than younger men. This may be due to age-related differences in the amount of fluid accumulating in the neck or upper airway collapsibility in response to intravenous fluid loading. These possibilities remain to be tested in future studies.

▶ This study draws on previous work from this group of investigators examining rostral fluid shift as a mechanism for upper airway obstruction in obstructive sleep apnea (OSA). In the previous study, these investigators reported that the Apnea Hypopnea Index (AHI) is strongly related to the amount of fluid displaced from the legs into the neck.[1] In this randomized single-blind double crossover study of 7 older and 10 younger men with AHI score < 10, a 22-mL/kg infusion of normal saline during 1 night resulted in an increase in neck circumference for both young and older men. However, in the older men, this infusion of saline also produced an increase in total AHI by 3-fold compared with the control night for older men (Fig 2 in the original article). This supports the investigators previous work that fluid loading may lead to the development of OSA.

The impact of this work may lie in the area of OSA and perioperative care. Previous research supports that patients with OSA have longer length of stay, serious complications, and unplanned intensive care unit transfers after surgery.[2] Surgical patients frequently receive intraoperative intravenous fluids. This may perhaps have negative consequences, but additional research is needed.

S. F. Jones, MD, FCCP, DABSM

References

1. Redolfi S, Yumino D, Ruttanaumpawan P, et al. Relationship between overnight rostral fluid shift and obstructive sleep apnea in nonobese men. *Am J Respir Crit Care Med.* 2009;179:241-246.
2. Kaw R, Pasupuleti V, Walker E, Ramaswamy A, Foldvary-Schafer N. Postoperative complications in patients with obstructive sleep apnea. *Chest.* 2012;141:436-441.

Pediatric Sleep-Disordered Breathing

Predictors of Obstructive Sleep Apnea Severity in Adenotonsillectomy Candidates

Weinstock TG, Rosen CL, Marcus CL, et al (Brigham and Women's Hosp and Beth Israel Deaconess Med Ctr, Boston, MA; Case Western Reserve Univ, Cleveland, OH; Univ of Pennsylvania, Philadelphia; et al)
Sleep 37:261-269, 2014

Study Objectives.—There is uncertainty over which characteristics increase obstructive sleep apnea syndrome (OSAS) severity in children. In candidates for adenotonsillectomy (AT), we evaluated the relationship of OSAS severity and age, sex, race, body mass index (BMI), environmental tobacco smoke (ETS), prematurity, socioeconomic variables, and comorbidities.

Design.—Cross-sectional screening and baseline data were analyzed from the Childhood Adenotonsillectomy Trial, a randomized, controlled, multicenter study evaluating AT versus medical management. Regression analysis assessed the relationship between the apnea hypopnea index (AHI) and risk factors obtained by direct measurement or questionnaire.

Setting.—Clinical referral setting.

Participants.—Children, ages 5 to 9.9 y with OSAS.

Measurements and Results.—Of the 1,244 children undergoing screening polysomnography, 464 (37%) were eligible ($2 \leq$ AHI < 30 or $1 \leq$ obstructive apnea index [OAI] < 20 and without severe oxygen desaturation) and randomized; 129 (10%) were eligible but were not randomized; 608 (49%) had AHI/OAI levels below entry criteria; and 43 (3%) had levels of OSAS that exceeded entry criteria. Among the randomized children, univariate analyses showed significant associations of AHI with race, BMI *z* score, environmental tobacco smoke (ETS), family income, and referral source, but not with other variables. After adjusting for potential confounders, African American race ($P = 0.003$) and ETS ($P = 0.026$) were each associated with an approximately 20% increase in AHI. After adjusting for these factors, obesity and other factors were not significant.

Conclusions.—Apnea hypopnea index level was significantly associated with race and environmental tobacco smoke, highlighting the potential effect of environmental factors, and possibly genetic factors, on pediatric obstructive sleep apnea syndrome severity. Efforts to reduce environmental tobacco smoke exposure may help reduce obstructive sleep apnea syndrome severity.

Clinical Trial Registration.—Clinicaltrials.gov (#NCT00560859).

▶ The Childhood Adenotonsillectomy Trial (CHAT) is a randomized controlled multicenter study evaluating adenotonsillectomy vs medical management in children. This study draws from that study sample and aims to find the risk factors for the presence and severity of OSA. It is important because it assesses the significance of each risk factor. Such knowledge would allow better screening tools in a clinical setting. Although in practice we see children who have histories of snoring, enlarged tonsils, asthma, allergies, eczema, obesity, and history of prematurity, it is difficult to know which of these factors are most predictive of OSA in children. In clinical practice, we perform sleep studies in children and find that some children who are loud snorers with enlarged tonsils do not have OSA and yet others who may have similar histories have significant OSA. In this study, half of the children who underwent polysomnography did not have OSA.

The characteristics of African-American race and environmental tobacco smoke were significantly associated and were the strongest predictors of the severity of the apnea hypopnea index in this study. These factors were significant and separate from obesity or presence of respiratory inflammation (from allergy or asthma) and from socioeconomic status. This finding highlights genetic predisposition and greater effect from environment on severity of OSA in children and weaker associations of symptoms and signs of OSA. It is not clear why African-American race and exposure to tobacco increases the severity, and additional research to explore these questions is needed. However, the findings of this study could direct screening efforts, referrals to sleep providers, and increase awareness to drive change and address preventable risk, such as tobacco exposure.

S. F. Jones, MD, FCCP, DABSM

8 Critical Care Medicine

Introduction

Each year I am amazed at the progress we are making in improving the care for our patients and in advanced medical science. We have accumulated some fascinating and useful reads. We start with a great article about how to line up the best view for laryngoscopy and intubation using the angle of the jaw. The last article disproves a common myth—that those with sepsis from cholecystitis improve from having a drain placed percutaneously when they are too ill for surgery. In between, there are more great articles on topical subjects that you will find great and enjoyable reading. I hope you enjoy them all as much as I did.

James A. Barker, MD, CPE, FACP, FCCP, FAASM

Sepsis

Preparing an ICU room to welcome a critically ill patient with Ebola virus disease

Pasquier P, Ficko C, Mérens A, et al (Bégin Military Teaching Hosp, Saint-Mandé, France)
Intensive Care Med 41:118-119, 2015

Background.—Hospitals are being equipped to manage the care of critically ill patients with Ebola virus disease. The specifics of what is needed for an Ebola virus disease-n-intensive care unit (EVD-ICU) differ from what is available in a regular ICU room.

Patient Equipment.—The EVD-ICU room is entered through an airlock, and negative air pressure is maintained. The pressure gradient increases from the airlock to the room. The equipment commonly found in an ICU room is present along with a field laboratory recovered with a pyramidal portable glove bag, a mobile system for obtaining radiographs, and a portable ultrasound machine. This equipment is dedicated to the patient throughout his or her stay in the room.

Healthcare Workers.—The safety of healthcare workers requires special equipment for the management of EVD patients. Their personal protective

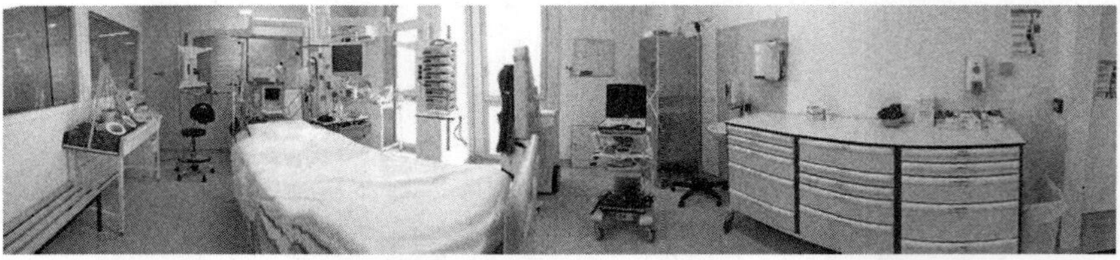

FIGURE 1.—A fully equipped EVD-ICU room. (With kind permission from Springer Science+Business Media. Pasquier P, Ficko C, Mérens A, et al. Preparing an ICU room to welcome a critically ill patient with Ebola virus disease. *Intensive Care Med.* 2015;41:118-119, with permission from Springer-Verlag Berlin Heidelberg and ESICM.)

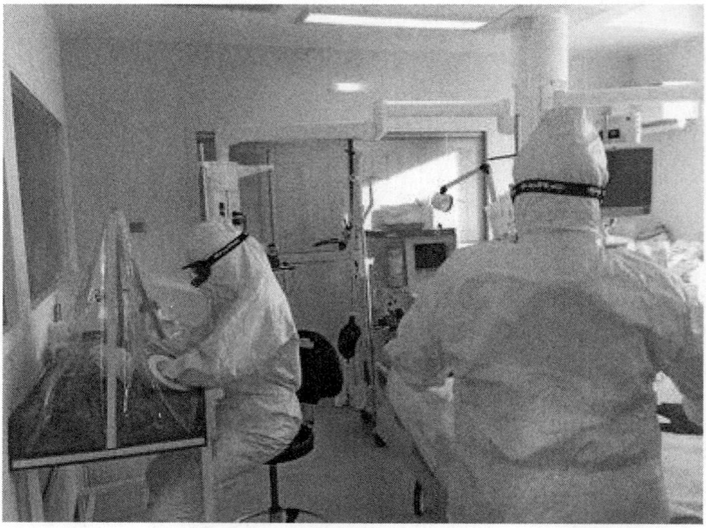

FIGURE 2.—Healthcare providers wearing PPE and training at a field laboratory recovered with a portable glove bag. (With kind permission from Springer Science+Business Media. Pasquier P, Ficko C, Mérens A, et al. Preparing an ICU room to welcome a critically ill patient with Ebola virus disease. *Intensive Care Med.* 2015;41:118-119, with permission from Springer-Verlag Berlin Heidelberg and ESICM.)

equipment includes a single-use impermeable gown, a hood, a face mask, goggles, two pairs of nitrile gloves, a pair of gloves with extended cuffs, and boots. In addition, specific equipment for the disposal of waste products is also available.

Conclusions.—The safe, appropriate management of EVD patients who require intensive care demands specific equipment in a dedicated ICU room. Both the patient and the healthcare provider must be accommodated (Figs 1 and 2).

▶ This is the reality in which we all now live. If your hospital has not invested the hours of preparation for Ebola or a similarly catastrophic outbreak, this short article will be of great use. Please review Figs 1 and 2, which outline the setup and personal protective equipment that will be needed.

J. A. Barker, MD, CPE, FACP, FCCP, FAASM

Diagnostic Characteristics of a Clinical Screening Tool in Combination With Measuring Bedside Lactate Level in Emergency Department Patients With Suspected Sepsis

Singer AJ, Taylor M, Domingo A, et al (Stony Brook Medicine, NY; et al)
Acad Emerg Med 21:853-857, 2014

Background.—Early identification of sepsis and initiation of aggressive treatment saves lives. However, the diagnosis of sepsis may be delayed in patients without overt deterioration. Clinical screening tools and lactate levels may help identify sepsis patients at risk for adverse outcomes.

Objectives.—The objective was to determine the diagnostic characteristics of a clinical screening tool in combination with measuring early bedside point-of-care (POC) lactate levels in emergency department (ED) patients with suspected sepsis.

Methods.—This was a prospective, observational study set at a suburban academic ED with an annual census of 90,000. A convenience sample of adult ED patients with suspected infection were screened with a sepsis screening tool for the presence of at least one of the following: temperature greater than 38°C or less than 36°C, heart rate greater than 90 beats/min, respiratory rate greater than 20 breaths/min, or altered mental status. Patients meeting criteria had bedside POC lactate testing following triage, which was immediately reported to the treating physician if ≥2.0 mmol/L. Demographic and clinical information, including lactate levels, ED interventions, and final diagnosis, were recorded. Outcomes included presence or absence of sepsis using the American College of Chest Physicians/Society of Critical Care Medicine consensus conference definitions and intensive care unit (ICU) admissions, use of vasopressors, and mortality. Diagnostic test characteristics were calculated using 2-by-2 tables with their 95% confidence intervals (CIs). The association between bedside lactate and ICU admissions, use of vasopressors, and mortality was determined using logistic regression.

Results.—A total of 258 patients were screened for sepsis. Their mean (± standard deviation [SD]) age was 64 (±19) years; 46% were female, and 82% were white. Lactate levels were 2.0 mmol/L or greater in 80 (31%) patients. Patients were confirmed to meet sepsis criteria in 208 patients (81%). The diagnostic characteristics for sepsis of the combined clinical screening tool and bedside lactates were sensitivity 34% (95% CI = 28% to 41%), specificity 82% (95% CI = 69% to 90%), positive predictive value 89% (95% CI = 80% to 94%), and negative predictive value 23% (95% CI = 17% to 30%). Bedside lactate levels were associated with sepsis severity ($p < 0.001$), ICU admission (odds ratio [OR] = 2.01; 95%

CI = 1.53 to 2.63), and need for vasopressors (OR = 1.54; 95% CI = 1.13 to 2.12).

Conclusions.—Use of a clinical screening tool in combination with early bedside POC lactates has moderate to good specificity but low sensitivity in adult ED patients with suspected sepsis. Elevated bedside lactate levels are associated with poor outcomes.

▶ This is a useful first-try study. However, my conclusion is different from the authors. I would argue that the clinical screening tool is too nonspecific to identify those patients who should then need lactate levels checked. Elevated lactate is specific that something bad is wrong with the system: underperfusion, sepsis, liver failure, or drug effect (such as metformin). In addition, the study size is too small for conclusions.

Adjustment of clinical screening criteria and measurement of lactate in a much larger population should be the next logical study. The hypothesis is worth further investigation.

J. A. Barker, MD, CPE, FACP, FCCP, FAASM

Bleeding complications of central venous catheterization in septic patients with abnormal hemostasis

Vinson DR, for the Kaiser Permanente CREST Network Investigators (The Permanente Med Group, Oakland, CA; et al)
Am J Emerg Med 32:737-742, 2014

Objectives.—Central venous catheterization (CVC) is thought to be relatively contraindicated in patients with thrombocytopenia or coagulopathy. We measured the 24-hour incidence of bleeding in septic emergency department (ED) patients undergoing CVC.

Methods.—This multicenter, retrospective cohort study included septic ED patients undergoing CVC with one of the following: platelets less than 100 000/μL, international normalized ratio at least 1.3, or partial thromboplastin time at least 35 seconds. Major bleeding included radiographically confirmed intrathoracic, mediastinal, or internal neck hemorrhage or line-related bleeding causing hemodynamic compromise. Minor bleeding included local oozing or superficial hematoma. Multivariable regression analysis was performed to determine the association between candidate variables and hemorrhagic complications.

Results.—Of the 936 cases, mean age was 68.1 years; 535 (57.2%) were male. Two or more qualifying laboratory abnormalities were present in 204 cases (21.8%). The proceduralists were predominately attendings (790; 84.4%). The initial veins were the internal jugular (n = 800; 85.5%), subclavian (n = 123; 13.1%), and femoral (n = 13; 1.4%). Initial access was successful in 872 cases (93.2%). We found one case (95% upper confidence limit: 0.6%) of major bleeding and 37 cases (4.0%; 95% confidence interval [CI], 2.8%-5.4%) of minor bleeding. Only failed

TABLE 1.—Distribution of Hemostatic Abnormalities in Patients Undergoing CVC

Hemostatic Abnormality	n = 936
INR level	n (%)
≥1.3	768 (82.1)
≥1.3 and <1.5	293 (31.3)
≥1.5 and <2.0	239 (25.5)
≥2.0 and <3.0[a]	139 (14.9)
≥3.0[a]	97 (10.4)
Platelet count (1000/μL)	
<100	317 (33.9)
≥75 and <100	146 (15.6)
≥50 and <75	100 (10.7)
≥20 and <50[a]	55 (5.9)
<20[a]	16 (1.7)
PTT ≥35 (s)	72 (7.7)
≥50[a]	17 (1.8)

[a]Moderate-to-severe hemostatic laboratory abnormality

TABLE 2.—Characteristics of Septic ED Patients Undergoing CVC

Patient Demographics	n = 936
Age, year mean (SD)	68.1 (14.9)
Sex, male (%)	535 (57.2)
Comorbidities	n (%)
Chronic kidney disease	280 (29.9)
Chronic liver disease	144 (15.4)
Congenital and acquired coagulation and qualitative platelet defects	42 (4.5)
Source of sepsis	
Pulmonary	363 (38.8)
Intraabdominal	187 (20.0)
Urinary	172 (18.4)
Skin/soft tissue	56 (6.0)
Other	45 (4.8)
Unclear	113 (12.1)
Initial ED laboratory values	
Hemoglobin (gm/dL)	
<8	79 (8.4)
≥8 <10	162 (17.3)
≥10	695 (74.3)
Creatinine clearance (mL/min)	
<30	310 (33.1)
≥30 <60	342 (36.5)
≥60	252 (26.9)
Not available	32 (3.4)
Serum lactate (mmol/L)	
<2.0	105 (11.2)
≥2.0 <4.0	233 (24.9)
≥4.0	598 (63.9)

access at the initial site was independently associated with hemorrhagic outcomes: adjusted odds ratio 8.2 (95% CI, 3.7-18.0).

Conclusions.—Major bleeding from CVC in ED patients with abnormal hemostasis is rare. Minor bleeding is uncommon and infrequently requires intervention. Successful catheterization on the initial attempt is associated with fewer hemorrhagic complications. These results can inform the risk/benefit calculus for CVC in this population (Tables 1 and 2).

▶ This is an important article. Many physicians worry and alter practice for this subgroup of patients—those with abnormal coagulation parameters yet who are acutely ill and in need of fluid resuscitation and thus central line placement. I am pleasantly surprised that only 1 of 936 patients had a major hemorrhagic complication. The other finding confirms my own previous clinical experience (and I suspect that of our readers): namely, placement of the lines will have many fewer complications if the first attempt is successful. In other words, line up the cue ball for the money ball shot. Use ultrasound and physical examination to find the most suitable anatomic location. Go for a compressible vessel in case local hemorrhage does occur. Use a seasoned physician to place the line.

This means an attending or senior resident will carefully examine the patient for a jugular or femoral line placement.

In an emergency, the operator can then proceed with cannulation without awaiting platelets or reversal of other coagulant factors. Table 1 demonstrates that many of these patients are quite coagulopathic (25% with international normalized ratio > 2.0! and 34% with platelets < 100 000). Table 2 likewise confirms that these are indeed quite ill patients, predominantly with kidney or liver disease. Only 11% had normal lactic acid levels.

This is a useful study for day-to-day care of these critically ill patients.

J. A. Barker, MD, CPE, FACP, FCCP, FAASM

Cholecystostomy offers no survival benefit in patients with acute acalculous cholecystitis and severe sepsis and shock

Anderson JE, Inui T, Talamini MA, et al (Univ of California San Diego; SUNY Stony Brook, NY)

J Surg Res 190:517-521, 2014

Background.—Acute acalculous cholecystitis is often managed with cholecystectomy or cholecystostomy, but data guiding surgical practice are lacking.

Materials and Methods.—Longitudinal analysis of the California Office of Statewide Health Planning and Development Patient Discharge Data was performed from 1995-2009. Patients with acute acalculous cholecystitis were identified by International Classification of Diseases 9 code. Cox proportional hazard analysis found predictors of time to death, adjusting for patient demographics, sepsis, shock, frailty, Charlson comorbidity index, length of stay, insurance status, teaching hospital status, and year.

Results.—Of 43,341 patients, 63.5% received a cholecystectomy, 2.8% received a cholecystostomy, and 1.2% received both. Overall, 30.4% of patients died, with higher mortality among patients with cholecystostomy (61.7%) or no procedure (42.0%) than cholecystectomy (23.0%). In patients with severe sepsis and shock, there was no difference in survival of patients with cholecystostomy versus no intervention (hazard ratio [HR] 1.13, $P = 0.256$), although patients with cholecystectomy (with or without prior cholecystostomy) had improved survival (HR 0.29, $P < 0.001$; HR 0.56, $P < 0.001$). Results were similar among patients on the ventilator >96 h.

Conclusions.—Although cholecystostomy offered no survival benefit for patients with severe sepsis and shock, cholecystectomy offered improved survival compared with patients without surgical management. Cholecystostomy may not benefit the sickest patients in whom cholecystectomy may never be considered.

▶ This actually comes up quite frequently. Severely ill patients develop acalculous cholecystitis but are deemed too ill for acute surgery, and therefore a percutaneous drainage is performed. Occasionally the gallbladder disintegrates, and a new problem presents itself. This large database suggests no improvement in survival by doing the tube drainage.

J. A. Barker, MD, CPE, FACP, FCCP, FAASM

Early intensive care unit-acquired hypernatremia in severe sepsis patients receiving 0.9% saline fluid resuscitation

Van de Louw A, Shaffer C, Schaefer E (Penn State Univ College of Medicine, Hershey, PA)

Acta Anaesthesiol Scand 58:1007-1014, 2014

Background.—Intensive care unit (ICU)-acquired hypernatremia is associated with increased mortality and ascribed to excessive sodium/insufficient free water intakes. We aimed to determine whether the volume of intravenous 0.9% saline fluid resuscitation was associated with hypernatremia in severe sepsis.

Methods.—We retrospectively reviewed the charts of patients admitted to our medical ICU over 1 year with severe sepsis, and recorded all fluid intakes and plasma sodium levels (Na_p) for 5 days along with clinical data. ΔNa_p was defined as the difference between maximal Na_p reached and initial Na_p. Hypernatremia was defined as $Na_p > 145$ mmoles/l.

Results.—Among 95 patients with severe sepsis, 29 developed hypernatremia within 5 days (31%), reaching a maximum Na_p of 149.1 ± 2.5 mmoles/l on average 3.8 ± 1.5 days after admission. For every 50-ml/kg increase in 0.9% saline intake for the first 48 h, the odds of hypernatremia were 1.61 times larger [confidence interval (CI): 0.98-2.62; $P = 0.06$] and the mean of ΔNa_p increased by 1.86 mmoles/l (CI: 0.86-2.86; $P < 0.001$). Compared with non-hypernatremic patients, hypernatremic patients received more 0.9% saline within the first 48 h (111 ± 50 ml/kg vs. 92 ± 42 ml/kg, $P < 0.05$) and more other fluids from 48 to 96 h (64 ± 38 ml/kg vs. 42 ± 24 ml/kg, $P < 0.05$). Patients developing hypernatremia had increased length of mechanical ventilation (12.0 ± 12.6 vs. 9.1 ± 7.2 days, $P < 0.05$) and ICU mortality (38.5% vs. 13%, $P < 0.01$).

Conclusions.—Early acquired hypernatremia is a frequent complication in severe sepsis patients and is associated with the volume of 0.9% saline received during the first 48 h of admission.

▶ It is always worthwhile to look at current practice to see if we are helping or harming patients. Current approaches to septic shock include aggressive volume resuscitation. This is most commonly done with normal saline. However, just as in patients with diabetic ketoacidosis, there is risk of raising both sodium and chloride. This may have deleterious effects. The authors here show correlation with increased ventilation days and worsened mortality. Clearly we don't want that!

Figure 3 nicely demonstrates the linear correlation between volume of normal saline given and rise in sodium. What is the solution? I am sure there are several reasonable possibilities such as changing solutions earlier (half normal saline, lactated Ringer's, colloids, and so on). Perhaps fluids could be reduced on day 2 of hospitalization.

These are important observations. Sepsis is common, and the physician's mantra should always be "first do no harm."

J. A. Barker, MD, CPE, FACP, FCCP, FAASM

Early Management of Severe Sepsis: Concepts and Controversies

Marik PE (Eastern Virginia Med School, Norfolk, VA)
Chest 145:1407-1418, 2014

Sepsis is among the most common reasons for admission to ICUs throughout the world, and it is believed to be the third most common cause of death in the United States. The pathogenetic mechanism and physiologic changes associated with sepsis are exceedingly complex, but our understanding is evolving rapidly. The major pathophysiologic changes in patients with septic shock include vasoplegic shock (distributive shock), myocardial depression, altered microvascular flow, and a diffuse endothelial injury. These pathophysiologic changes play a central role in the management of sepsis. The early management of patients with severe sepsis and septic shock centers on the administration of antibiotics, IV fluids, and vasoactive agents, followed by source control. However, the specific approach to the resuscitation of patients with septic shock remains highly controversial. This review provides a practical and physiologic-based approach to the early management of sepsis and explores the controversies surrounding the management of this complex condition.

▶ Dr Marik lays out the current controversies of sepsis management in a thoughtful and clear-cut article. He differs somewhat from the Surviving Sepsis leadership and publications but outlines his rationale and backs it up with literature support. This is a useful read for all intensivists.

J. A. Barker, MD, CPE, FACP, FCCP, FAASM

Airway

Angular change in the line of vision to the larynx: implications for determining the laryngoscopic view

Park S, Jeong J, Cha S, et al (Seoul Natl Univ Bundang Hosp, Korea)
Can J Anaesth 61:433-440, 2014

Background.—We measured the angular change from the line of vision to the larynx around the upper incisors under defined laryngoscopic forces and investigated its association with the laryngoscopic view.

Methods.—Laryngoscopy was performed under general anesthesia with muscle paralysis in male patients with a difficult laryngoscopy (DLG, n = 11) and in male patients matched for age and body mass index with an easy laryngoscopy (ELG, n = 11). A Macintosh blade #3 was used for the procedure. The line of vision was marked on lateral photographs during laryngoscopy by simultaneously delineating two straight lines: a line from the upper incisors to the lowest surface of the laryngoscope blade and a line from the upper incisors to the thyroid notch. The angle difference, defined as the angle between those two lines, was measured at laryngoscopic forces of 10-50 N.

Results.—The angle difference was significantly greater in the DLG than in the ELG at 50 N [median, 18.0° (range, 16.5-21.0°) vs 12.0° (12.0-13.5°), respectively; $P < 0.001$] and at lower forces (10-40 N; $P \leq 0.001$). A higher Cormack-Lehane grade was associated with a greater angle difference at 50 N ($P < 0.001$).

Conclusions.—Compared with ELG, DLG is associated with a larger angle difference, i.e., a larger gap between the underside of the blade and the thyroid notch at all laryngoscopic forces (10-50 N). The concept of angle difference, based on the angular change in the line of vision around the upper incisors, may provide a new approach to understanding DLG. This study was registered with the Clinical Research Information Service, registration number KCT0000433.

▶ Numerous methods have been used to predict a difficult airway. However, none are perfect. These authors discuss the anatomy and approaches very nicely. In addition, the technique described shows considerable promise as a predictive model. See Fig 3 in the original article to better visualize the angles and technique itself. Every intensivist should learn these anatomic pearls to avoid a missed or difficult intubation in the future.

J. A. Barker, MD, CPE, FACP, FCCP, FAASM

Difficult Airway Management for Novice Physicians: A Randomized Trial Comparing Direct and Video-Assisted Laryngoscopy

Ambrosio A, Pfannenstiel T, Bach K, et al (Naval Med Ctr San Diego, CA)
Otolaryngol Head Neck Surg 150:775-778, 2014

Objectives.—To detect a difference in (1) intubation success and (2) successful intubation times between novice physicians using a Macintosh-style or video-assisted laryngoscope on a difficult airway manikin.

Study Design.—Prospective randomized trial.

Setting.—Academic, tertiary medical center.

Methods.—Forty first-year residents across a variety of disciplines with fewer than 5 total live intubations were recruited for the study. Testing took place during orientation prior to commencement of clinical duties. The entire group was provided training by faculty otolaryngologists and anesthesiologists using both laryngoscope types on a manikin airway simulator in a standard intubating scenario. Subjects were then randomized into 2 testing groups, using either a Macintosh laryngoscope or video-assisted laryngoscope in a difficult intubation scenario. The difficult airway simulation entailed oral cavity/oropharyngeal obstruction using inflation of the tongue, as well as cervical spine immobilization with a rigid collar preventing extension and elevation of the head and limiting oral cavity opening. Success was defined as a confirmed endotracheal intubation by the testing instructor in 120 seconds or less.

Results.—The Macintosh laryngoscope group ($n = 19$) had an intubation success rate of 47.4% with a mean intubation time of 69.0 seconds (95% confidence interval [CI]: 52.7, 85.2). The video-assisted group ($n = 21$) demonstrated a significantly higher success rate of 100% ($P < .0001$) and a decreased mean intubation time of 23.1 seconds (95% CI: 18.4, 27.8; $P < .0001$). The mean difference in success rate between groups was 52.6% (95% CI: 30.0%, 75.3%).

Conclusions.—Novice physicians with little to no prior intubation experience showed significantly higher intubation success with lower intubation times using a video-assisted laryngoscope in a difficult airway manikin simulator.

▶ Video laryngoscopy for intubation should now be the standard in teaching hospitals, which this study confirms. One hundred percent success in half the time compared with under 50% success could mean the difference between life and death for a patient. In addition, the mentor can see what the learner is doing both to instruct and to ensure the proper placement of the endotracheal tube.

This simple study is useful as well as elegant.

J. A. Barker, MD, CPE, FACP, FCCP, FAASM

Acute Respiratory Disorder Syndrome

Acute respiratory distress attributed to sirolimus in solid organ transplant recipients

Wang WL, Yu LX (Tianjin First Central Hosp, China)
Am J Emerg Med 33:124.e1-124.e4, 2015

Pulmonary toxicity has frequently been recognized as a potentially serious complication associated with sirolimus therapy. It consists of a wide spectrum of syndromes most characterized by the presence of lymphocytic alveolitis and lymphocytic interstitial pneumonitis. The most commonly presenting symptoms are fever and dyspnea. Chest computed tomography generally reveals bilateral, patchy, or diffuse alveolointerstitial infiltrates. The discontinuation or dose reduction of sirolimus usually leads in most cases to a good outcome with complete clinical and radiologic resolution. However, to establish a diagnosis is difficult because of the absence of specific diagnostic criteria, and in rare cases, it could be fatal or life threatening when the diagnosis was delayed. Here, we reported 2 severe cases of acute respiratory distress attributed to the therapy of sirolimus in solid organ transplant recipients. Although the diagnostic course was difficult, withdrawal of sirolimus and temporary administration of steroids eventually resulted in a rapid recovery in both 2 patients. In addition, possible mechanisms, clinical characteristics, approach to diagnosis, and treatment strategies of sirolimus-induced pulmonary toxicity were also discussed in this article.

▶ Acute respiratory distress syndrome (ARDS) is, as its name indicates, a syndrome. There are many putative causes. Sirolimus should now be added to that list. This is important in these days of complex medicine when solid organ transplants are commonly done. Rather than acute rejection or *Pneumocystis* pneumonia, ARDS will now have to be added to the list of differential diagnoses for acute hypoxemic respiratory failure after transplant.

J. A. Barker, MD, CPE, FACP, FCCP, FAASM

Acute Respiratory Failure

A 42-Year-Old Farmer From Bangladesh With Respiratory Failure, Septic Arthritis, and Multiple Cavitating Consolidations

AlShati MH, Joshi RM (Al-Adan Hosp, Ahmadi, Kuwait)
Chest 146:e56-e59, 2014

A 42-year-old man was directly admitted to the ICU with respiratory failure and hypotension. Two weeks prior and just after returning from

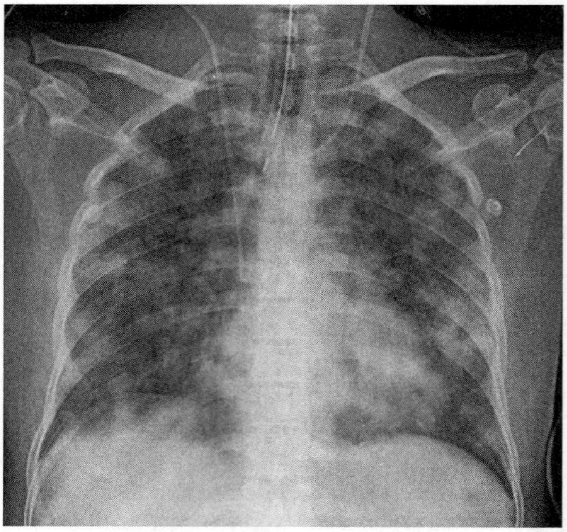

FIGURE 1.—Plain posteroanterior chest radiograph showing multifocal cavitating consolidations. Endotracheal tube and right and left internal jugular central lines are also evident. (Reprinted from AlShati MH, Joshi RM. A 42-year-old farmer from bangladesh with respiratory failure, septic arthritis, and multiple cavitating consolidations. *Chest.* 2014;146:e56-e59, © 2014, American College of Chest Physicians.)

Bangladesh, he presented to a polyclinic with fever, right knee pain, and generalized aches, for which he received oral antibiotics. He was a farmer, had diabetes, never smoked, and consumed alcohol occasionally (Fig 1).

▶ Travel history is paramount. That much is clear to all of us—in this new age of pandemics such as ebola virus disease.

Melioidosis is a disease we all study and that shows up on examinations. Occasionally, it may be seen in real life. It had previously been classified as a *Pseudomonas* infection. However, the antibiotic sensitivity pattern and other microbiologic characteristics certainly confirm the placement of it in the *Burkholderia* genus.

Not all cavitating nodules are squamous cell lung cancers or endocarditis from *Staphylococcus aureus*! Look closely at Fig 1.

J. A. Barker, MD, CPE, FACP, FCCP, FAASM

Acute Lung Injury

A Quality Improvement Project Sustainably Decreased Time to Onset of Active Physical Therapy Intervention in Patients with Acute Lung Injury

Dinglas VD, Parker AM, Reddy DRS, et al (Johns Hopkins Univ School of Medicine, Baltimore, MD; Mayo Clinic, Rochester, MN)
Ann Am Thorac Soc 11:1230-1238, 2014

Rationale.—Rehabilitation started early during an intensive care unit (ICU) stay is associated with improved outcomes and is the basis for many quality improvement (QI) projects showing important changes in practice. However, little evidence exists regarding whether such changes are sustainable in real-world practice.

Objectives.—To evaluate the sustained effect of a quality improvement project on the timing of initiation of active physical therapy intervention in patients with acute lung injury (ALI).

Methods.—This was a pre–post evaluation using prospectively collected data involving consecutive patients with ALI admitted pre–quality improvement (October 2004–April 2007, n = 120) versus post–quality improvement (July 2009–July 2012, n = 123) from a single medical ICU.

Measurements and Main Results.—The primary outcome was time to first active physical therapy intervention, defined as strengthening, mobility, or cycle ergometry exercises. Among ICU survivors, more patients in the post–quality improvement versus pre–quality improvement group received physical therapy in the ICU (89% vs. 24%, $P < 0.001$) and were able to stand, transfer, or ambulate during physical therapy in the ICU (64% vs. 7%, $P < 0.001$). Among all patients in the post–quality improvement versus pre–quality improvement group, there was a shorter median (interquartile range) time to first physical therapy (4 [2, 6] vs. 11 d [6, 29], $P < 0.001$) and a greater median (interquartile range) proportion of ICU days with physical therapy after initiation (50% [33, 67%] vs. 18% [4, 47%], $P = 0.003$). In multivariable regression analysis, the post–quality improvement period was associated with shorter time to physical therapy (adjusted hazard ratio [95% confidence interval], 8.38 [4.98, 14.11], $P < 0.001$), with this association significant for each of the 5 years during the post–quality improvement period. The following variables were independently associated with a longer time to physical therapy: higher Sequential Organ Failure Assessment score (0.93 [0.89, 0.97]), higher FI_{O2} (0.86 [0.75, 0.99] for each 10% increase), use of an opioid infusion (0.47 [0.25, 0.89]), and deep sedation (0.24 [0.12, 0.46]).

Conclusions.—In this single-site, pre–post analysis of patients with ALI, an early rehabilitation quality improvement project was independently associated with a substantial decrease in the time to initiation of active physical therapy intervention that was sustained over 5 years. Over the entire pre–post period, severity of illness and sedation were independently associated with a longer time to initiation of active physical therapy intervention in the ICU.

▶ Quality improvement is particularly difficult to sustain. This study demonstrates "hard-wiring" movement to early physical therapy in intensive care unit patients. Review of Table 2 in the original article shows just how different this approach was for pre- and postintervention for actual patients. Although this seems simple, there are significant implications. For example, much less sedation and paralysis is used when patients are planned for early mobility. And other studies have shown a mortality benefit to early mobility as well as other more obvious benefits such as decrease in pressure ulcer and deep vein thrombosis risk. The movement to early mobility continues to build!

J. A. Barker, MD, CPE, FACP, FCCP, FAASM

Trauma

Association of head, thoracic and abdominal trauma with delayed diagnosis of co-existing injuries in critical trauma patients

Lee W-C, Chen C-W, Lin Y-K, et al (Kaohsiung Med Univ Hosp, Kaohsiung, Taiwan)

Injury 45:1429-1434, 2014

Background.—Management of critically injured patients is usually complicated and challenging. A structured team approach with comprehensive survey is warranted. However, delayed diagnosis of co-existing injuries that are less severe or occult might still occur, despite a standard thorough approach coupled with advances in image intervention. Clinicians are easily distracted or occupied by the more obvious or threatening conditions. We hypothesised that the major area of injured body regions might contribute to this unwanted condition.

Methods.—A retrospective study of all trauma patients admitted to our surgical intensive care units (ICU) was performed to survey the incidence of delayed diagnosis of injury (DDI) and the association between main body region injured and possibility of DDI. Demographic data and main body regions injured were compared and statistically analysed between patients with and without DDI.

Results.—During the two-year study period, a total 976 trauma patients admitted to our surgical ICU were included in this study. The incidence of DDI was 12.1% (118/976). Patients with DDI had higher percentages of thoracic, abdominal, and pelvic injuries (30.5%, 16.1%, and 7.6% respectively) than the non-DDI group (14.7%, 7.5%, and 3.0% respectively) ($p < 0.001$, 0.003, and 0.024 respectively). A logistic regression model demonstrated that head (odds ratio = 1.99; 95% CI = 1.20–3.31), thoracic (odds ratio = 2.44; 95% CI = 1.55–3.86), and abdominal injuries (odds ratio = 2.38; 95% CI = 1.28–4.42) were independently associated with increasing DDI in patients admitted to the surgical ICU.

Discussion.—In conclusion, critical trauma patients admitted to the surgical ICU with these categories of injuries were more likely to have DDI. Clinicians should pay more attention to patients admitted due to injuries in these regions. More detailed and dedicated secondary and tertiary surveys should be given, with more frequent and careful re-evaluation (Table 3).

▶ Traumatologists pride themselves in a thorough approach to these complex and severely injured patients. They use checklists and primary, secondary, and tertiary survey techniques to minimize missed injuries. Despite this organized and systematic approach, they can and do still miss important injuries. Table 3

TABLE 3.—Independent Risk Factors[a] Associated with Delayed Diagnosis

Factor	Odds Ratio	p Value	95% Confidence Interval
Head injury	1.99	0.007	1.20–3.31
Thoracic injury	2.44	<0.001	1.55–3.86
Abdominal injury	2.38	0.006	1.28–4.42
Soft tissue injury	1.73	0.054	1.00–3.03

[a]The risk factors included in the logistic regression model were head injury, thoracic injury, abdominal injury, and soft tissue injury.

indicates that a trouble spot is the presence of a major injury to head, thorax, abdomen, or soft tissue. In those patients, tunnel vision can develop, and thus important injuries may have delayed diagnosis. These could, of course, be catastrophic events, such as an aorta tear or splenic hemorrhage. Perhaps repeat secondary and tertiary surveys should always be done after initial stabilization.

In supporting surgeons, I found the same findings to be true. As an internist intensivist, it is our call to be comprehensive and thorough. However, our surgical colleagues have the training to then evaluate traumatic injuries. It is truly a team sport.

J. A. Barker, MD, CPE, FACP, FCCP, FAASM

Air Transport of Patients with Pneumothorax: Is Tube Thoracostomy Required Before Flight?

Braude D, Tutera D, Tawil I, et al (Univ of New Mexico Health Science Ctr, Albuquerque)

Air Med J 33:152-156, 2014

Objective.—It is conventionally thought that patients with pneumothorax (PTX) require tube thoracostomy (TT) before air medical transport (AMT), especially in unpressurized rotor-wing (RW) aircraft, to prevent deterioration from expansion of the PTX or development of tension PTX. We hypothesize that patients with PTX transported without TT tolerate RW AMT without serious deterioration, as defined by hypotension, hypoxemia, respiratory distress, intubation, bag valve mask ventilation, needle thoracostomy (NT), or cardiac arrest during transport.

Methods.—We conducted a retrospective review of a case-series of trauma patients transported to a single Level 1 trauma center via RW with confirmed PTX and no TT. Using standardized abstraction forms, we reviewed charts for signs of deterioration. Those patients identified as having clinical deterioration were independently reviewed for the likelihood that the clinical deterioration was a direct consequence of PTX.

Results.—During the study period, 66 patients with confirmed PTX underwent RW AMT with an average altitude gain of 1890 feet, an average barometric pressure 586-600 mm Hg, and average flight duration of 28 minutes. All patients received oxygen therapy; 14/66 patients (21%) were supported with positive pressure ventilation. Eleven of 66 patients (17%) had NT placed before flight and 4/66 (6%) had NT placed during flight. Four of 66 patients (6% CI 0.3-11.7) may have deteriorated during AMT as a result of PTX; all were successfully managed with NT.

Conclusions.—In this series, 6% of patients with PTX deteriorated as result of AMT without TT, yet all patients were managed successfully with NT. Routine placement of TT in patients with PTX before RW AMT may not be necessary. Further prospective evaluation is warranted.

▶ Standard dogma is that patients with pneumothoraces should not fly (nor dive!). However, these authors present useful information that contradicts the dogma. This does have important implications for trauma patients. For example, perhaps they can transport directly to the Level 1 trauma center rather than have a chest tube placed at a first-stop hospital or in the field (which will not always be possible). More information is needed, but this is a useful contribution.

J. A. Barker, MD, CPE, FACP, FCCP, FAASM

Non Invasive Ventilation

Efficacy and Safety of Early Dexmedetomidine During Noninvasive Ventilation for Patients with Acute Respiratory Failure: A Randomized, Double-Blind, Placebo-Controlled Pilot Study

Devlin JW, Al-Qadheeb NS, Chi A, et al (Northeastern Univ, Boston, MA; Tufts Med Ctr, Boston, MA)
Chest 145:1204-1212, 2014

Background.—Successful application of noninvasive ventilation (NIV) for acute respiratory failure (ARF) requires patient cooperation and comfort. The efficacy and safety of early IV dexmedetomidine when added to protocolized, as-needed IV midazolam and fentanyl remain unclear.

Methods.—Adults with ARF and within 8 h of starting NIV were randomized to receive IV dexmedetomidine (0.2 μg/kg/h titrated every 30 min to 0.7 μg/kg/h to maintain a Sedation-Agitation Scale [SAS] score of 3 to 4) or placebo in a double-blind fashion up to 72 h, until NIV was stopped for ≥ 2 h, or until intubation. Patients with agitation (SAS ≥ 5) or pain (visual analog scale ≥ 5 of 10 cm) 15 min after each dexmedetomidine and placebo increase could receive IV midazolam 0.5 to 1.0 mg or IV fentanyl 25 to 50 μg, respectively, at a minimum interval of every 3 h.

Results.—The dexmedetomidine (n = 16) and placebo (n = 17) groups were similar at baseline. Use of early dexmedetomidine did not improve NIV tolerance (score, 1 of 4; OR, 1.44; 95% CI, 0.44-4.70; P = .54) nor, vs placebo, led to a greater median (interquartile range) percent time either tolerating NIV (99% [61%-100%] vs 67% [40%-100%], *P* =.56) or remaining at the desired sedation level (SAS score = 3 or 4, 100% [86%-100%] vs 100% [100%-100%], *P* =.28), or fewer intubations (*P* =.79). Although use of dexmedetomidine was associated with a greater duration of NIV vs placebo (37 [16-72] vs 12 [4-22] h, *P* =.03), the total ventilation duration (NIV + invasive) was similar (3.3 [2-4] days vs 3.8 [2-5] days, *P* =.52). More patients receiving dexmedetomidine had one or more episodes of deep sedation vs placebo (SAS ≤ 2, 25% vs 0%, *P* =.04). Use of midazolam (*P* =.40) and episodes of either severe bradycardia (heart rate ≤ 50 beats/min, *P* =.18) or hypotension (systolic BP ≤ 90 mm Hg, *P* =.64) were similar.

Conclusions.—Initiating dexmedetomidine soon after NIV initiation in patients with ARF neither improves NIV tolerance nor helps to maintain sedation at a desired goal. Randomized, multicenter trials targeting patients with initial intolerance are needed to further elucidate the role for dexmedetomidine in this population.

Trial Registry.—ClinicalTrials.gov; No: NCT00871624; URL: www.clinicaltrials.gov.

▶ This is a common practice at present, yet there is little evidence to confirm its efficacy. This study indicates that other alternatives should be pursued for sedation in patients on noninvasive ventilation. No efficacy was demonstrated in this nice study.

J. A. Barker, MD, CPE, FACP, FCCP, FAASM

Severe Pneumonia

Excluding infection through procalcitonin testing improves outcomes of congestive heart failure patients presenting with acute respiratory symptoms: Results from the randomized ProHOSP trial

Schuetz P, for the ProHOSP Study Group (Univ Dept of Medicine, Aarau, Switzerland; et al)

Int J Cardiol 175:464-472, 2014

Background/Objectives.—We sought to determine whether exclusion of infection and antibiotic stewardship with the infection biomarker procalcitonin improves outcomes in congestive heart failure (CHF) patients presenting to emergency departments with respiratory symptoms and suspicion of respiratory infection.

Methods.—We performed a secondary analysis of patients with a past medical history of CHF formerly included in a Swiss multicenter randomized-controlled trial. The trial compared antibiotic stewardship according to a procalcitonin algorithm or state-of-the-art guidelines (controls). The primary endpoint was a 30-day adverse outcome (death, intensive care unit admission); the secondary endpoints included a 30-day antibiotic exposure.

Results.—In the 110/233 analyzed patients (47.2%) with low initial procalcitonin (<0.25 μg/L), suggesting the absence of systemic bacterial infection, those randomized to procalcitonin guidance (n = 50) had a significantly lower adverse outcome rate compared to controls (n = 60): 4% vs. 20% (absolute difference −16.0%, 95% confidence interval (CI) −28.4% to −3.6%, $P = 0.01$), and significantly reduced antibiotic exposure [days] (mean 3.7 ± 4.0 vs. 6.5 ± 4.4, difference−2.8 [95% CI, −4.4 to −1.2], $P < 0.01$). When initial procalcitonin was ≥0.25 μg/L, procalcitonin-guided patients had significantly reduced antibiotic exposure due to early stop of therapy without any difference in adverse outcomes (25.8% vs. 24.6%, difference [95% CI] 1.2% [−14.5% to 16.9%, $P = 0.88$]).

Conclusions.—CHF patients presenting to the emergency department with respiratory symptoms and suspicion for respiratory infection had decreased antibiotic exposure and improved outcomes when procalcitonin measurement was used to exclude bacterial infection and guide antibiotic treatment. These data provide further evidence for the potential harmful effects of antibiotic / fluid treatment when used instead of diuretics and heart failure medication in clinically symptomatic CHF patients without underlying infection.

▶ Is it heart failure or pneumonia? This is a frequent question for the pulmonologist. Procalcitonin measurement can be helpful when applied in a logical approach as outlined here. Congestive heart failure does not improve with antibiotics!

J. A. Barker, MD, CPE, FACP, FCCP, FAASM

Pulmonary Hypertension

Catheter-Directed Thrombolytic Intervention Is Effective for Patients with Massive and Submassive Pulmonary Embolism

Akin H, Al-Jubouri M, Assi Z, et al (Jobst Vascular Inst, Toledo, OH)
Ann Vasc Surg 28:1589-1594, 2014

Background.—Massive pulmonary embolism (MPE) is a significant cause of mortality and, with submassive pulmonary embolism (SPE), is associated with chronic thromboembolic pulmonary hypertension, resulting in ongoing patient morbidity. Standard treatment is anticoagulation, although systemic thrombolytic therapy has been shown to reduce early mortality in patients with MPE and improve cardiopulmonary hemodynamics in patients with SPE. However, systemic lysis is associated with significant bleeding risk. Early reports of catheter-directed techniques (CDT) suggest favorable outcomes in patients with MPE and SPE with reduced risk of hemorrhage. The purpose of this study is to evaluate efficacy and safety outcomes in MPE and SPE patients treated with CDT.

Methods.—Seventeen patients treated with CDT for MPE and SPE were clinically and hemodynamically evaluated. Patients were grouped by severity of pulmonary embolism: MPE ($n = 5$) or SPE ($n = 12$). Pre- and post-interventional measures were assessed, including pulmonary artery pressures (PAPs), cardiac biomarkers, tricuspid regurgitation, right ventricular (RV) dilatation, and systolic function. Nine patients had contraindications to systemic thrombolytic therapy.

Results.—PAP was elevated in 94% at presentation. The average dose of recombinant tissue plasminogen activator (rt-PA) was 31 mg; 44 mg in MPE and 26 mg in SPE. Pre- and post-intervention PAPs were recorded in 13 patients. All demonstrated an acute reduction in post-treatment PAP, averaging 37%. At presentation, all MPE and 10 (83%) SPE patients showed both RV dilatation and reduced function on echocardiography, which normalized in 76% (13/ 17) and improved in 24% (4/17) after CDT. Patients who demonstrated left ventricle underfilling before CDT (2 [40%] MPE and 2 [20%] SPE) normalized after CDT. All MPE and 11 (92%) SPE patients had tricuspid regurgitation on echocardiography pretreatment, which resolved in 60% and 58% of MPE and SPE patients, respectively. One delayed mortality occurred in an MPE patient who was hypotensive and hypoxic at presentation. There was one puncture site bleed.

Conclusions.—CDT was successful in the acute management of patients with MPE and SPE. CDT rapidly restores cardiopulmonary hemodynamics using reduced doses of rt-PA. These observations suggest that CDT should be considered in MPE and SPE patients to rapidly restore cardiopulmonary hemodynamics, reduce acute morbidity and mortality, reduce bleeding complications, and potentially avoid long-term morbidity.

▶ This procedure is now commonly performed by interventional radiologists. It is reassuring to know that it is indeed safe and effective for those patients who need it.

J. A. Barker, MD, CPE, FACP, FCCP, FAASM

Miscellaneous

Critical care responsibility in health care reform: What would Osler say?

Moore EE, Moore HB (Denver Health Med Ctr, CO)

J Trauma Acute Care Surg 76:1507-1509, 2014

Background.—The costs of health care in the United States now account for about 18% of the gross domestic product. However, US global health care among the 34 Organization for Economic Co-operation and Development (OECD) countries now ranks 26th for life expectancy and healthy life expectancy, which are 78.7 years and 68.1 years, respectively. In principle the Patient Protection and Affordable Care Act was designed to address the crisis but progress will rely on active participation by all healthcare system stakeholders. Forty-two percent of the expenditures are on hospitals and other care facilities, 30% on professional services,

13% on prescription drugs and equipment, 7% on administrative costs, 6% on investment, and 3% on public health.

Analysis of Health Concerns.—The main risk factors identified by the US Burden of Health Collaborators for poor health status are dietary composition, tobacco smoking, hypertension, high body mass index, and physical inactivity. These risks are unlikely to be altered in the near future even with the current emphasis on preventive care. Doctors' choices in managing these conditions and their adverse consequences are a key factor in controlling healthcare costs. However, most physicians believe that trial lawyers, health insurance companies, health systems, and pharmaceutical and/or device manufacturers should shoulder most of the blame, with just over a third seeing practicing physicians as having a major role. However, the third-party payment system is responsible for providing unneeded tests, drugs, or procedures that waste dollars.

Value-Based Care.—In value-based care, limited resources are balanced against the care of individual patients. In educating physicians, this philosophy must be furthered or physicians' autonomy in patient care decisions will be lost to management plans dictated by healthcare system administrators and politicians.

Intensivists can begin to control health care expenditures. For example, use of the intensive care unit (ICU) during a patient's last month of life consumes considerable resources. With the expanded ability to understand the basic mechanisms of disease and related organ dysfunction, clinicians and researchers have developed more sophisticated and costly diagnostic and treatment modalities. Evidence-based medicine and its related management guidelines and algorithms should be used to determine cost-effective care, although it must be tempered by appropriate point-of-care decision making. The need for diagnostic tests should be based on whether or not the result will change patient management and what the change may be. Therapeutic interventions should also be assessed for their cost-benefit value. Low-cost technology should be used when appropriate. For example, the use of bedside contrast-enhanced ultrasound may help identify organ-specific disease and guide therapy. Endoscopic guided percutaneous tracheostomy and gastrostomy should become the standard. The transition to palliative care should be based on evidence and the family counseled about futile care so they feel less guilt when they need to decide about abandoning heroic efforts to prolong life.

Conclusions.—Intensivists can contribute to a more cost-effective approach to health care. The current cost of healthcare in the United States is unsustainable.

▶ Osler's words remain true today. I think he would be shocked at our use of resources.

Note also that, despite healthcare being easily the highest expense of the US population, we in the United States rank only 26th as far as life expectancy or healthy life expectancy is concerned. Because much of healthcare cost is incurred in the last few months of life and 20% of those dying have been in intensive care units, there is real opportunity for intensivists to bend the cost curve. Care won't be worsened.

J. A. Barker, MD, CPE, FACP, FCCP, FAASM

Copper removal strategies for Wilson's disease crisis in the ICU

Reynolds HV, Talekar CR, Bellapart J, et al (Royal Brisbane and Women's Hosp, Herston, Queensland, Australia)

Anaesth Intensive Care 42:253-257, 2014

Wilson's disease is a rare, inherited, autosomal recessive disorder of copper metabolism which leads to an accumulation of copper in body tissues. If a patient develops a Wilson's crisis, mortality can approach 100%. The treatment of such patients is mostly organ support but a possible treatment goal is to try to rapidly remove copper from their system. We performed a literature search on methods for de-coppering strategies for patients in intensive care with known Wilson's disease. We found 11 case reports where therapeutic plasma exchange was used and six case reports where various forms of albumin dialysis were used as techniques for rapidly reducing serum copper levels. To date, the case reports are encouraging that therapeutic plasma exchange and albumin dialysis can either delay or prevent the need for liver transplantation in patients with fulminant hepatic failure due to Wilson's disease. However, these case reports are mainly in the paediatric or young adult population, thus further studies in adults are warranted.

▶ There are zebras, and then there are albino zebras! Acute Wilson's disease may be in the albino category. These authors have nicely summarized a creative approach for those future cases.

J. A. Barker, MD, CPE, FACP, FCCP, FAASM

A randomised controlled trial comparing incentive spirometry with the Acapella® device for physiotherapy after thoracoscopic lung resection surgery

Cho YJ, Ryu H, Lee J, et al (Seoul Natl Univ Hosp, South Korea)

Anaesthesia 69:891-898, 2014

Lung resection surgery has been associated with numerous postoperative complications. Seventy-eight patients scheduled for elective video-assisted thoracoscopic lung resection were randomly assigned to receive standard postoperative care with incentive spirometry or standard care plus positive vibratory expiratory pressure treatment using the Acapella® device. There was no significant difference between incentive spirometry and the Acapella device in the primary outcome, forced expiratory volume in 1 s, on the third postoperative day, mean (SD) 53% (16%) vs 59% (18%) respectively, $p = 0.113$. Patients treated with both devices simultaneously found incentive spirometry to be less comfortable compared with the Acapella device, using a numeric rating scale from 1 to 5 with lower scores indicating higher comfort, median (IQR [range]) 3 (2–3 [2–4]) vs 1 (1–2 [1–3]) respectively, $p < 0.001$. In addition, 37/39 patients (95%) stated a clear preference for the Acapella device. Postoperative treatment with the Acapella device did not improve pulmonary function after thoracoscopic lung resection surgery compared with incentive spirometry, but it may be more comfortable to use.

▶ Incentive spirometry is the lung expansion technique of choice in many hospitals, especially in postoperative patients. However, recent studies have shown that it is primarily effective in young healthy patients and thus equivalent in that group to deep breath and walking. This study shows another take. In postoperative thoracotomy patients, is a positive pressure device superior vs intracostal? The results show no difference. However, the study numbers are small, and we are not entirely sure as to the "illness" or "acuity" of the patients. Thus, I would caution generalizing from these data. More studies will follow, I hope.

J. A. Barker, MD, CPE, FACP, FCCP, FAASM

Characteristics and Outcomes of Patients Admitted to the Acute Palliative Care Unit From the Emergency Center

Shin SH, Hui D, Chisholm GB, et al (Univ of Texas M. D. Anderson Cancer Ctr, Houston; et al)

J Pain Symptom Manage 47:1028-1034, 2014

Context.—Most patients admitted to acute palliative care units (APCUs) are transferred from inpatient oncology units. We hypothesized that patients admitted to APCUs from emergency centers (ECs) have symptom burdens and outcomes that differ from those of transferred inpatients.

Objectives.—The purpose of this retrospective cohort study was to compare the symptom burdens and survival rate of patients admitted to an APCU from an EC with those of inpatients transferred to the APCU.

Methods.—Among the 2568 patients admitted to our APCU between September 1, 2003 and August 31, 2008, 312 (12%) were EC patients. We randomly selected 300 inpatients transferred to the APCU as controls (The outcome data were unavailable for two patients). We retrieved data on patient demographics, cancer diagnosis, Edmonton Symptom Assessment System scores, discharge outcomes, and overall survival from time of admission to the APCU.

Results.—The EC patients had higher rates of pain, fatigue, nausea, and insomnia and were less likely to be delirious. They were more than twice as likely to be discharged alive than transferred inpatients. Kaplan-Meier plot tests for productlimit survival estimate from admission to APCU for EC patients and inpatients were statistically significant (median survival 34 vs. 31 days, $P < 0.0001$). In multivariate analysis, EC admission (odds ratio [OR] = 1.8593, 95% confidence interval [CI] 1.1532–2.9961), dyspnea (OR = 0.8533, 95% CI 0.7892–0.9211), well-being (OR = 1.1192, 95% CI 1.0234–1.2257), and delirium (OR = 0.3942, 95% CI 0.2443–0.6351) were independently associated with being discharged alive.

Conclusion.—The EC patients have a higher acute symptom burden and are more likely to be discharged alive than transferred inpatients. The APCU was successful at managing symptoms and facilitating the discharge of both inpatients and EC patients to the community although the patients had severe symptoms on admission.

▶ Inpatient care continues to evolve in creative and fascinating ways. Acute referral to an inpatient palliative care site as opposed to an intensive care unit (ICU) could lead to many positive outcomes, such as enhanced patient satisfaction and better resource utilization. (Many authorities would estimate Medical ICU patient admissions as having 10% to 25% nonsurvivable illnesses.) Also of note here is that the emergency center—admitted palliative care patients have improved symptoms and also may survive to discharge.

J. A. Barker, MD, CPE, FACP, FCCP, FAASM

A Health System-Based Critical Care Program with a Novel Tele-ICU: Implementation, Cost, and Structure Details

Fortis S, Weinert C, Bushinski R, et al (Univ of Minnesota, Minneapolis)

J Am Coll Surg 219:676-683, 2014

Background.—Improving the efficiency of critical care service is needed as the shortfall of intensivists is increasing. Standardizing clinical practice, telemedicine, and organizing critical care service at a health system level improve outcomes. We developed a health system Critical Care Program based at an academic medical center. The main feature of our program is an intensivist who shares on-site and telemedicine clinical responsibilities. Tele-ICU facilitates the standardization of high-quality critical care across the system. A common electronic medical record made the communications among the ICUs feasible. Combining faculty from medical and surgical critical care divisions increased the productivity of intensivists.

Study Design.—We retrospectively reviewed the administrative database data from 2011 and 2012, including mean census, number of transfers, age, sex, case mix index, mortality, readmissions, and financial data.

Results.—The Critical Care program has 106 adult ICU beds; 54 of those beds can be managed remotely using tele-ICU based at the main University hospital. The mean midnight census of the system for 2012 was

69.44 and total patient-days were 34,406. The capital cost of the tele-ICU was $1,186,220. The annual operational cost is $1,250,112 or $23,150 per monitored ICU-bed. Unadjusted mortality was 6.5% before and 4.9% after implementation ($p < 0.0002$).

Conclusions.—We describe a novel health system level ICU program built using "off the shelf" technology based on a large University medical center and a tele-ICU with a full degree of treatment authority across the system.

▶ Electronic intensive care unit (ICU) programs seem like the wave of the future. There is automatic monitoring of many more patients than can be achieved with "usual" staffing. Indeed, it is almost a population health model applied to the sickest of patients. However, logistics and politics can be complex, and then there is cost. Cost of implementation is a very real and often a rate-limiting step. Reimbursement is the elephant in the room as well. It is actually more efficient to staff > 100 ICU patients at night with a single attending than to have 3 to 5 in-house physicians. However, telemedicine reimbursement has been slow to catch on, and thus the work may be worthwhile but not reimbursed.

This multihospital, multi-ICU academic system has nicely laid out its progression to an integrated tele-ICU system. Of note, there is integrated critical care cross coverage that spans historical surgical and medical boundaries. It also appears that a less expensive software solution was developed compared with some current systems.

If an academic practice can develop this level of integration and organization, it would seem that electronic ICUs can be replicated in almost any venue. The real questions that remain are: (1) Do quality and mortality improve? and (2) Is it really cost-effective? I hope follow-up studies address these fundamental questions.

J. A. Barker, MD, CPE, FACP, FCCP, FAASM

Dying with Dignity in the Intensive Care Unit

Cook D, Rocker G (Univ, Hamilton, Ontario; Dalhousie Univ, Halifax, Nova Scotia, Canada)

N Engl J Med 370:2506-2514, 2014

Background.—Intensive care units (ICUs) are traditionally designed to reduce morbidity and mortality related to critical illness, support organ function, and restore the patient to health. However, ICUs are not strangers to death, with an estimated one in five deaths in the United States occurring in a critical care setting. With this in mind, it is important for ICU clinicians to be able to allow patients to die with dignity, recognizing the intrinsic, unconditional quality of human worth and maintaining physical comfort, autonomy, meaning, preparedness, and connections with others. The components of dying with dignity and the implications for clinicians were outlined.

Components of a Dignified Death.—Attitudes, behaviors, compassion, and dialogue comprise the ABCDs of dignity-preserving care for patients. The goal is to care for patients in a way that fits with their values even when they cannot speak for themselves. Palliative care can be extended to family members as well. The attitudes of clinicians should reflect respect for the patient and family as well as compassion. It is important to elicit patient values through the use of engaging, deferential questions and then structure a framework through which to express empathy while sharing information that will prepare the patient for final decision making. Communication should be clear and open during end-of-life care.

Preferences for decision-making vary between families, but the clinician should clarify the preferences and engage in the process accordingly. Prognostic information must be valid so that all concerned will understand the course ahead and be prepared. Clinicians should be aware that families tend to expect patients will survive even dire circumstances more often than physicians do. Families also may show an optimism bias, interpreting grim news as a positive statement. The clinician should respect the family's choice to hope while maintaining a realistic view. They should analyze each situation and tailor their language choice and approach to the patient's and family's preferred decision-making model, understand interpersonal relationships, and avoid overemphasizing any particular point of view.

Clinician Roles.—The palliative approach is based on providing culturally and spiritually sensitive care for the patient. Both verbal and nonverbal communication can be powerful in end-of-life decision-making processes. A spiritual framework is often used to interpret the patient's illness, purpose in life, death, suffering, and destiny. A mnemonic for gathering information about spiritual issues is SPIRIT, which is acknowledgement of a spiritual belief system, the patient's personal involvement with this system, integration with a spiritual community, rituals, implications for medical care, and terminal events planning. Personalized care includes sensitivity to faith-based preferences for discussions and decision-making and the influence of spirituality on coping. Chaplains provide an indispensable service in this area.

Some clinicians who have views about advanced life support that do not align with those of the patient will experience moral distress. Vicarious traumatization can occur with repeated empathic engagement with sadness and loss. Clinicians should be aware of emotional withdrawal or lability and take steps to address the problem. Possibilities include informal debriefing or case-based rounds, local meetings with professionals, modified work assignments, and formal bereavement counseling.

The mnemonic VALUE frames five objectives of communication between clinician and family in a proactive conference to set forth the plan for palliative care: value and appreciate the concerns family members express, acknowledge the emotions they are experiencing, listen to their concerns, understand who the patient was before the illness by asking questions, and elicit questions from members of the family. Caregivers who use this proactive conference approach are less negatively affected and experience less anxiety, depression, and symptoms of post-traumatic stress within 90 days of the patient's death.

Conclusions.—The guiding principles of palliative care in the ICU are providing care so the patient can die with dignity. This includes providing the patient with freedom to engage in reflection, connections with survivors, and peaceful surroundings during the final days or hours of life. In addition, the clinician should be prepared to support bereaved family members after the patient's death.

▶ This is a fantastic article and a must read for all intensivists, in my opinion. Why? Because 20% of those dying in the United States are in an intensive care unit or have been in one. Besides, the issues of palliation and comfort care vs aggressive high-technology critical care are daily concerns we all face.

Table 1 in the original article provides an excellent framework for Dying with Dignity, ABCD: Attitude, Behavior, Compassion, Dialogue.

Fig 1 in the original article shows visually the difference in a critical care approach and a palliative care approach. Note the increased time and effort at life end by palliative practitioners and that care (for the family) continues after death. Table 3 in the original article then gives a nice outline of preparation for withdrawal of life support. The focus is clearly patient- and family-centric. The formalization of the process drives the critical care team back to that patient-centric focus that we all must strive for.

There are many practical and useful insights outlined here. Read on!

J. A. Barker, MD, CPE, FACP, FCCP, FAASM

Brain Death and Islam: The Interface of Religion, Culture, History, Law, and Modern Medicine

Miller AC, Ziad-Miller A, Elamin EM (Natl Inst of Health, Bethesda, MD; New York Law School; James A. Haley Veteran's Hosp and Univ of South Florida, Tampa, FL)

Chest 146:1092-1101, 2014

How one defines death may vary. It is important for clinicians to recognize those aspects of a patient's religious beliefs that may directly influence medical care and how such practices may interface with local laws governing the determination of death. Debate continues about the validity and certainty of brain death criteria within Islamic traditions. A search of PubMed, Scopus, EMBASE, Web of Science, PsycNet, Sociological Abstracts, DIALOGUE ProQuest, Lexus Nexus, Google, and applicable religious texts was conducted to address the question of whether brain death is accepted as true death among Islamic scholars and clinicians and to discuss how divergent opinions may affect clinical care. The results of the literature review inform this discussion. Brain death has been acknowledged as representing true death by many Muslim scholars and medical organizations, including the Islamic Fiqh Academies of the Organization of the Islamic Conference and the Muslim World League, the Islamic Medical Association of North America, and other faith-based medical organizations as well as legal rulings by multiple Islamic nations. However, consensus in the Muslim world is not unanimous, and a sizable minority accepts death by cardiopulmonary criteria only.

▶ Death is relative, in a sense. Cultural and religious beliefs significantly affect one's response to life and to death. Although the morals and ethics predominant in the United States are based on Judeo-Christian tenets, in our pluralistic society, there are many other religions. This useful article outlines the variety of thought in current Islamic thinking and practice in the context of brain death.

J. A. Barker, MD, CPE, FACP, FCCP, FAASM

Imaging

Double-lung point sign in traumatic pneumothorax

Aspler A, Pivetta E, Stone MB (Brigham and Women's Hosp, Boston, MA)

Am J Emerg Med 32:819.e1-819.e2, 2014

Lung ultrasound has emerged as a rapid and accurate screening tool for pneumothorax. The lung point sign, a sonographic representation of the point on the chest wall where the pleural layers readhere, is 100% specific to confirm the diagnosis. Double lung point sign for a single pneumothorax is extremely unusual and has only been reported twice in the literature.

A 49-year-old woman was transported to the emergency department (ED) intubated and sedated with severe head injury. She remained

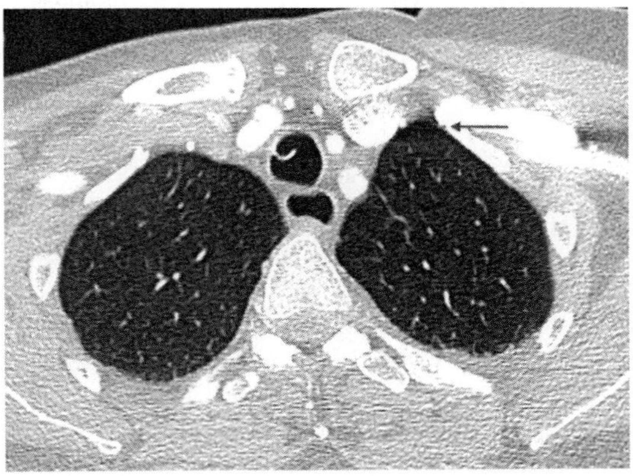

FIGURE.—Chest CT image of left anterior pneumothorax with associated contusion. (Reprinted from the American Journal of Emergency Medicine. Aspler A, Pivetta E, Stone MB. Double-lung point sign in traumatic pneumothorax. *Am J Emerg Med.* 2014;32:819.e1-819.e2, Copyright 2014, with permission from Elsevier.)

hemodynamically stable without respiratory compromise throughout her ED course. Chest computed tomography was notable for an anterior left pneumothorax with underlying pulmonary contusion. Bedside ultrasound of this region revealed a double lung point sign.

Our case report is the first to confirm association of the double lung point sign with a single pneumothorax on corresponding computed tomographic imaging (Fig).

▶ Ultrasound of the chest is becoming standard in critical care. This case nicely illustrates the correlation of computed tomography scan findings and ultrasound. See the subtle but real pneumothorax in the Fig. Double lung point sign is an important chest ultrasound finding. We all need to continuously improve our ultrasound skills and knowledge, as illustrated here.

J. A. Barker, MD, CPE, FACP, FCCP, FAASM

Article Index

Chapter 1: Asthma, Allergy, and Cystic Fibrosis

Chapter 2: Chronic Obstructive Pulmonary Disease

Chapter 3: Lung Cancer

Chapter 6: Lung Transplantation

Chapter 7: Sleep Disorders

Author Index